Redesigning Nursing Care Delivery

TRANSFORMING OUR FUTURE

Redesigning Nursing Care Delivery

TRANSFORMING OUR FUTURE

DOMINICK L. FLAREY, PhD, MBA, RN, C, CNAA, CHE

Administrator and Chief Operating Officer,
Youngstown Osteopathic Hospital
Youngstown, Ohio
and
Executive Consultant
to the national health care practice of
Coopers & Lybrand Consulting
Chicago, Illinois

J. B. Lippincott Company
Philadelphia

Sponsoring Editor: Jennifer E. Brogan
Coordinating Editorial Assistant: Danielle J. DiPalma
Project Editor: Karen S. Huffman
Indexer: Patricia Perrier
Cover Designer: Richard Spencer
Interior Designer: Arlene Putterman
Design Coordinator: Melissa Olson
Production Manager: Helen Ewan
Production Coordinator: Robert Randall
Compositor: Pine Tree Composition, Inc.
Printer/Binder: R.R. Donnelley & Sons Company

1   3   5   6   4   2
∞ This paper meets the requirements of ANSI/NISO Z39.48–1992 (Permanence of paper).

Library of Congress Cataloging-in-Publication Data

Flarey, Dominick L.
    Redesigning nursing care delivery : transforming our future /
Dominick L. Flarey
      p. cm.
    Includes bibliographical references and index.
    ISBN 0–397–55132–0
    1. Nursing services—Administration—Case studies.
2. Organizational change—Case studies. 3. Nursing services—
Administration. I. Title.
RT89.F54   1995
362.1′73′068—dc20   94-7894
                                                              CIP

Any procedure or practice described in this book should be applied by the health-care
practitioner under appropriate supervision in accordance with professional standards of care
used with regard to the unique circumstances that apply in each practice situation. Care has
been taken to confirm the accuracy of information presented and to describe generally
accepted practices. However, the authors, editors, and publisher cannot accept any
responsibility for errors or omissions or for any consequences from application of the
information in this book and make no warranty, express or implied, with respect to the
contents of the book.

Every effort has been made to ensure drug selections and dosages are in accordance with
current recommendations and practice. Because of ongoing research, changes in
government regulations and the constant flow of information on drug therapy, reactions and
interactions, the reader is cautioned to check the package insert for each drug for
indications, dosages, warnings, and precautions, particularly if the drug is new or
infrequently used.

CONTRIBUTORS

RELLA ADAMS, PhD, RN, CNAA
Senior Vice President of Nursing
Valley Baptist Medical Center
Harlingen, TX

LESLIE J. AJL, RN, MS, CS
Psychiatric Liaison Nurse
Beth Israel Hospital
Boston, MA

RHONDA ANDERSON, RN, MPA, CNAA, FAAN
Administrator
Hartford Hospital
Hartford, CT

MAIA GRUBER BAKER, RN, MSN
Administrative Director of Nursing
Valley Baptist Medical Center
Harlingen, TX

SUSAN L. BECK, PhD, RN
Research Associate Professor
University of Utah
College of Nursing
Project Director
University Hospital's Program to Improve Patient Care
Salt Lake City, UT

SUZANNE SMITH BLANCETT, EdD, RN, FAAN
Editor-in-Chief
Journal of Nursing Administration (JONA)
J. B. Lippincott
Philadelphia, PA

CAROL BOSTON, JD, MS, RN
Senior Consultant
The Hay Group
Chicago, IL

ERNESTINA BRIONES, MSN, RN
Administrative Assistant
Doctoral Candidate
University of Houston
Valley Baptist Medical Center
Harlingen, TX

LINDA BIRCH BUNKERS, MEd, RN
Nursing Administrator
Education, Research and Development
Sioux Valley Hospital
Sioux Falls, SD

DOREEN DANN, BSN, CNA
Vice President
Clinical Services/Chief Nurse Executive
St. Jude Medical Center
Fullerton, CA

VICKI DEBACA, RN, MSN, DNS candidate
Mercy Health Care, San Diego
San Diego, CA

MARY ANN DIMOLA, RN, MA
Director of Education
St. Vincent's Health System
Jacksonville, FL
Independent Consultant
Bethesda, MD

SISTER EILEEN DONOGHUE, RN, MSN
Director
Patient Care Redesign Project
St. Vincent's Medical Center
Jacksonville, FL

LAURA J. DUPRAT
Project Coordinator
Integrated Clinical Practice
Beth Israel Hospital
Boston, MA

RUBEN D. FERNANDEZ, RN, BSN, MA, PhD candidate
Vice President
Newark Beth Israel Medical Center
Newark, NJ

MARY L. FISHER, PhD, RN, CNAA
Associate Professor
Indiana University School of Nursing
Senior Administrative Consultant
St. Vincent's Health Services
Indianapolis, IN

DOMINICK L. FLAREY, PhD, MBA, RN, C, CNAA, CHE
Administrator and Chief Operating Officer
Youngstown Osteopathic Hospital
Youngstown, OH
Executive Consultant
Coopers & Lybrand Consulting
Chicago, IL

MARYANN F. FRALIC, RN, DrPH, FAAN
Vice President for Nursing
The Johns Hopkins Hospital
Adjunct Professor and Associate in Administration
Johns Hopkins University School of Nursing
Adjunct Professor
Department of Health Policy and Management
Johns Hopkins University School of Hygiene and Public Health
Baltimore, MD

PAMELA GENTZSCH, RN, MSN, OCN
Director
Professional Practice/Oncology Services
St. Jude Medical Center
Fullerton, CA

S. JO GIBSON, MS, RN, CCRN
Clinical Nurse Specialist and Director for Case Management
Sioux Valley Hospital
Sioux Falls, SD

LISA MARIE EDLIN GRAY, MSHA
Medical Information Systems Coordinator/Nursing Administration
Valley Baptist Medical Center
Harlingen, TX

SANDRA HAZEN, RN, BSN
Nursing Manager
St. Vincent's Medical Center
Jacksonville, FL

GEORGE J. HEBERT, RN, BSN, MA
Assistant Director
Christ Hospital School of Nursing
Jersey City, NJ

MARIA HILL, RN, BSN, MS
Senior Consultant
The Center for Case Management, Inc.
South Natick, MA

CYNTHIA HINOJOSA-ALARCÓN, RN, MSN, CNA
Director of Nursing Education
Valley Baptist Medical Center
Harlingen, TX

MARILYN HOBBS, RN, BSN, MBA
Director
Cardiac and Metabolic Services
St. Jude Medical Center
Fullerton, CA

SUSAN B. JESKA, RN, MBA, EdD
Associate Director/Director Education Services
University of Minnesota Hospital and Clinic
Minneapolis, MN

RICHARD JONES, MS, RN
Nursing Administrator
Adult Specialty Care Services
Sioux Valley Hospital
Sioux Falls, SD

TERRY KACMARYNSKI, RN, BSN
Vincentian Project Educator
St. Vincent's Health System/St. Vincent's Medical Center
Jacksonville, FL

EILEEN M. KEEFE, RN, BSN
Clinical Nurse
Beth Israel Hospital
Boston, MA

CHERYL L. KINNEAR, RN, BSN
Program Manager
University of Utah Hospital
Program to Improve Patient Care
Salt Lake City, UT

JOELLEN KOERNER, PhD, RN, FAAN
Vice President Patient Services
Sioux Valley Hospital
Sioux Valley, SD

MARY K. KOHLES, RN, MSW
Deputy Director
Strengthening Hospital Nursing Program
A National Program co-sponsored by The Robert Wood
  Johnson Foundation and the Pew Charitable Trusts
St. Anthony's Health Care Foundation
St. Petersburg, FL

KATHRYN GRANGER KUWIK, RN, MSN
Director of Medical-Surgical Nursing
St. Vincent's Medical Center
Jacksonville, FL

PATRICIA M. LYDON, RN, BSN, MSN
Clinical Nurse Manager
Beth Israel Hospital
Boston, MA

MARY JANE MADDEN, PhD, RN
Assistant Professor
University of Minnesota
Minneapolis, MN
Principal
Lawrenz, Madden, and Associates Inc.
St. Paul, MN

ANITA MAHONY, BHS, RN
IPCS Coordinator/Assistant to the Vice President
St. Jude Medical Center
Fullerton, CA

MAUREEN P. MCCAUSLAND, DNSc, RN, FAAN
Associate Vice President for Nursing
Beth Israel Hospital
Boston, MA

BARBARA A. MILLER, RN
Director
Medical-Surgical Rehabilitation Nursing
St. Jude Medical Center
Fullerton, CA

BECKY NELSON, RN, MS
Nursing Administrator for Critical Care Services
Sioux Valley Hospital
Sioux Falls, SD

M. LYNNE O'DAY, RN, BSN, MHA
Vice President, Operations
St. Vincent Hospital and Health Care Center, Inc.
Indianapolis, IN

CAROL PIERSON, RN, MSN
Director Clinical Education, Community Outreach, Senior Services
St. Jude Medical Center
Fullerton, CA

PEGGY J. REILEY, RN, MSN, MSPH
Director of Quality Assurance and Development for Nursing
Beth Israel Hospital
Boston, MA

JOANNE RIGGS, MA, RN
Director
Nursing Standard Assurance and Research
Newark Beth Israel Medical Center
Newark, NJ

NELLIE C. ROBINSON, MS, RN
Assistant Dean for Clinical Services
Howard University
College of Nursing
Assistant Executive Director
Patient Care Services
Chief Nursing Officer
Howard University Hospital
Washington, DC

KALEEN SANTEMA, RN
Nursing Administrator
Women and Children Services
Sioux Valley Hospital
Sioux Falls, SD

LINDA SCHARF, RN, DNS, CNAA
Vice President, Nursing
Millard Fillmore Health System
Buffalo, NY

NANCY SHENDELL-FALIK, RN, MA
Assistant Vice President, Nursing
Robert Wood Johnson University Hospital
New Brunswick, NJ

ROXANE B. SPITZER-LEHMAN, PhD, MBA, RN, MA, FAAN
Visiting Professor, College of Business, University of Colorado
Associate Professor, University of Southern California
Assistant Professor, Vanderbilt University
Assistant Professor, Texas Tech School of Nursing
National Advisor Medicus Systems
CEO S L Associates
San Diego, CA

CHERYL B. STETLER, PhD, RN, FAAN
Project Director
Patient-Centered Redesign Program
Hartford Hospital
Hartford, CT

JOLENE TORNABENI, MA, RN, CNAA, CHE
Vice President, INOVA Health System
Administrator/CEO
Fairfax Hospital
Falls Church, VA

KATHERINE W. VESTAL, PhD, RN, FAAN
National Director
Work Transformation Services
The Hay Group
Dallas, TX

PAM ARMSTRONG WARNER, RN, CPHQ
Director of Quality Improvement
Valley Baptist Medical Center
Harlingen, TX

KATHY R. WILDE, RN, MA
Assistant Director
Strategic Planning
University of Minnesota Hospital and Clinic
Minneapolis, MN

FOREWORD

This foreword was written the day after President Clinton unveiled his plan for a reformed health care system. The goal of his system is affordable, accessible health care for every American. Through his proposal for radical redesign of the system, inefficiency, waste, and cost would be reduced. An assumed by-product is increased provider satisfaction, productivity, and availability for providing care. While what will remain of the President's vision for reform, after lobbying by special interest groups, is highly speculative, one fact is certain—it will never again be business as usual in health care.

Concerned for years about the issues the President is trying to address nationally, savvy health care administrators have been designing programs to address system-wide problems. Of note has been the leadership of nurses in these efforts. Nurse pioneers gave us primary nursing, case management, differentiated practice, shared governance, and self-managed units. Nurses lead the way in experimenting with approaches to care delivery that held the promise of increasing patient and staff satisfaction, improving operations' efficiency, decreasing cost, and improving patient care outcomes.

This book is a tribute to nursing and those nursing leaders who dared to undertake the difficult task of redesigning, restructuring, and reengineering a system in trouble. In its pages, we see the creativity, the perseverance, the power, and the intelligence of nurses as they help lead complex organizations through significant change. We feel pride when we read what these nurses, in collaboration with their colleagues, dreamed possible and then were able to accomplish; we see again that nurses have the knowledge, skills, talent, and will to profoundly effect the lives of our organizations, staff, and consumers.

For the many nurse leaders who have not experienced significant paradigm shifts, redesign, or role transformation, this book is a guide. In its pages, readers will find many approaches to redesign based on differing staff and organizational cultures, demographics, and financial imperatives; methods for effectively measuring outcomes; and caveats and recommendations. For those who are overwhelmed by what lies ahead, this book provides support and guidance and the belief that significant paradigm shifts can occur. For those already in the implementation process of redesign, the book contains valuable ideas for fine-tuning as well as evaluating your efforts.

In significant projects such as those described in this book, one must always remember that work is only accomplished by people and that goals are reached because at least one person had an unwavering belief that things could be different. While all the contributors to this book, most of whom I know personally, are to be commended for their significant undertaking, I want to single out the editor and primary author, Dr. Dominick Flarey.

From our early relationship in which I was a mentor to Dominick, to our relationship today in which we learn and share equally, I am continually amazed by Dominick's ability to take risks, trust people, put failure and success in perspective, and to inspire and motivate others to excellence. Dominick personifies the transformational leader who will take us into the 21st century with vision and pragmatism. This book, its editor, and the nurse leaders who tell their stories through its pages inspire confidence and hope that nursing is, and surely will remain, the keystone of the health care delivery system.

Suzanne Smith Blancett, *EdD, RN, FAAN*
Editor-in-Chief
Journal of Nursing Administration (JONA)
Philadelphia, PA

PREFACE

This book is about dreams and visions and the nurses who made them come true. It is about a journey through a time of revolution in our health care system. As we stand at the door of reform, our professional future may seem uncertain. How we will emerge and what the system will look like are somewhat speculative. The challenge before us is to recreate our profession and our practice so that nursing will emerge strong and empowered in this new era.

More importantly, this book is about the transformation of a profession that has withstood the test of time; that has emerged as a winner time and time again in a system of constant change and turbulence. Transformation is never complete; it is constantly evolving. This work provides a foundation for all that will come after it, in the quest for a profession to transform itself.

Redesigning care delivery systems is both complex and challenging. It requires an enormous commitment to time and self. Throughout the pages of this book, today's nurse leaders tell the story of their personal experiences, sharing their talents and methodologies, so that others may benefit from their pioneering efforts. These leaders willingly gave of their time to bring this project to fruition. They believe that their work will live on and provide the foundation for the future transformation of our profession and practice.

As you read of their experiences and journeys through this time of great uncertainty, you will be amazed at their display of exemplary leadership and proud of their successes and contributions to the care of people. As you read their stories you will come to realize that it is the nursing leadership who has taken the reigns and is reforming our health care system, long before our government took action.

It is the hope of my colleagues and me that this work will serve as a new beginning in nursing leadership and practice; motivating others to greater levels of success in redesigning delivery systems. If in some small way this work serves to continue the transformation of nursing practice and makes a difference to those we serve—then we will have contributed greatly and realized our mission.

This work is a product of many professionals coming together in the hope of making a difference. First and foremost, I would like to acknowledge and publicly thank all of the contributors of this book who gave their time to make this vision a reality. I was most honored to work with each one of them. They taught me what nursing leadership is all about and for that I will be forever grateful.

There are several others whom I must single out and acknowledge for all of their help and support with this project. I thank Dr. Suzanne Smith Blancett, RN, FAAN, for her constant support and motivation. She taught me the art of writing and then encouraged me to accomplish more than I ever thought possible. This book would not have materialized had it not been for her insistence that I too could turn dreams into reality. Thank you, Suzanne.

A special thank you to Dr. Katherine Vestal, RN, FAAN, renowned expert and leader in redesign, for taking time out of her busy schedule to write the prologue to this book. Kathy is a real role model for me; she exemplifies what executive leadership is all about. She also unselfishly imparts her knowledge so that others may learn and grow.

My sincerest thanks to Mary Kay Kohles, RN, MSW, Deputy Director of the Strengthening Hospital Nursing Program. This work would never have been published were it not for Mary's help and support. She willingly assisted me in seeking out contributors to this book who pioneered delivery system redesign. Her dedication to the transformation of nursing practice is to be commended.

I would also like to thank my friends and colleagues who provided overwhelming support and encouragement during this project. A special thank you to nursing administration at the Youngstown Osteopathic Hospital, who give me the support I need to keep trying. To Mark, who mentored me during my earlier years as an executive and encouraged me to follow my dreams. To Weiss and Susan, for always believing that I could make a difference.

Finally, I would like to acknowledge and thank my new colleagues of the health care consulting practice of Coopers & Lybrand. They are dedicated professionals who work hard every day to assist health care organizations to realize their dreams for transformation and success. I am honored to work with the best practice in health care consulting. To Bob and Mary Kay; thank you for this opportunity.

This book is dedicated to the memory of all those nursing leaders who have gone before us. Through their hard work and efforts, nursing can continue on the journey to transformation.

Dominick L. Flarey, *PhD, MBA, RN, C, CNAA, CHE*

PROLOGUE

In the beginning there was someone who needed care to heal. Then there were nurses, hospitals, and health care systems. Tracing the evolution of patient care delivery would require focusing on the many heroes, many pioneers, and many stories of valiant efforts on the road to continually improve the services provided to take care of people who want and deserve health. This evolution would also chronicle the false starts, the failures, and the misguided attempts to find answers for complicated and often controversial problems. Somewhere between the triumphs and the disappointments we find the present health care delivery system that provides care for people today.

No one would dispute the need to constantly redesign and redefine our health care delivery system. Certainly in the face of major social reform of health care there is a mandate to produce improved results at lower cost. But even if this mandate were not looming, the need would still exist. We still have not found "the best" ways to deliver health care services to people.

Nursing has a history of providing leadership in redesigning nursing practice, usually in ways that promote significant organizational change. The evolution of nursing practice through many generations of care delivery changes provides interesting testimony about the progressive nature of nurses. Conversely, this same history provides evidence that the prior changes have often taken place within the insular world of nursing, seldom reaching out to capture the interdisciplinary opportunities to improve overall delivery of care. The reasons for the previous history of isolationism are immaterial at this point; they must be overcome in order to truly reform health care for people.

Restructuring care delivery involves redesigning systems, processes, and people's jobs in ways that improve the outcomes for patients and other customers. Our efforts and our attention are focused on the things that make the most difference, and those that produce results more economically. Concurrently, restructuring supports the development of high quality work environments in which to practice. The quality of worklife improvements will then support the work we do to care for patients; it is a two-way street. Change of this magnitude cannot be accomplished by any profession in isolation, but requires the interdisciplinary integration of thought, creativity, and development to redesign the basic flow of work, to achieve exceptional outcomes needed by patients.

The amount of work redesign taking place has been minimally reflected in the literature. Perhaps we are all so busy "doing" that there is little time to report. Or perhaps we are all so scared about the radical nature of changes that we are waiting for the final analysis before we go public. This book will provide one of the first efforts to pull together both the theories and the practices of work redesign. The in-depth review of available literature on the topic will help you understand the multifaceted nature of redesigning an organization. The pragmatic accounts from the field of those actually making changes will help you learn from the pioneering efforts of others.

Above all, this book with its wealth of information, will underscore an important fact—that work redesign is *both* an art and a science. It is a messy process that defies rules and raises anxiety. It is the ultimate challenge for health care leaders today and is not for the faint of heart. It is fun. It is hard. It is strategy that requires thinking at 50,000 feet. It is implementing change that requires being in the weeds to make things happen. It is an opportunity to play on a team and reduce isolationism. It is time to rise to a level of professionalism that nurses have always wanted to practice. It is time to focus on results and not allow obstacles to stand in your way.

Is it necessary? Yes. This book will make it happen.

Katherine W. Vestal, RN, PhD, FAAN

CONTENTS

Part 1
Delivery Systems Redesign: Theories and Methodologies

Chapter 1

Planning for Redesign: The Journey to Transformation

DOMINICK L. FLAREY

> *It was the best of times,*
> *It was the worst of times...*
> *—Charles Dickens*

"It was the age of wisdom, it was the age of foolishness, it was the epoch of belief, it was the epoch of incredulity,...it was the spring of hope, it was the winter of despair, we had everything before us, we had nothing before us..." So wrote Charles Dickens in the opening of his 1859 literary classic, *A Tale of Two Cities.* His story is about revolution. Dickens was born in 1812, at the time of the Industrial Revolution. It seems fitting that he who had experienced the reality of revolution would later write a story about the French Revolution.

I believe the famous opening to this classic work sums up what Dickens perceived a revolution to be: a difficult time of change that provides an opportunity for significant growth and transformation. We live today within a revolution in our health care system, an unprecedented time of reform. If Dickens were alive today, he would probably agree that it seems to be the worst of times, but he would also say it is the best of times, because revolution provides the greatest opportunity to bring about positive change, growth, and transformation.

As we enter the age of health care reform, only one thing is certain—change. This change will occur rapidly and will transform health care and our practice in ways we can not yet imagine (Flarey, 1993). "Reform will change the role of nursing more dramatically than that of any other health care profession" (Sherer, 1993a). To prepare for these changes, nurse leaders must plan now to successfully meet the challenges ahead. It is critical that we examine closely what our business is and how it will change in the age of reform.

■ REDESIGN FOR CHANGE

Redesign is a very significant undertaking in nursing and health care administration (Tonges, 1992). Despite its prevalence, there is much confusion as to what redesign actually is and what it means. Many definitions abound, each seemingly born from individual perceptions of some type of change in nursing and health care. Some commonly included elements of redesign are a restructuring of roles, a change in the way work is accomplished, a change or restructure of systems in health care, a reshaping of behavior on the part of workers, development of a "seamless" work-flow pattern in organizations, a shift in business operations, and a restructuring of work processes (Madden & Lawrenz, 1990; Skeggs, Vestal, & Wolter, 1991; Spitzer-Lehmann, 1993; Porter-O'Grady, 1993; Lathrop, 1993).

For purposes of this discussion, redesign is defined broadly, encompassing the major premises of nursing and health care leaders who are pioneering these initiatives. Redesign is a radical departure from the norm, involving the creation of new and innovative methods, means, and structures for successfully meeting the changing paradigms in a system. It entails changes in people, work processes, cultures, services and products, communication patterns, attitudes and behaviors, rewards, and systems thinking and integration. Its purpose is to transform systems in order to respond effectively to a real revolution. Redesign, then, is an evolving methodology focused on producing fundamental and radical changes within a system. Its sole purpose is to ensure survival in a threatened environment.

The impetus for redesigning nursing care delivery originated at the same time as the prospective payment system, in 1983. This new system mandated that we design care delivery to be affordable while also maintaining quality and reducing length of stay. Out of this era came newer delivery systems and strategies that proved successful for the time. A second major impetus was the national nursing shortage of several years ago. Here, we witnessed an escalation in redesign activities as nurse leaders were faced with scarce resources and rising costs related to the use of agency personnel, the development of recruitment and retention programs, and the rapid increase in nurses' pay and wage decompression.

The impetus to redesign care delivery today is different, as are the critical issues we face: the increasing expense of a professional work force; a consistent decline in inpatient census; a shift to outpatient services; further declines in reimbursements; more stringent quality-of-care mandates; mergers and acquisitions; managed competition; integrated service networks; a change to a primarily managed care system; physician–hospital organizations; and a capitated payment system. These forces mandate that nurse leaders redesign the delivery of our primary product—patient care.

In a reformed health care system, "nurses will be leaders in almost everything surrounding patient care" (Sherer, 1993b). The need for redesign is more critical today than ever before. We have yet to fully maximize our resources and integrate services appropriately into the delivery of care. Many inefficiencies and systems problems exist that prevent the delivery of high-quality, cost-effective service and innovations in care delivery.

As nursing leaders pioneer the redesign of care delivery, it is essential to have a good understanding of these problems and issues. This knowledge and insight is valuable for planning redesign initiatives and creating visions of a new, redesigned system. Understanding the current delivery systems provides a solid foundation for all successive planning. The following are a few of the current realities. They are but a few of the many signs and symptoms of a health care system in trouble.

Registered nurses (RNs) spend the majority of their time on indirect care activities. One comprehensive study demonstrated that only 42% of an RN's time is spent providing direct care (Quist, 1992).

Only 16 cents of every health care dollar is allocated for patient care; 14 cents of the dollar is spent for scheduling and coordinating services, and 29 cents is spent on documentation (Brider, 1992).

"In today's hospital, direct care for patients accounts for less than 25% of hospital personnel expenditures" (Lathrop, 1992).

During an average 4-day hospital stay, one patient may interact with approximately 60 different employees (Lathrop, 1992).

Health care staff today are not multiskilled; rather, they are over-specialized.

In most current delivery systems, patient care is designed around various specialized departments. Services are centralized and far removed from the patient (Sherer, 1993c).

Most health care organizations still have traditional pay and reward systems that are not linked to customer expectations (Eubanks, 1992).

Up to 65% of non-nursing tasks currently performed by nurses could easily be reallocated to more technical personnel (Henderson & Williams, 1991).

Patients perceive the health care delivery system much differently than do health care providers (Gerteis, Levitan, Daley, & DelBanco, 1993).

"The average hospital requires about 4 hours to process and deliver a routine service" (Lathrop, 1993).

Hospitals are overburdened with management staff. A typical 300-bed hospital has on staff at least 80 department heads and senior managers (Lathrop, 1993).

A large number of our hospitals are having serious financial difficulties (Wilson, 1992). Costs are out of control and are not being managed effectively.

It has been said that "the heart of patient care delivery is nursing" (Henderson & Williams, 1991). Nurse leaders are taking the initiatives to redesign and transform our health care delivery systems (Vestal & Flannery, 1993). To be successful, nurse executives and managers must become visionary and transformational leaders and emphasize the importance of planning if they are to prevail. Attempts to redesign care delivery will be futile unless sufficient time and resources are allocated for planning.

■PLANNING FOR REDESIGN

Planning is the cornerstone of redesign. Planning for redesign is a major undertaking; little has been published about it, and few methodologies exist. Nurse leaders have the knowledge and skills required to plan redesign projects. It is essential that we establish ourselves as leaders in redesign and develop sound methodologies to guide others in this critical process. Such an initiative will guarantee our own successes in a reformed health care system and will be the driving force for the ongoing transformation of nursing practice.

One method of planning which is highly advocated for redesign projects is termed interactive planning. This method, supported by Ackoff (1981), regards the past, present, and future equally and is rooted in the system's age. The interactive concept of planning may be simply described as "the design of a desirable future and the invention of ways to bring it about" (Ackoff, 1981).

To plan interactively, nurse leaders must become "interactivists." This means becoming proactivists: those who are unwilling to return to previous states and will not accept things as they are. Ackoff (1981) describes the critical attributes and beliefs of interactivists as follows.

1. They rely on experiments rather than experience to seek out solutions.
2. They rely on experience to reveal problems.
3. Their major focus is on improving performance over time.
4. They believe that planners frequently fail to address the right problems because they are not fully aware of what they are striving for.
5. They engage in normative planning, with an emphasis on the selection of goals, objectives, and ideals.
6. They assert that planning is indefinite.

To become interactivists, we must change our thinking and relinquish older beliefs about management and the planning process. We must be transformational leaders, with a focus on creating visions and providing the leadership necessary to achieve what often seems impossible. In short, we must learn to plan backward, from the dream to its actuating steps. This may seem like a radical departure from what we have been taught regarding planning. In fact, it is. It is a dynamic, systems-oriented process which is highly effective in producing desired results; it requires a real commitment to change and a great deal of effort and time.

Ackoff's (1981) interactive planning methodology comprises five key phases, which are presented in Display 1-1. From the foundation of these phases, a solid methodology for planning delivery system redesign emerges. The following discussion highlights the key components of the planning process for redesign. These components correlate with Ackoff's model of interactive planning.

Systems Thinking and Integration
To plan effectively, we must undergo a radical shift in our thinking from an emphasis on parts to consideration of the entire system (Senge, 1990). For too long the major components of care delivery have been compartmentalized, segregated, and centralized into departments with poor integration and interrelationships. The threats that result from this type of thinking include critical inefficiencies within the system, such as poor control of costs and productivity, substandard quality, and customer and employee dissatis-

---

DISPLAY 1-1   Ackoff's Phases of Interactive Planning

PHASE 1. FORMULATE THE MESS
Identify systems of threats and opportunities facing the organization.

PHASE 2. ENDS PLANNING
Determine the ends to be pursued; envision the desired future.

PHASE 3. MEANS PLANNING
Determine the means by which the ends are to be pursued; invent the means to your desirable future.

PHASE 4. RESOURCE PLANNING
Determine what resources will be needed and how to obtain them for your desired future.

PHASE 5. DESIGN OF IMPLEMENTATION AND CONTROL
Determine who is to do what, when, and how to manage the implementation.

Adapted from Ackoff, R. (1981). *Creating the Corporate Future*. New York: John Wiley.

---

faction. A major goal of any redesign effort must be integration. A lack of integration now becomes the opportunity for effective systems redesign.

Redesign cannot be only a nursing agenda. Such a focus is destined to fail. "When viewing health care organizations as a system, the evaluation of new nursing structures must be examined within the context of the whole organization" (Hatler & Malloch, 1992). The challenge to nurse leaders is to redesign delivery systems in an integrated fashion. This means developing an organization-wide perspective and integrating all departments into one systems redesign. All customers of the organization must also be integrated into planning for redesign.

The best way to plan for an integrated systems redesign is to include those who work in the system. Twenty years ago, Peter Drucker said that workers' knowledge, experience, and needs are critical resources to planning. They must be included from the start and integrated into the overall planning process. If the workers' knowledge and imagination are not tapped in the planning process, change and transformation will not be realized (Drucker, 1974). Despite this wise advice, we still view planning as a management responsibility and right. A fundamental change—a commitment to include everyone within the system and served by the system in the planning process—is key to successfully redesigning care delivery systems.

An organization's staff and customers can provide insights into the threats and opportunities that face the organization. One strategy to elicit their participation is the use of surveys and focus groups regarding perceptions of the system, its inefficiencies, and opportunities for change. Integrated planning must include patients as well as workers. Since patients perceive the system differently than caregivers do, they are often better able to identify inefficiencies within the system (Gerteis, Levitan, Daley, & DelBanco, 1993).

Visions and Outcomes

Nurse leaders must provide visionary leadership for the planning of redesign. One of the first and most important elements in planning is to envision outcomes (Hatler & Malloch, 1992). Outcomes should focus on the overall transformation of the nursing profession. Systems redesign is not just about cost-effectiveness, productivity, work restructuring, and quality; rather, it involves a total transformation of the system, including those who work within it and are served by it. Display 1-2 details five visionary outcomes for the growth and transformation of professional nursing practice through systems redesign. These outcomes serve as critical indicators for the planning process as well as measures of success. Although not all-inclusive, they serve as a sample of goals to be attained in the overall, broad transformation of practice.

In planning for redesign, it is essential that visions of the new, transformed system be articulated. Visions should be realistic and at the same time uninhibited. A revolution requires that we develop emotionally exciting visions (Tichy & Sherman, 1993). Visions must be created together (Fisher, 1993). "A vision is a group effort. It is what we believe to be important. It is a work in progress, an architectural rendering that constantly gets modified" (Tichy & Sherman, 1993).

Once visions are defined, they must be well communicated to everyone in the organization and continually reinforced. Those who do not acknowl-

---

DISPLAY 1-2   Visionary Outcomes for the Transformation of Nursing Practice Through Redesign

1. *Omnicompetence:* Staff develop an unlimited ability to satisfy their own desires for transformation as well as the desires of others. This is a meta-ideal which implies the ability to perform effectively (Ackoff, 1981). There is increased job satisfaction, customer satisfaction, and effectiveness of care delivery.
2. *Metanoia:* Staff exhibit a "shift of mind" toward integration of care delivery within a systems framework. This shift of mind also focuses on the imperative for continuous learning. Staff transform the system into a learning organization, and through learning recreate themselves and their profession (Senge, 1990).
3. *Empowerment:* New leadership styles empower staff to become self-directed. Staff are encouraged to lead the system to new and greater levels of excellence that benefit everyone (Belasco & Stayer, 1993).
4. *Completeness:* Staff move beyond quality management to prevention. A "zero defects" philosophy becomes operational. Everyone is committed to delivering care in the right way at all times. There is a solid belief in the basic premise of completeness; whole systems make up an organization and must be treated as such (Crosby, 1992).
5. *Reform:* Nurses are leaders in the transformation of health care delivery. Nurses will emerge as the primary deliverers of health services in a reformed system.

edge the visions tend to resist change and cling to the old ways of doing things (Anderson, 1993). Visions for each organization are unique, because they are formulated within the context of the organization's goal and objectives for a transformed system. The establishment of visions and outcomes serves as the foundation for all successive planning in redesign.

Model of Care

In planning for redesign, it is imperative that a model of care be defined. Models of care are uniquely designed around an individual organization's mission and philosophy as well as its availability of resources. Many models of care have been developed and widely publicized. Some of the newer models include case management systems, theory-based models, patient-centered care, multidisciplinary team models, work-flow models, and service unit models (Spitzer-Lehmann & Yahn, 1992; Madden & Lawrenz, 1990; Fritz, 1992; Lathrop, 1993).

The type of model selected is not important. What is important is that the new model be an original design for the organization, rather than a reproduction of a published model. Developing a model of care requires intense planning and the collective, creative imaginations of the staff and customers. When planning for model redesign, the following points should be considered.

1. Model design should be planned with the organization's culture, climate, values, customers, product lines, and fiscal standing in mind.
2. Care delivery models should be outcome-oriented (Tonges, 1992).
3. The model should maximize the proportion of professional nurses' time spent in direct patient care.
4. The model should be designed with three major goals in mind: a) to improve the quality of care delivered; b) to manage the cost of care effectively; and c) to improve the work life of the staff (Skeggs, Vestal, & Wolter, 1991).
5. Care delivery protocols, such as critical paths, should be designed into the model to enhance quality, integrate services, reduce length of stay, and effectively manage resources (Lumsdon & Hagland, 1993).
6. The model of care should be affordable and, at the same time, efficient and effective.
7. Customers should be partners in the design process (Jacob, 1993).
8. The model should provide the necessary support services for nurses to deliver high-quality patient care (Yancer, 1990).
9. Technology should be incorporated into the design for added effectiveness and efficiency of work processes within the system.
10. Staffing patterns should be realigned in a qualitative and financially sound manner (Smeltzer, Formella, & Beebe, 1993).

One necessity in planning is to realize that redesign is ongoing. In an age of reform, our health care system will become heavily focused on managed care. By the end of this decade, 90% of Americans will be in some type of managed care plan (Smith, 1993). We will see the rapid emergence of community networks, integrated systems, and physician–hospital organizations. The redesign of care delivery must recognize, acknowledge, and include these emerging systems of care.

Role Redesign

A major imperative to delivery system redesign is redesigning caregiver roles. Significant time must be given to this dimension of redesign, since it is critical to the overall success of the project. Role redesign must be carried out collaboratively with all personnel who provide patient care. The attention given to this component of redesign is often the first test of the organization's willingness and ability to remove barriers between departments and begin integration of the system.

To plan effectively for role redesign, it is useful to first examine some important trends that will reshape the workplace of the future: 1) companies will be smaller and employ fewer people; 2) technicians will become the elite workers; 3) vertical division of labor will be replaced by horizontal structures; and 4) work will continually be redefined (Kiechel, 1993).

The redesign of roles in patient care delivery must also be unique to the organization. Roles must be examined for their usefulness and value. One powerful question that should be posed for each role and its corresponding tasks is, "Is what you're doing useful enough for someone to pay money for it?" (Jacob, 1993). Other questions are, How can the role be redesigned to add value to the overall system? and How can work processes be restructured to enhance productivity, improve quality, reduce expenses, and increase job satisfaction of the staff?

A few major imperatives to consider when redesigning roles include the following.

Restructure roles to support patient care and provide integration of services at the bedside (Spitzer-Lehmann & Yahn, 1992).

Encourage all staff to become multiskilled; caregivers from all disciplines should be integrated on the unit and report to one unit manager (Sheedy, 1993).

Cross-train all staff to provide direct and indirect components of care.

Redesign the role of the professional nurse to focus on cognitive, highly skilled tasks (Spitzer-Lehmann & Yahn, 1992).

Redesign care delivery by facilitating and building teams of caregivers (Naubauer, 1993).

Design newer roles that are focused heavily on the technical components of care.

Redesign roles with a focus on health care team partnerships.

Quality

Quality must be planned and integrated into all components of a redesigned delivery system. A comprehensive continuous quality improvement (CQI) program can be designed into the system. In a recent survey of organizations involved in redesign, 43% of respondents asserted that CQI is a logical outgrowth of redesign. Quality is enhanced through a redesign effort because productivity is increased and greater quality outcomes in patient care are realized (Sherer, 1993c).

CQI initiatives should be unit-based, and they should be fully integrated into an organization-wide program. The focus should shift from department quality assurance issues to customer service issues. Each unit can be designed as a service unit, functioning as a customer and supplier to other service units (Fritz, 1992).

In planning for quality, attention should be given to the analysis of medical and nursing protocols. Critical path variances should be routinely analyzed to identify inefficiencies in the system, leading to further redesign or reengineering. A comprehensive assessment of patient outcomes is also critical to the accurate evaluation of a redesigned system. In a managed care environment, the documentation of patient outcomes will be essential and will impact heavily on the organization's ability to acquire network contracts and retain them (Aston, 1993).

It is also necessary to move beyond total quality management to a zero-defects philosophy. This requires developing strategies and initiatives to build prevention into the redesigned system, a newer philosophy called "completeness" (Crosby, 1992). Also, the use of statistical tools and analysis will become more important in the future as we analyze processes and redesign them for zero defects. Nurse leaders must plan now to acquire these important skills (Flarey, 1993b).

Costs

In planning for redesign, affordability must be a governing factor. Each organization must assess its financial standing and ability to provide the resources necessary to realize the vision. One projection estimated that in 1993, $940 billion would be spent on health care in this country (Smith, 1993). Health care spending is out of control, and a reformed system will mandate more effective management of costs. Declining reimbursements will adversely affect an organization's ability to redesign.

To deal with the coming financial issues, it is necessary to build cost savings into care delivery redesign. One way is to meticulously cost out the current delivery of care. Some recent studies reveal that up to 75% of a registered nurse's time is spent in nonclinical, indirect care activities (Brider, 1992). Not only is this a waste of professional, highly skilled resources, but it will be unaffordable in a reformed system. Planning should focus, then, on redesigning roles and work processes to deliver care in the most cost-effective way. Nurses have the ability to move patients through the care system cost-effectively (Sherer, 1993b), and they should be empowered to practice in an economically responsible way. Other strategies to control and manage the organization's financial resources include enhancements to charging systems, such as automation, that serve to maximize revenues; new product lines and ventures for revenue enhancement; downsizing; management restructuring; and competing successfully in the market for managed care contracts.

Management Redesign

Redesigned delivery systems require that the structure and roles of management be concomitantly redesigned. Management's primary role in redesign is to clearly communicate the organization's visions for transformation and provide the leadership necessary to realize them. This can be adequately supported by redesigning management roles for greater levels of leadership, with less emphasis on the traditional elements of management.

To this end, executive leadership must support and guide the transformation of management roles. This can be accomplished by planning for major paradigm shifts in the roles. These shifts include moving from manager to leader; director to coach; boss to mentor; participatory management to self-governance; quality assurance to continuous quality improvement; nursing perspective to organizational perspective; clinical audits to research; turf protection to collaboration; control to partnerships; planning to strategic vision; vertical management to horizontal management; budgeting to fiscal accountability; status quo to innovation; and from a nursing focus to a product line focus (Flarey, 1993a). Successful shifts to these new paradigms will ensure the transformational leadership required to successfully redesign care delivery and move the organization closer to realizing its visions.

Newer management structures must also be evaluated in the planning process. It will be common in a reformed system for nurse managers to provide leadership for more than one unit. With the move to patient-focused care and multiskilled workers, matrix relationships between nurse managers and other department managers will be commonplace. Such relationships should be planned and agreed to early on in the redesign process. Many of the following departments will report to nursing in the future: home care, infection control, social services, utilization review, physical therapy, occupational therapy, pharmacy, housekeeping, and dietary services (Sherer, 1993b). These new reporting structures will drive the redesign of management roles.

Education

Intense planning for education is a critical component in the overall planning process. Newer models of care and role redesign require that everyone in the organization be trained at the appropriate skill levels. Education topics should also include the visions, goals, and objectives of the redesign process, the economics of care, skills for quality improvements, and health care reform and managed care networks. Sufficient time and resources must be allocated for training and education. Education of physicians and other customers of the organization on the redesign of care delivery must also be a priority. Plans should also include mechanisms for evaluating learning and skills credentialing for newer care delivery roles.

Compensation

New systems require new programs for rewards and compensation. Plans must be formulated for appropriately compensating those in redesigned roles that require greater skill levels. Redesigned systems will be heavily focused on teams, but most current models of pay and performance reward individuals and not teams (Eubanks, 1992). More innovative compensation plans will reward team performance. The way performance is assessed will change to fit a redesigned system. Incentives and rewards should acknowledge some of the following achievements: (1) meeting quality-of-care outcomes, (2) effective cost management, (3) quality initiatives, (4) enhanced customer satisfaction, and (5) revenue generation.

▰CONCLUSION

"The year 2000 will dawn on a Saturday, perfect for nursing recollections of the nineties and soberly contemplating the era ahead" (Kiechel, 1993). What will our health care system look like? Will nursing survive? How will nursing change in this new era? Although the answers to these questions may be speculative, nurses can expect to emerge strong and empowered, as the primary providers of patient care in a reformed system of networks and partnerships, within a prevention and wellness model.

However, this transformation will not occur by itself. It will come to pass because, years earlier, facing a revolution in health care, professional nurse leaders had a vision of what could be, and worked hard to see their dreams become reality. As a result, nurse leaders will be recognized as leaders in systems redesign, and it will be evident that through our strategic planning and leadership, our health care delivery system and our profession have been transformed.

▰REFERENCES

Ackoff, R. (1981). *Creating the corporate future.* New York: Wiley.
Anderson, H. (1993, February 5). New planning models. *Hospitals,* pp. 20–22.
Aston, G. (1993). Employees bear brunt of hospital push to streamline operations. *American Hospital Association News, 29*(1), 1, 5.
Belasco, J. & Stayer, R. (1993). *Flight of the Buffalo.* New York: Warner.
Brider, P. (1992, September). The move to patient-focused care. *American Journal of Nursing,* pp. 26–33.
Crosby, P. (1992). *Completeness: Quality for the 21st century.* New York: Dutton.
Dickens, C. (1988). *A Tale of Two Cities.* New York: Tom Doherty.
Drucker, P. (1974). *Management: Tasks, responsibilities, practices.* New York: Harper & Row.
Eubanks, P. (1992, October). Work redesign calls for new pay and performance plans. *Hospitals,* pp. 56–60.
Fisher, K. (1993). *Leading self-directed work teams.* New York: McGraw-Hill.
Flarey, D. (1993a). The changing role of the nurse manager: Redesign for the 1990s and beyond. *Seminars for Nurse Managers, 1*(1), 41–48.
Flarey, D. (1993b). Quality improvement through data analysis: Concepts and applications. *Journal of Nursing Administration, 23*(11), 21–30.
Fritz, L. (1992). Changing the structure of daily operations: The work-flow model of the future. *Healthcare Executive, 7*(4), 24–26.
Gerteis, M., Levitan, S., Daley, J., & DelBanco, T. (Eds.). (1993). *Through the patients' eyes: Understanding and promoting patient-centered care.* San Francisco: Jossey-Bass.
Hatler, C. & Malloch, K. (1992). Delivery system redesign: Making it worth your while. In C. Wilson (Ed.), *Building new nursing organizations: Visions and realities* pp. 163–185. Gaithersburg: Aspen.

14 Redesigning Nursing Care Delivery

Henderson, J. & Williams, J. (1991). The people side of patient care redesign. *Healthcare Forum Journal, 34*(4), 44–49.

Jacob, R. (1993). Beyond quality and value. *Fortune, 128*(13), 8–11.

Kiechel, W. (1993). How we will work in the year 2000. *Fortune, 127*(10), 39–52.

Lathrop, J. (1992). The patient-focused hospital. *Healthcare Forum Journal,* May/June, 76–78.

Lathrop, J. (1993). *Restructuring health care: The patient-focused paradigm.* San Francisco: Jossey-Bass.

Lumsdon, K. & Hagland, M. (1993, October 20). Mapping care. *Hospitals & Health Networks,* pp. 34–40.

Madden, M. J. & Lawrenz, E. (1990). Work redesign. In G. Mayer, M. Madden, & E. Lawrenz (Eds.), *Patient care delivery models.* Rockville, MD: Aspen.

Naubauer, J. (1993). Redesign: Managing role changes and building new teams. *Seminars for Nurse Managers, 1*(1), 26–32.

Porter-O'Grady, T. (1993). Work redesign: Fact, fiction, and foible. *Seminars for Nurse Managers, 1*(1), 8–15.

Quist, B. (1992). Work sampling nursing units. *Nursing Management, 23*(9), 50–51.

Senge, P. (1990). *The fifth discipline: The art and practice of the learning organization.* New York: Doubleday.

Sheedy, S. (1993). The head nurse role in redesign. *Journal of Nursing Administration, 23*(7/8), 14–15.

Sherer, J. (1993a). Health care reform: Nursing's vision of change. *Hospitals, 20,* 20–25.

Sherer, J. (1993b, April 20). Next steps for nursing. *Hospitals & Health Networks,* pp. 26–28.

Sherer, J. (1993c, February 5). Putting Patients First. *Hospitals,* pp. 14–18.

Skeggs, L., Vestal, K., & Wolter, R. (1991). *Redesigning care delivery* [Video Tape 1]. Chicago: American Organization of Nurse Executives.

Smeltzer, C., Formella, N., & Beebe, H. (1993). Work restructuring: The process of decision making. *Nursing Economics, 11*(4), 215–222.

Smith, L. (1993). The coming health care shakeout. *Fortune, 127*(10), 70–75.

Spitzer-Lehmann, R. (1993). Front-line ambassador. *Health Management Quarterly, 15*(2), 11–15.

Spitzer-Lehmann, R. & Yahn, K. (1992). Patient needs drive an integrated approach to care. *Nursing Management, 23*(8), 30–32.

Tichy, N. & Sherman, S. (1993). *Control your destiny or someone else will.* New York: Doubleday.

Tonges, M. (1992). Work designs: Sociotechnical systems for patient care delivery. *Nursing Management, 23*(1), 27–31.

Vestal, K. & Flannery, T. (1993, April). *Leadership for work transformation: Keys to success.* Paper presented at the 26th annual meeting of the American Organization of Nurse Executives. Orlando, FL.

Wilson, C. (1992). *Building new nursing organizations: Visions and realities.* Gaithersburg: Aspen.

Yancer, D. (1990). Redesigning the work. *Aspen's Advisor for Nurse Executives, 5*(8), 4–5.

Chapter 2

Redesigning Nursing Care Delivery: From Theory to Implementation

NELLIE C. ROBINSON

American business is entering the 21st century with companies structured and designed during the 19th century (Hammer and Champy, 1993). Accelerated worldwide changes and the increasing complexities of today's market demand the redesign of work processes, structures, and organizational cultures in order to become more customer-focused and thereby ensure success and survival in the competitive world of the 1990s and beyond.

Few industries face the formidable challenges that confront health care and the nursing profession. Spiraling health care costs, widespread consumer pessimism, and shrinking resources have fueled the need for health care reform. The fundamental rethinking and radical redesign of the industry will achieve dramatic changes in measures of performance such as cost, quality, and service. "As health care moves into a competitive environment, hospitals will be pressed to create and maintain a competitive edge to survive. Core clinical staff, such as registered nurses, are a key component to increasing quality, understanding patient care needs and balancing cost in a reformed health care system" (Prescott, 1993).

The current health care environment offers unparalleled opportunities for hospitals and nursing services to redesign nursing care delivery toward high-quality, cost-effective care that will strengthen institutional alignment with current and future customers. As members of the largest clinical discipline within the health care industry, nurses also have a professional responsibility to assist in the redesign of institutional health care delivery systems to address core issues of access, competition, choice, quality, cost, and security while meeting the individualized needs of patients and families.

▄WORK REDESIGN

Redesigning nursing care means rethinking and changing the policies, work processes, and relationships required to deliver care and bring a high level of satisfaction to customers. Redesign does not mean rearranging current systems to achieve incremental improvements but rather indicates rad-

Flarey, D: REDESIGNING NURSING CARE DELIVERY: Transforming Our Future
© 1995, J. B. Lippincott Company

ical restructure and reinvention to facilitate significant redirection and measurable improvements in customer services.

A variety of redesign and reengineering techniques and methods have been successfully applied in business and in the health care industry. Common elements of these successful redesign efforts include:

- Leadership commitment to organizational change;
- Clearly delegated responsibility, accountability, and empowerment that encourages creativity and innovation;
- Multidisciplinary redesign teams consisting of insiders, outsiders, management, and front-line employees;
- A customer-focused approach to redesign;
- Defined methods for incorporating the voice of the customer;
- Recognition and reward; and
- Measurement strategies.

Regardless of changes in national health policy, most of us are engaged at the organizational level, and there exists enormous opportunity for contribution to the reinvention of how work is done at the point of service. Health care reform will not take place in the White House or in the halls of Congress; for the majority of us, the changes will be realized at the bedside. Through the process of redesign, nurses have the opportunity to participate in planning the inevitable changes rather than being victims of such changes.

▄ THEORY-BASED WORK REDESIGN

The rapid rate of change, the chaotic environment, and the complexity of issues currently facing health care institutions and nursing have the potential to create reactive responses. Nursing services experiencing a sense of urgency and pressure to respond may develop task-oriented approaches to restructuring work, roles, and relationships. This approach could be short-sighted and may undermine core values and principles of nursing care. As nursing recreates the future through redesign and responds to the mandate for managed competition, managed care, high quality, and cost efficiency, it is imperative that the response be coordinated, systematic, and formalized and that it be developed and implemented based on careful consideration of professional, ethical, financial, and sociotechnical principles.

According to Fernandez and Wheeler, a theory-based approach to work redesign "provides the structure for understanding all the practice components of nursing service delivery. It lays the foundation for nursing practice by providing a framework that organizes knowledge and the delivery of care based on that knowledge, thus creating a bridge between nursing theory and nursing practice" (Fernandez and Wheeler, 1990). The development and implementation of theory-based models in the practice arena has implications for further research and the potential to contribute significantly to bridging the gap between theory and practice in nursing.

Developing a theoretical base for redesigning nursing care entails the identification, purposeful examination, and clear articulation of beliefs and values relevant to patients, nursing, health care, management, education, and nursing care. These values must be formulated into a specific philosophy of care that can be used to direct the development of a conceptual framework that will strengthen professional nursing practice and guide nursing care delivery within the institution.

A conceptual framework is a network of interrelated concepts, constructs, and definitions relevant to a discipline. A nursing conceptual framework for work redesign must address guiding themes for all major areas related to structure, practice, relationships, care delivery, resources, development, and research. The conceptual framework for theory-based redesign provides

- A system for organizing existing knowledge;
- A common language for nursing staff;
- A structure for decision-making;
- A structure for the generation of new knowledge;
- Guidance for nursing actions within the practice setting; and
- A system that facilitates the translation of values and philosophy into practice.

■ A PATIENT-CENTERED FRAMEWORK FOR RESTRUCTURING CARE

A patient-centered framework for restructuring care can facilitate the redesign of delivery systems that will rebuild trust and confidence in quality of service, meet customer expectations, and allow for considerations to be given to human and financial resource limitations.

Rationale for a Patient-Centered Framework

In the complex network of the hospital system, the patient provides the impetus for integration of all health care services and is the catalyst for reshaping and strengthening professional practice. Defining and putting into effect a framework that places the patient at the center of all operations is therefore the appropriate means of achieving high-quality services, cost-efficiency, and satisfaction among patients, nurses, and physicians. In 1961, Abdellah and colleagues stated that hospitals and community services should be tailored to meet patient care needs (Abdellah, Beland, Martin, & Matheney, 1961). This observation is still valid in hospitals today.

A patient-centered approach does not require the discarding of values; rather, it reshapes and strengthens professional practice within the goal of improving patient care delivery. In addition, this approach fosters collaboration within the health care team, since the patient provides the focus for all health care providers to develop and achieve common goals. The product of nursing services is patient care. The most important stakeholder is the patient. It is therefore a logical conclusion that a patient-centered framework for care will facilitate the desired changes while maintaining core values.

The Patient-Centered Framework

In a patient-centered environment, the patient is the primary focus of nursing care activities. Staff and services are organized around the needs of patients, and emphasis is placed on meeting individualized patient care needs. Patients and families can be conceptually incorporated into the organizational structure of the Division of Nursing. Figure 2-1 illustrates the nontraditional inverted pyramid, with patients occupying the broadest point, followed by direct caregivers, who are supported in turn by nursing management and administrative staff. This empowerment of patients and direct caregivers demonstrates the core value of the patient-centered framework. Nursing practice operates through a value system of patient-centeredness, and actions are consistently performed within the context of the system.

The value-based, patient-centered framework is composed of four interrelated constructs, each supported by lower level concepts (Fig. 2-2). These constructs and their related concepts serve to unify the practice of nursing and provide the model through which the patient-centered care delivery system becomes operational. The constructs further serve as guiding themes that frame and drive the development of group goals. The four constructs are as follows.

1. *A Patient-Centered Environment.* The major construct in this value-based system is the patient-centered environment, which is central to the framework and is depicted at the center of the diagram in Figure 2-2. Inherent to this construct is the position of the patient as the focal point within the system. This construct recognizes that the quality of health care services that are delivered is directly related to

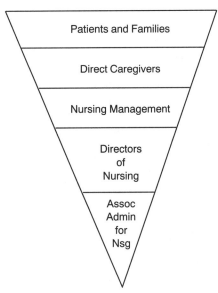

FIGURE 2-1 Conceptual illustration of division of nursing organizational chart.

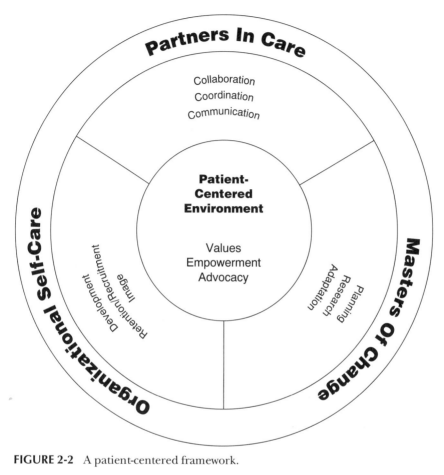

FIGURE 2-2 A patient-centered framework.

the commitment of an organization to meet the health care needs of the patient. Therefore, this basic belief dictates the integration of patient care needs into the design and delivery of all services.

2. *Organizational Self-Care.* Denoted here is the institution's priority concern with the need for support and care for its constituent health care providers; this is an essential element of an institution's ability to provide patient-centered care. Usually, the benefits associated with organizational self-care far exceed the investments often required, and these benefits contribute positively to the long-range health and viability of the institution.

3. *Partners in Care.* This construct acknowledges the interdependent roles of health care professionals. The element emphasizes the need for communication and collaboration among all health care providers, patients, and families in order to achieve desired outcomes.

4. *Masters of Change.* To succeed in today's health care environment,

institutions must acknowledge that change is inevitable and continuous. Integrated within the patient-centered framework is the realization of the dynamics of this change within the health care industry. As change agents, each individual health care provider should participate in defining and achieving goals, realizing that change is the catalyst for organizational as well as personal development.

The conceptual representation of the patient-centered framework (see Fig. 2-2) delineates each major construct. It is important to note that the elements of the system are not mutually exclusive but interdependent. The patient-centered framework is strengthened by the dynamic relations among the patient-centered environment and the other three supporting constructs.

The patient-centered framework demonstrates a unique model that unites these four vital constructs. These constructs, when coordinated under a single system, articulate the key values important to patients and families, professional nursing, all other health care providers, and the health care industry. In addition, these four major constructs provide the basis for the development of goals and strategies from which specific objectives are achieved.

■ PUTTING THE FRAMEWORK INTO EFFECT

The patient-centered care delivery system (Table 2-1), demonstrates the linkage between the conceptual and operational components of the process by translating the framework into measurable goals and related strategies for restructuring. This further demonstrates the unifying and supportive relationships that must exist between the patient-centered framework and the institutional objectives that support care, partnerships, and change.

Implementing the patient-centered care delivery system involves the development of specific behavioral objectives and associated evaluation methodology to support the goals and strategies outlined in the system. The patient-centered care delivery system encompasses individual patient/family services and nonclinical support, and the organizing principles of managed care and case management are used to structure the way work is organized and processed (Zander, 1990). All levels of nursing staff should contribute to the achievement of patient care outcomes, and multidisciplinary teams should plan activities and programs around patient care needs. The system incorporates a number of management tools and techniques that enhance development and facilitate participation in the redesign process.

A commitment to excellence in nursing practice and to professional growth and development of nursing staff is a key area of focus in seeking to optimize the quality of patient care services and enhance the market position of any institution. At the District of Columbia General Hospital, the current economic pressures, the emphasis on cost containment, quality-of-care outcomes, and productivity, and the need to contribute to the fiscal health of the organization were factors that fostered the creation and implementation of a new philosophy of patient-centeredness. The need to re-

TABLE 2-1 A Patient-Centered Care Delivery System

	Patient-Centered Environment	Organizational Self-Care	Partners in Care	Masters of Change
Major Constructs	Patient-Centered Environment	Organizational Self-Care	Partners in Care	Masters of Change
Related Concepts	Values Advocacy Empowerment	Development Retention/ Recruitment	Collaboration Coordination Communication	Planning Research Adaptation
Goals	Establish a high-quality outcome-oriented, fiscally-responsive Patient-Centered Care environment.	Create an environment that is attractive to professional practice.	Coordinate goal-directed patient care activities through effective communication and professional collaboration.	Motivate staff to participate as change agents as the process of patient-centeredness evolves
Strategies	Clarification and Communication of Values and Beliefs Patient-Centered Care Delivery Method Decentralization Quality Improvements Cost Containment	Role Clarification Work Redesign Professional Development Organizational Development Retention and Recruitment Recognition and Reward	Patient and Family Involvement Clinical Partnerships Interdisciplinary Problem Solving and Decision Making Peer Review Participative Management	Multidisciplinary Interactive Planning Risk Taking Creativity Measurement and Evaluation Research

structure had become evident through bed closures, decreased staff morale, and a high turnover of registered nurses. The development of a patient-centered approach to restructuring care also grew out of the needs to create a basis for strategic planning, to develop a common language, to develop realistic initiatives based on identified patient care needs, and to develop a system through which both patients and staff could be empowered.

The conceptual basis for the patient-centered framework was presented to one group of nursing administrative staff at an off-site retreat. Deliberations and discussions during the initial retreat led to a clear articulation of the status of nursing and an assessment of the issues related to the practice environment. The patient-centered framework was presented to all levels of nursing personnel, physicians, hospital management, and administrators to ensure understanding, gain input, and encourage support for implementation. The patient-centered framework was validated as the system that would guide nursing practice development as well as divisional planning.

A subsequent series of meetings among administrative, management, and unit staff members were held to further describe and define areas of focus and to elicit input for enhancement and program planning. A second off-site retreat was convened with the management staff and members of the unit-level staff. Using assessment data, projecting a desired future, and holding the four major constructs of the framework as guiding themes, the group formulated a comprehensive design for a patient-centered care delivery system (see Table 2-1).

The Division of Nursing has since developed a shared understanding of the framework, formulated unifying objectives for each construct, and devised priority listings of initiatives for implementation. The framework created a vision that expressed the beliefs and values of the Division of Nursing as they relate to the patient as central focus, the importance of the caregiver, commitment to high-quality services, and the importance of patient, nurse, and physician interaction and satisfaction with care. Putting the framework into practice became the primary focus for the Division of Nursing, and the four major constructs formed the basis for its application to the restructuring process.

Creating the Patient-Centered Environment

The most important element in successfully creating a patient-centered environment was the development of a defined direction—a mission that would reflect the overall basic philosophy, values, beliefs, and priorities of patient-centered care delivery and nursing practice. In addition, organizational structure, quality improvement programs, and the method of care delivery required examination and redesign to facilitate the goals of a patient-centered environment.

Organizational Self-Care

While the patient-centered framework emphasizes patients and the clinical components of care, it also illustrates the importance of other elements of hospital life in achieving patient-centered care. Support of the caregivers is a vital element in successfully applying the concept of patient-centeredness.

Work redesign, organizational development, retention and recruitment, and recognition and reward were key elements of organizational self-care found to be of vital importance in supporting the clinical component.

Partners in Care

Focusing on the work of patient care required a multidisciplinary approach, in contrast to the narrower vision of solving problems within individual departments. As the focal point of the patient-centered framework, the patient provided the impetus for the development of new interdisciplinary relationships based on a shared commitment to patient care. The partners in care construct was applied to a restructuring process by means of patient and family focus groups, interdisciplinary planning, implementation of restructuring processes at the unit level, and increased lateral communication among first-line managers.

Masters of Change

The rapid rate of change in health care dictates the need for nurse leaders to muster their inherent strength as planners and change agents in the hospital setting. The phrase "plan or be planned for" was translated into the need for nurses to be actively involved in planning and decision-making activities related to patient care delivery. The involvement of all levels of staff on committees and the use of tools such as nominal group technique, responsibility charting, and project planning afforded enthusiastic participation in the change process.

Application of the patient-centered framework to practice required an investment in planning, professional development, multidisciplinary communication, and involvement. Participation in the planning grant for the project, "Strengthening Hospital Nursing: A Program to Improve Patient Care," sponsored by The Robert Wood Johnson Foundation and The Pew Charitable Trusts, helped facilitate multidisciplinary interactive planning efforts related to conceptualizing and implementing the patient-centered framework.

■PRELIMINARY RESULTS

Hospital response to the patient-centered framework and the subsequent development and implementation of the patient-centered care delivery system has been positive. The multidisciplinary approach to patient care planning and problem-solving has resulted in a new collaborative relationship among all departments.

Research and evaluation methodologies were varied and focused on explication of objectives in behavioral terms, on identification of questions of concern to patients, staff, and administration, on a variety of qualitative and quantitative study designs, and on a balance between objective and subjective measures (Waltz, Chambers, & Hechenberger, 1989). Content analysis of structured patient and staff focus groups provided invaluable data on the attitudes and perceptions of patients, their families, and nurses and their needs in terms of the patient-centered approach to restructuring care. Retrospective and cross-sectional management information data from a variety of sources—including admission, discharge, and length-of-stay records, documentation in the medical record, and quality assurance data analysis—provided descriptive quantitative findings to support framework implementation.

Initial research and evaluation data reflect the total impact of the patient-centered framework on patient care and staff responsiveness. Turnover among registered nurses decreased from 33% to 19%; the overall length of stay for managed care patients decreased by 1 to 4 days; and quality assurance indices reflect a 55% improvement in documentation of discharge planning, a 57% increase in implementation of patient teaching, and a 70% increase in individualized patient care planning. There is further evidence of decreased patient readmission (from 40% to less than 1% on one obstetric-gynecologic unit), increased patient and family involvement, and increased patient, nurse, and physician satisfaction with care.

To improve patient care in today's complex health care environment, nursing must take the leadership in examining beliefs and values and in articulating a vision to guide patient care. These beliefs and values must be structured into a framework for practice. The patient-centered framework is simple, providing a common language for all levels of staff and health care disciplines.

This framework has been adopted and translated into a model for practice. Expansion, further development, and research of the patient-centered framework is ongoing. Research and evaluation related to the full impact of this value-based system on the restructuring process is needed. The preliminary findings, however, demonstrate the feasibility of such a comprehensive plan in an acute care hospital confronted with the challenges of providing high-quality, cost-effective care.

■ A GUIDE TO REDESIGNING NURSING CARE: FROM THEORY TO IMPLEMENTATION

Table 2-2 presents a guide that has been developed to provide a road map for restructuring. It outlines five phases essential to the redesign of nursing care and incorporates the process from theory to implementation as follows.

> *Phase I—Visionary* outlines the theoretical base that is fundamental to the redesign of nursing care.
>
> *Phase II—Assessment and Planning* facilitates internal and external scanning of the organization and builds consensus while further providing for clarification of concepts.
>
> *Phase III—Design and Development* affords the translation of theory to practical application through the development of strategies, goals, and objectives.
>
> *Phase IV—Implementation* indicates that practices are implemented according to the theory and plans developed. This phase affords true integration and application of work redesign.

TABLE 2-2   A Guide to Redesigning Nursing Care: From Theory to Implementation

Phase I–Visionary
1. Clarify beliefs and values.
2. Formulate a philosophy of care.
3. Define mission.
4. Develop conceptual framework.
5. Identify strategic advantage.
6. Determine institutional readiness.
7. Establish a multidisciplinary steering committee.
8. Build shared vision.

Phase II–Assessment and Planning
1. Perform internal and external organizational assessment.
2. Identify and collect data based on staffing, patient, physician, and nurse satisfaction with care and services, skill mix, quality indicators, length of stay, operating cost, and collaborative initiatives.
3. Identify stake-holders.
4. Seek commitment, build trust, solicit input, accommodate changes, build consensus.
5. Define infrastructure.
6. Educate management.
7. Plan resources.
8. Facilitate interactive planning.

Phase III–Design and Development
1. Communicate with all levels of nursing, staff, physicians, management, and administration.
2. Build support for change effort.
3. Define specific goals, objectives, and strategies.
4. Select or develop a care delivery model.
5. Define investment strategy.
6. Establish criteria for selection of start up unit(s).
7. Establish multidisciplinary teams.
8. Educate teams.
9. Develop action plans.
10. Redesign work.
11. Develop policies, standards, and practice guidelines.
12. Develop critical pathways.
13. Examine human resource issues.
14. Examine labor/management issues.
15. Develop position descriptions and associated performance appraisal criteria.
16. Redesign facility (if applicable).
17. Validate customer alignment with redesign plans.

Phase IV–Implementation
1. Educate and inform all staff.
2. Renovate facility (if applicable).
3. Start up unit(s).
4. Apply new methodologies.
5. Create feedback discussion loop for staff and customers.
6. Develop recognition and reward system.

Phase V–Evaluation and Research
1. Identify key processes and outcomes for measurement and evaluation.
2. Design research methodology.
3. Collect data.
4. Identify opportunities for quality improvement.
5. Apply research techniques and provide information and feedback to guide redesign implementation.

Phase V—Evaluation and Research enables the documentation of the current situation and facilitates the development of new knowledge regarding the change process.

The phases of this guide are not mutually exclusive but are interrelated. Since no one system is appropriate for all settings, each reader should explore the process of redesigning nursing care and adjust the guide to achieve the goals of his or her institutional program.

SUMMARY

A combination of factors has led to the challenges facing health care and nursing today. In redesigning its future, nurses must take leadership in examining beliefs and values and formulating a philosophy of care. To ensure a comprehensive and formalized process, it is necessary to articulate a vision and to plan, develop, design, and implement theory-based, patient-centered systems as a foundation and a structure to guide changes in nursing practice and patient care within institutions.

REFERENCES

Abdellah, F. G., Beland, I. L., Martin, A., & Matheney, R. V. (1961). *Patient-centered approaches to nursing.* New York: MacMillan.

Fernandez, R. D. & Wheeler, J. I. (1990). Organizing a nursing system through theory-based practice. In G. Mayer, G. Madden, & E. Lawrenz (Eds.), *Patient care delivery models.* Rockville, MD: Aspen.

Graham, P., Constantini, S., Balick, B., Bedor, B., Hooke, M., Papin, D., et al. (1987). Operationalizing a nursing philosophy. *The Journal of Nursing Administration. 17*(3), 14–18.

Hammer, M. & Champy, J. (1993). *Reengineering the corporation, a manifesto for business revolution.* New York: Harper Business.

Lombardi, D.N. (1992). *Progressive health care management strategies.* Chicago: American Hospital.

Prescott, P.A. (1993). Nursing: An important component of hospital survival under a reformed health care system. *Nursing Economics, 22*(4), 192–198.

Robinson, N.C. (1991). A patient-centered framework for restructuring care. *The Journal of Nursing Administration, 21*(9).

Waltz, F. C., Chambers, S. B., & Hechenberger, N. B. (1989). *Strategic planning, marketing and evaluation for nursing education and service.* New York: National League for Nursing.

Zander, K. (1990). Managed care and nursing management. In G. G. Mayer, M. J. Madden, & E. Lawrenz (Eds.), *Patient care delivery models* (37–61). Rockville, MD: Aspen.

Chapter 3

The Strengthening Hospital Nursing Program: Restructuring for a Patient-Centered Health Care Delivery System

MARY K. KOHLES

Imagination, dreams, innovations, visions, and other inspirational terms are components of the language of those planning and implementing the future generation of health care delivery systems. Strengthening Hospital Nursing: A Program to Improve Patient Care (SHNP) (Strengthening Hospital Nursing Program, 1992) encourages its participants not only to dream but to turn those dreams into actions. It is through those actions that the participants are bringing about a system of care in hospitals and multihospital systems that is based on the understanding that the patient is the reason such organizations exist. The actions of SHNP participants bring together nontraditional partners such as payors, policymakers, educational institutions, unions, care providers, and health care administrators. Their actions are resulting in an integrated, patient-centered health care system that is sensitive to patient concerns and the patient's understanding of how to use that system. Their actions acknowledge that accountability resides with all stakeholders within the health care environment and the community they serve.

▄ WHAT THE PROGRAM IS ABOUT

The SHNP program is about collaboration, commitment, and interdependent relationships. It is about using human resources appropriately, supporting cost-effectiveness and care efficacy, and championing continuous quality improvement. The program emphasizes solidarity among disciplines (ie, among nurses, physicians, support staff, and other professionals) from all levels of the organization and focuses on finding new ways to get work done by building on a shared vision of what the institution may one day be

(National Program Office, 1992).* The SHNP design is based on a continuum of care in which patient's needs are identified. The patient's needs are addressed as conveniently and efficiently as possible by care providers working together.

▬THE SPONSORING FOUNDATIONS

The SHNP was developed by The Robert Wood Johnson Foundation and The Pew Charitable Trusts in the mid-1980s. The 1980s were plagued by a shortage of nurses and other key professionals, changes in reimbursement, advances in biomedical technology, and alterations in the profile of hospitalized patients. Nurses provide much of the complex care needed by hospitalized patients, and the presenting factors caused an imbalance in supply and demand. The sponsoring foundations desired to strengthen the usage of nursing resources in an increasingly complex patient care environment. They recognized that only through institution-wide restructuring is it possible to address problems that deter nurses and other professionals from providing optimal patient care services.

Understanding hospital traditions, the Foundation and the Trusts in August 1988 challenged nursing leaders and their executive colleagues to take a risk, shift their paradigms, and use their imaginations to create a vision for their future. SHNP was conceived to provide that challenge. Because of the magnitude of that challenge, the grant was awarded in two phases. In phase one, 80 hospitals or hospital consortia, representing 211 hospitals in 42 states and the District of Columbia, were selected to receive one-year planning grants of up to $50,000. During the planning year, grantees completed a detailed five-year blueprint for restructuring the workplace to promote a patient-centered care delivery system. In October 1990, phase two of the grant program began; 20 hospitals or consortia with the most promising organizational and operational designs from phase one were selected to receive five-year implementation grants for up to $1,000,000. The 20 grantees represent 68 hospitals in 19 states and the District of Columbia. Nineteen of the 20 grantees continue in their implementation phase, which ends October 1995 (National Program Office, 1992).

▬PROGRAM OBJECTIVES

The program seeks to improve patient care by addressing the following objectives:

- To foster the development of innovative, institution-wide systems for strengthening patient care through the coordinated efforts of all patient care providers, including nurses, physicians, support staff, and other professionals;

---

*The National Program Office at St. Anthony's Hospital in St. Petersburg, Florida, under the direction of Barbara A. Donaho, RN, MA, FAAN, provides technical and administrative assistance to the grantees. The program office collects ongoing data on project activities and will assess the implementation phase of the program.

- To create work environments that optimally use nursing resources and improve care in a cost-effective and efficient manner; and
- To establish patterns of service delivery that promote satisfaction among patients, nurses, physicians, and other staff.

▬ CONSISTENT THEMES: FACTORS FOR SUCCESS

Although the restructuring projects for the grantees are diverse, there are consistent themes. The following themes are considered factors for success and served as the basis for the selection of the implementation projects.

- The hospital or consortium has a substantive, shared vision known by affected stakeholders at all levels of the organization.
- Executive management, board of trustees, and key medical staff representatives are committed and actively involved. SHNP has learned that strength, commitment, and involvement by key leadership is imperative to sustain the innovative project over time.
- The change process is interactive, involving individuals from many different levels and departments within and, at times, outside the hospital. The change process strives for interdependent relationships and a seamless system of health care across care settings—acute, home, long-term, wellness, and preventive care.
- The patient care delivery archetypes are patient-centered, meaning that the delivery of service is designed to meet the needs of the patient rather than the needs of a department or discipline. Patient services take place in the environment most germane to the patient, and services are delivered by the most appropriate care provider.
- Decision-making is pushed to the level of the organization closest to the patient and, when appropriate, involves the patient or the patient's family.
- The hospital has undergone a shift in organizational culture, and is open to continuous learning, improving, and adapting. The hospital acknowledges the economic, legal, and competitive struggles that it faces in the future. It is prepared to view the struggles as opportunities through partnerships with employees, physicians, payors, policymakers, and the community.

▬ DEVELOPMENT OF A VITAL COMPONENT

The SHNP educational sessions and workshops attended by the grantees were a vital part of their development as change agents. The chief executive officers, nurse executives, chief financial officers, medical staff representatives, trustee representatives, and project staff members from each grant project attended educational sessions as a team. The first educational session, in April 1989, presented the work of Russell L. Ackoff, PhD, founder of the Philadelphia-based consultant firm, Interact, The Institute for Interactive Management. Ackoff discussed his theories and techniques for an interactive planning model. Ackoff's model promotes an interdisciplinary process through which organizational leaders and employees at all levels of the organization envision their idealized future. Using system-age tools rather than machine-age thinking, the organization involves many disciplines and their leaders in inventing ways to approximate that future (Ackoff, 1981).

In an effort to continue the learning process and provide pragmatic tools for organizational change, grantee teams attended a two-day workshop held at the University of Pennsylvania's Leonard Davis Institute of Health Economics in Philadelphia. Under the direction of Sheldon Rovin, DDS, MS, Associate Director of the Institute, the teams learned nominal group technique—a process which is interactive, nonthreatening, and, by its design, guaranteed to provide equal time and consideration to all participants regardless of their organizational status (National Program Office, 1992). They learned stakeholder mapping, a systematic tool used to identify the key players, and responsibility charting, a method of determining the levels of responsibility of the stakeholders. They learned the importance of recording minutes and journalizing their stories for a historical record of their innovations. Their notes and anecdotes became the basis of their revision processes, facilitating their learning about what worked and what didn't. The notes and anecdotes also serve as groundwork for their publications and presentations.

The second educational program, building on Ackoff's work, featured Peter M. Senge, PhD, founding partner of Innovation Associates in Farmington, Massachusetts. Creating an ideal future requires building a shared vision among the people involved, according to Senge. He stressed that the hospital does not have to reach total agreement on what the organization should do, but people must agree on what the hospital is about—the hospital's mission and objectives (Senge, 1990). Senge discussed characteristics of a learning organization. Learning is a process whereby people within an organization improve their effectiveness by adapting to change (Senge, 1990).

The third educational session teamed up Donald N. Lombardi, PhD, the principal partner of CHR/InterVista, Inc., of New Jersey, and Thomas N. Gilmore, PhD, Vice President, Center For Applied Research, in Philadelphia. The grant projects were again represented by the chief executive officers, nurse executives, medical staff representatives, trustee representatives, and project staff, along with the chief financial officers and leaders of other departments such as information systems, human resources, and management engineering.

Lombardi began the third session with his work in value-driven management. According to Lombardi, value-driven management is the basis of progressive management—a term he used to describe the management activities and strategies of an effective health care manager at any level of an organization (Lombardi, 1992). He focused on the management of human resources, delineating specific situations that confront managers. He provided the audience alternatives for achieving higher levels of performance by using value-driven strategies (Lombardi, 1992).

Gilmore, building on Lombardi's work, provided the grantee teams an opportunity to think about the dilemmas of institutionalizing innovations. Through interactive dialogue within the grantee teams, Gilmore asked the teams to think about the tension that exists between parallel (ad hoc) structures developed to generate new ideas and the ongoing operational structures used to carry out business as usual. He emphasized that innovation requires freedom from existing organizational structures. Ideas coming from many sources—health care consumers, community leaders, care providers, and new organizational leaders and staff—need a structure in which to germinate and evolve. Ad hoc structures are often put in place to allow for the development of those new ideas, plan for implementation, set targets, and monitor performance. These ad hoc structures can bring drawbacks and dangers, especially if the desired end result is a new organizational culture. The resulting tension requires energy, attention, and commitment from key leadership to enable the emergence of an enduring change (Gilmore & Krantz, 1991).

▬ BUILDING A SHARED VISION

Building a shared vision by organizational members requires an alliance among key stakeholders involved at all levels of the organization. Though the process may not start at the executive level, at some point, executive management has to take ownership and become a part of the collective "we" that is responsible for moving it forward. The executive team conducts an educational assessment to determine what resources and means are needed to support the process. They are responsible for weighing the resource demands for change against the organizational priorities. The executive team also determines whether the base budget can support the innovation.

Part of the resource demands will be for development programs for management and staff. Costs to the organization for development will vary depending on what is needed to get people empowered to do the right thing without asking for permission. If the organization has a mindset that it is consultants or executive staff who solve problems and they want to move to a mindset of collaboration across lines of hierarchy, the developmental cost will be in proportion to degree of that mind shift. The cost may be high; the value added to the organization may not be realized for years to come. The executive leadership and trustee commitment required may seem like a leap of faith. However, they are necessary if the desired result is a new organizational culture.

▬ INTERNAL AND EXTERNAL BARRIERS

As part of the national program's application process, grantees identified internal and external barriers that interfered with the ability for hospital leaders and caregivers to provide patient care services. Phase one and phase two grantees highlighted inadequate nursing resources, nursing practice deficits, insufficient departmental support services, unmet compensation and benefits needs, lack of nursing management participation in hospital-wide decision-making, and job dissatisfaction as internal barriers to their work. The external barriers included supply-and-demand imbalance of nurses, limitations imposed by reimbursement and other regulatory issues, variations in regional demographic patterns, and difficulties in recruiting health care workers.

The importance of a given barrier varied with the type of hospital. For example, urban hospitals identified the lack of a unified model of delivery for patient care as the most significant internal barrier and variations in regional demographics as the most important external barrier. Rural hospitals identified low compensation and benefit levels for nurses and other health professionals as their priority internal barrier and difficulties in recruitment of health care workers as their most important external barrier. Teaching hospitals saw the lack of a unified model for delivery of patient care as their top internal barrier; they did not mention any particular external barrier as the most significant. Community hospitals identified insufficient departmental support services as their top-ranked internal barrier and supply-and-demand imbalance of nurses as their most significant external barrier (National Program Office, 1992; Aiken & Fagin, 1992).

Since the hospitals have systematically implemented strategies to restructure their internal environments, their internal barriers have shifted to issues that are more influenced by economic, legal, and other conditions pertinent to their survival in an era of managed care and integrated delivery systems. The external barriers for the most part have remained constant. However, potential issues resulting from health care reform are causing leaders to direct their energies beyond the hospital boundaries to the local, regional, and national levels.

▬LESSONS LEARNED

Learning is an essential component of the national program. Sharing that learning is an expectation. A key finding is the issue of funding. The sponsoring foundations recognized that other hospitals may not be given supporting funds to restructure; lessons learned must be articulated in order to prevent other organizations from experiencing some unnecessary expenses. The grantees have a responsibility to help others consider where to invest and what the value-added result of that investment will be. The most meaningful lesson learned is that the template for future solutions is the process, not the outcome. This lesson comes with knowledge that each health care setting has its own internal and external factors to consider. Processes for innovation will be similar, but the desired outcomes will fit each unique environment. Some other lessons learned are included in the following list.

- Plan for significant up-front development time for affected stakeholders, including senior, middle, and line management, trustees, key physicians, and grass roots staff.
- Involve physicians early on; change is pertinent to them and impacts their practice with patients.

- Involve key departments, such as information systems and financial and human resources, in the planning and implementation of innovations.
- Develop community linkages, emphasizing the continuum of patient care services.
- Include payors and policymakers in a timely manner, to broaden the impact of change. Many of the grantees are now linking with their local and state legislators.
- Understand the competencies of all disciplines, recognizing the unique talents that each person brings to the change process.
- Integrate trustee-approved restructuring as part of the strategic plan.
- Develop measurements to demonstrate the cost impact of institution-wide restructuring and the return on the organization's investment (Kohles & Donaho, 1992).

▬EVALUATION DESIGN

The restructuring approach for each hospital or hospital consortium is different. An organization chooses a particular project for change based on its own perceived needs and culture, the population it serves, and the diversity inside its walls. Because the projects are different, the critical indicators demonstrating effectiveness differ among the grantees. The evaluation design, however, has commonalities. The design is based on the principles of action-learning or action research. The SHNP grantees quickly learned that the research design had to adapt to a changing environment, produce useful knowledge derived from real world practice, and allow for a better understanding of restructuring efforts. Experimental design alone is not adequate, because it requires too many controls and does not readily support a fluid, dynamic process.

After work teams or task forces define what it is they want to achieve by their efforts, they develop indicators by which to gauge their work and results (Kohles & Donaho, 1992). They use case studies, interviews, surveys, meeting minutes, anecdotal stories, and operational management reports as their data sources. Often, there are no national standards with which to compare their work. They are the pacesetters, establishing their own internal trends with which to compare over time. Hospital leaders have found during the evaluation process that financial systems and information systems must change in order to be responsive to the data elements required to capture effective cost information in support of innovations.

▬COMMUNITY OUTREACH

The SHNP grantees have embraced interdisciplinary, collaborative, interdependent relationships as they design care delivery systems that meet the needs of the patients and families they serve. Through those relationships, they are connecting with elementary schools, high schools, community colleges, and universities to jointly plan for the preparation of the health care worker for the 21st century. The grantees are communicating their concerns with payors, policymakers, and, at times, legislators to address issues that interfere with a patient-centered care delivery system—a delivery system that is convenient, efficient, and cost-effective, and provides services across many care settings. They are also working with community wellness and prevention services, churches, and other service agencies. The grantees recognize their role and are taking initiatives to improve the health status of the communities they serve. They are embracing a seamless health care system—a system that will be limited only by the imaginations of the health care providers, community leaders, and other stakeholders working collaboratively and interdependently.

The views expressed in this chapter are solely those of the author; official endorsement by The Robert Wood Johnson Foundation or The Pew Charitable Trusts is not intended and should not be inferred.

▄ REFERENCES

Ackoff, R. (1981). *Creating the corporate future.* New York: John Wiley.

Aiken, L. & Fagin, C. (1992). *Charting nursing's future agenda for the 1990s.* Philadelphia: Lippincott.

Gilmore, T. & Krantz, J. (1991). Innovation in the public sector: Dilemmas in the use of ad hoc processes. *Journal of Policy Analysis and Management, 10*(3), 455–468.

Kohles, M. & Donaho, B. (1992). Twenty grantees seek transformation: From discipline-driven, compartmentalized entities to patient-driven, unified care systems. *Strategies for Health Care Excellence, 5*(11), 1–12.

Lombardi, D. (1992). *Progressive health care management strategies.* Chicago: American Hospital.

Strengthening Hospital Nursing Program, National Program Office. (1992). *Strengthening Hospital Nursing: A program to improve patient care.* St. Petersburg, FL: The Robert Wood Johnson Foundation and The Pew Charitable Trusts.

Senge, P. (1990). *The fifth discipline: The art and practice of the learning organization.* New York: Doubleday.

Chapter 4

Integrating Quality Into Care Delivery System Redesign

MARYANN F. FRALIC   DOMINICK L. FLAREY

You either get better or you get worse; you never stay the same.
—*Lou Holtz*

These pragmatic words of Lou Holtz echo the realities of the rapid-fire change and transformation occurring in our health care environment. This overwhelming transformation demands that nursing administrators quickly move forward in redesigning nursing and patient care delivery systems. Failure to forge ahead aggressively will result in stagnation and even the demise of organizations. The emerging new systems of health care dictate the changes needed to survive and grow in these unprecedented times. Our challenge is to clearly understand these mandates and redesign our operations for the successful transformation of health care organizations.

Along with the federal mandate for health care policy reform, we are already experiencing a revolution in health care delivery at the state and local levels. What is needed for institutions to be successful in this volatile new environment is a revolutionized delivery system in which costs are managed and quality and value of health services to consumers become the organization's mission (Bowles, 1993).

In redesigning care delivery systems, two crucial realities exist: 1) finance will drive the system and the way in which care is structured and delivered, and 2) quality is not negotiable; it is paramount. Quality standards are highly influenced by consumer expectations and external regulatory requirements. These standards must be measured and met, but the quest for quality must be properly balanced with the mandate for cost management: the two are inseparable.

Peter Drucker, considered to be the father of management science, believes that a "cost crunch" should always be used as an opportunity to rethink and redesign operations. To accept this challenge, constant and accelerated learning is required. We cannot have all of the skills today that we will need in order to be successful for the rest of our professional lifetimes; these skills must be acquired continually.

Three major executive skills are essential to success now and in the future. First, we must welcome change and we must become masters of change. Those who can manage change will emerge winners in this next era

Flarey, D: REDESIGNING NURSING CARE DELIVERY: Transforming Our Future
© 1995, J. B. Lippincott Company

of health care. Second, we must become quality experts. We must learn quality, live quality, and integrate quality into our organization's belief system and all professional work systems. Last, we must become quantitatively expert and financially astute. Managing costs is no longer the domain of the finance department. Nurse executives, nurse managers, and professional staff must acquire financial skills and apply them routinely to the way care is organized and delivered. As our health care system is transformed, nurses also will assume new responsibilities for revenue generation and enhancements (Finkler & Kovner, 1993). Nurse executives must ensure that all staff are properly educated in the importance of prudent financial management.

▰ MASTERING CHANGE FOR REDESIGN

Without question, the escalating costs of health care in our society are driving reform. Reform, in turn, is influencing major changes in the way we deliver care. Other major driving forces for delivery system redesign are the rapid changes occurring both within the profession and from market forces.

Since the major national nursing shortage several years ago, great strides have been made in enhancing the image of nursing and its power base within organizations and society. Professional nurses are accorded more responsibility related to professional practice and low-level technical care tasks have been shifted to other workers. When the supply of nurses was low and demand was great, this economic reality was the fundamental driving force stimulating the development of methodologies for role and delivery system redesign.

Today, the nurse manpower market is decidedly better. Two major trends popularized during the era of limited supply were responsible for improving the market: 1) the significant increases in salaries combined with wage decompression, and 2) new and innovative staffing and scheduling systems. These strategies brought many nurses into nursing schools or back into the market, resulting in more and higher-paid nurses. The relatively inexpensive nurse of yesterday has been replaced with the relatively expensive nurse of today. However, the system today cannot afford unlimited numbers of newly hired nurses at expensive rates. In simple terms, it cannot be "the old numbers at the new rate." This new reality may be termed the availability/affordability dilemma. This dilemma is great, and is the impetus driving new and highly innovative redesign projects today.

As the unit price per nurse increases, we must look very carefully at how each nurse's skills are being used. It is certain that as reimbursement continues to decrease within our health care system, we will have fewer resources available to us. We must develop systems that use fewer nurses but improve the quality of care delivered. This mandates that we examine with greater intensity what nurses are doing in the care delivery process. This examination and analysis are the crux of redesign.

Redesign, then, is examining the way in which patient care is delivered and reorganizing that process to achieve cost-effective, quality outcomes despite limited resources. It requires complex system analysis and rethinking that is goal-driven and task-managed (Barnum, 1991). As Barnum observes, it requires weaving together quality and quantity in a complex "dance" of diversely prepared caregivers (Barnum, 1991). Redesign is not simply the reassignment of people; it is a genuine change in the structure of jobs and the work people are doing (Hackman & Oldham, 1980). Successful redesign requires two important imperatives: unequivocal top-down support, and a broad-based, bottom-up enthusiasm.

Key Elements
The work of delivery system redesign, regardless of the model used, must contain the following key elements: 1) it must achieve the desired patient outcomes (quality is the first imperative; if the process is not good for patients, then it cannot be beneficial to the system); 2) it must contribute to staff satisfaction, retention, and productivity; and 3) it must contribute to the financial integrity of the organization (Robert Wood Johnson University Hospital Nursing Division, Hallmark Characteristics of the ProACT™ Model). These principles should guide all system redesign projects.

Uniqueness
Each organization's design must be unique. What works for one organization does not necessarily work for another. Health care executives must develop systems based on their own internal operations, and address the uniqueness of their own realities, goals, mission, resources, and limitations.

Participation of All Departments
Another important component of any delivery system redesign project is the imperative that it be an organization-wide endeavor. The core product of health care organizations is patient care. All staff, departments, and systems must work together to achieve this output. Redesign cannot simply be a nursing department project. It is necessary that everyone in the organization understand and contribute to the work of redesign. Such an imperative will eliminate barriers between departments, help realize a strategic vision for the organization, and aid in creating an environment of collaboration among members working synergistically to achieve mutually agreed goals.

■ THE ROBERT WOOD JOHNSON UNIVERSITY HOSPITAL EXPERIENCE
In 1987, Robert Wood Johnson University Hospital (RWJUH) was experiencing many of the same pressures and realities as other health care organizations across the country. Faced with a critical nursing shortage and a hostile state reimbursement system, nursing administrators led the way in a major delivery system redesign project. Through a work analysis, they determined that 42% of what professional registered nurses were doing was indirect work, half of which was wholly appropriate and half of which could safely be delegated to unlicensed, technical support staff. It became neces-

sary to analyze, change, and manage the patient care delivery system to ensure organizational viability and success.

The major goals of the redesign project were: 1) to reduce the number of registered nurse staff while delivering care that meets institutional and professional standards of quality and 2) to provide attractive roles for all hospital staff involved in supportive care (Robert Wood Johnson University Hospital Nursing Division, ProACT™ Guidelines). After defining these goals, the project design team developed a needs analysis approach and asked the following key questions: 1) What does the organization need?, 2) What do patients need?, and 3) What does nursing need?

Defining goals and focusing on the needs of the entire operation allowed for the development of axioms that could provide the structural foundation for delivery system redesign. These axioms are as follows:

The model should be designed to maximize revenue.

The model must be designed to ensure high quality patient care.

The model must be designed to maximize patient throughput for appropriate utilization of the organization's resources.

The model must be designed in concert with the organization's objectives, philosophy, and mission.

Patient care is the direct work of the organization; all else is support work.

Nursing is a practice discipline; it is a core element to the direct work of the organization.

Nursing leadership's responsibility is to develop systems and supports that structure the delivery of care and make it satisfying for nurses practicing at the bedside.

The organization's overall role is to deliver high-quality, cost-effective care to the community.

The major imperatives of the redesign project are to restructure the work and to organize the patient's stay for effectiveness and efficiency.

The major goal of the redesign model is to ensure the continued success and growth of the organization by providing patient care that is both affordable and high quality.

■ THE PROFESSIONALLY ADVANCED CARE TEAM (PROACT ™) MODEL

The result of the project team's work was the development of the Professionally Advanced Care Team (ProACT™) model. This model was developed with full institutional support, and the outcomes met the defined objectives. The ProACT™ model was one of the country's first delivery system redesign projects. Previous publications provide details of the model structure, process, and outcomes (Tonges, 1990; Tonges, 1989a; Tonges, 1989b; Brett & Tonges, 1990; Ritter, Fralic, Tonges, & McCormac, 1992; Fralic, 1992).

In designing the model, four hallmark objectives were defined by the development team: 1) reduce hospital length of stay, 2) minimize the cost of delivering care, 3) maximize reimbursement, and 4) attain optimal clinical outcomes. These objectives provided the framework for role and work redesign and continue to drive the model as it continually evolves.

As the model was developed, distinct patient care roles emerged (Display 4-1).

In evaluating the model, the organization focused on four major success factors. The model had to be 1) attainable, 2) affordable, 3) sustainable, and 4) valued and valuable.

In retrospective analysis and evaluation, it was determined that the ProACT ™ model did meet the defined objectives and the identified success factors. The model is successful because it is designed around two critical features: high quality care and cost effectiveness.

The overall evaluation of the quality initiative in the ProACT™ model has been overwhelmingly positive. The bottom line is that quality of care and service have steadily improved as a result of the multiple mechanisms in place. This has occurred simply because the care team as a whole evaluates its practice, and the team is empowered to correct and improve the clinical care of patients. Another significant factor in the success of the quality initiative is that the entire organization is involved in and committed to improving quality. If the nursing division were alone in promoting quality, the outcomes would not be as significant.

■ QUALITY IN REDESIGN

The work of patient care redesign fits smoothly into the health care industry's transition from a quality assurance focus to a Total Quality Management/Continuous Quality Improvement (TQM/CQI) philosophy; it

---

DISPLAY 4-1   *ProACT™ Model: Patient Care Roles*

1. *Primary Nurse:* is the registered nurse who has primary responsibility for overseeing the delivery of nursing care by means of the nursing process. Provides the professional component of care, ensures quality, and manages care at the bedside.
2. *Clinical Care Manager:* merges high quality clinical management with aggressive business management. Provides nurse case management, works with critical paths, and focuses on quality/cost by intense collaboration with the patient/family, medical staff, other professionals, support services, and the community.
3. *Licensed Practical Nurses and Nursing Aides:* are supervised to provide technical and supportive nursing care in a quality and cost-efficient manner.
4. *Support Service Host/Hostess:* provides nonclinical support services at the unit level to relieve the nursing staff of non-nursing duties. Provides support services that contribute to high-quality outcomes.

will also fit into the next generation of quality enhancement activities. Work and system redesign are integral components of an organization's constant assessment of quality and must be structured as such. Multiple approaches are needed to vigilantly track quality in an organization, several of which are discussed here.

Continuous Quality Improvement

A redesigned delivery system should be, in essence, CQI in action. CQI is an ongoing process focused on initiatives to drive varying degrees of improvements in systems and processes, particularly as they relate to meeting customer needs. It is imperative that clinical indicators be established and measured both before and after implementation of the redesigned system. The defined indicators should be measured at specific periods after implementation, and then periodically within an established, ongoing time frame (Brett & Tonges, 1990). Data collection and display tools should be used to provide clear indices of quality outcomes in care and in system processes (Leebov & Ersoz, 1991).

All members of the care team must participate in the process that constantly seeks to enhance quality, including medical staff, house staff, nursing administration, other professionals, and members of all ancillary support services. When evaluating quality of care, an effective process is one that is unit-based. Each unit is unique in its structure and process; for example, in the mix of diagnoses, physicians, length of stay, leadership, patient acuity, geographic location, and preparation and experience of the staff. A unit-based approach provides a community of peers who can readily challenge one another as professionals and collectively develop critical thinking about their practice (Driever, 1991). It is always good practice to directly involve those who deliver patient care when evaluating that care.

Critical Paths

One of the most effective tools for integrating quality into care delivery system redesign are "critical paths," or clinical protocols, designed specifically for tracking a planned clinical course for patients. Besides guiding the process of quality care, critical paths provide an excellent adjunct to other methods for improving cost-effectiveness in care delivery. Designed according to the average and expected lengths of stay, their use in clinical practice greatly facilitates cost management of care. In 1863, Florence Nightingale stated, "In all hospitals the patient must not stay a day longer than is absolutely necessary" (Baly, 1991). Long ago, she echoed the belief that quality care must be delivered within an appropriate time frame, in a cost-effective manner, and without overutilization of resources. That always represents true quality for patients and organizations. Critical paths have proven to be a successful measurement instrument toward that end, and they will continue to grow in importance in the future.

A critical path is simply a diagram of the work processes involved in delivering care (Leebov & Ersoz, 1991). Care maps are more elaborate pathways focused on definable patient outcomes; these outcomes coincide with the defined case interventions detailed on the corresponding critical path (Zander, 1992). Analyzing critical path and care map variances allows for an intense assessment of quality in care delivery. A variance exists whenever a patient does not progress as anticipated. The purpose of variance analysis is to detail what works and what does not work in the delivery of care (Wood, Bailey, & Tilkemeier, 1992).

Variance analysis also helps an organization to identify and act on needs that are unexpected. Four distinct types of variances can be assessed: 1) variances of patient/family origin, 2) variances of hospital origin, 3) variances of community origin, and 4) variances of clinician origin (Zander, 1992). Each patient's critical path can be reviewed at discharge for documented variances, both positive and negative. It is important to identify what went well and what did not. Origins of the variances are identified and categorized. These data are then collected and aggregated. Aggregations of the identified variances can then be channeled through the quality assessment process. An analysis of variance aggregations allows the team to discuss changes in the patient care process that will decrease variations from the critical path (Zander, 1992). Variance analysis also provides a means in which to assess the appropriateness of the defined path and allow for revisions that are more realistic for patients and for the institution.

The use of critical paths in care delivery system redesign supports the TQM imperative. The major components of critical paths emulate and converge with six of Dr. E. W. Demmings' principles of TQM. Table 4-1 clearly presents this concept.

The Professional Practice Analyst

There are other essential components that are used to assure that quality has been implemented at RWJUH. A rotating position for the professional nursing staff was developed to monitor and integrate quality improvements. This position, "the professional practice analyst," is allocated for each unit (Fralic, Kowalski, & Llewellyn, 1991). A staff nurse is elected to the position by his or her peers and serves a one- or two-year term. This nurse spends 1

TABLE 4-1   Correlation Between TQM and Critical Paths

TQM PRINCIPLE	CRITICAL PATHS
1. Definition of quality	Sets process goals
2. Consumer orientation	Paths are patient-specific (diagnosis-related groups)
3. Work process focus	Define services required
4. Preventative systems	Variance analysis and corrective action
8. Management by fact	Document problems and corrective actions
9. Continuous improvement	Ongoing reviews, modifications, and research

From Zander, K. (1992). Critical pathways. In M. Melum & M. Sinioris, *Total Quality Management: The health care pioneers* (p. 313). Chicago: American Hospital.

day per month on the unit monitoring quality, dressing in business clothes to designate his or her different function on that day.

The professional practice analyst performs the following imperative quality assessment actions: interviews patients and families to ascertain perceptions and satisfaction with care, interviews staff to assess the level of satisfaction with the system, reviews charts and assesses outcomes of specified clinical indicators, and examines unit-specific quality issues. After collecting all quality-related data, the Nursing Systems Department collates the information and returns it to the professional practice analyst for interpretation. Once monthly, all professional practice analysts meet and compare unit results. Identified problems are then reviewed with the staff of each unit. Significant issues are forwarded to the Nursing Division's quality committee. The committee, in turn, applies all of the standard principles of rigorous quality monitoring to further redesign processes that lead to problem resolution and greater achievements in quality outcomes.

The Role of the Nurse Manager

The nurse manager plays a critical role in the quality process. The Nursing Division, through its Nursing Systems Department, provides data through an aggregated information system called the Qual-dex system. With Qual-dex, quality parameters and cost parameters are reported, both contributing to the measure of unit performance. The system provides information to nurse managers through a unit-based analysis of quality and cost. Key data related to quality process and standards outcomes, patient- and unit-related incidents, infection rates, patient days, patient acuity, and patient satisfaction survey reports are collated. The system also provides critical data regarding budget compliance, budget related to workload, and staffing format and costs. This provides nurse managers with useful, timely, and organized data that can drive unit-based decisions about clinical and financial performance. Effective decision support systems are essential to high-quality performance.

Benchmarking

A current trend that is likely to be integrated into quality programs for care delivery system redesign is benchmarking. "Benchmarking requires the establishment of an agreed upon quality measurement, followed by a widespread search for the best performance to be measured against" (Caldwell, 1993). Hospitals with redesigned delivery systems can develop strategies to benchmark with one another and refine and improve processes based on their practice. How this information will be disseminated and shared will need to be determined. In 1994, the Joint Commission on Accreditation of Health Care Organizations will begin providing consumers with quality-related performance information on hospitals. Many hospitals will be moving quickly to improve their performance outcomes (Bergman, 1993) by benchmarking against published data. Benchmarking will prove to be a very effective strategy for raising standards related to outcomes, service, and cost-effectiveness in the new health care system.

▄ MANAGING COSTS IN REDESIGN

Case studies have repeatedly shown that the best way to contain costs is to improve quality (Bowles, 1993). This supports the premise that investments in quality reap financial rewards for the institution. Cost and quality go hand in hand. They can never be separated; they exist as an equation. Management's challenge is to keep the equation balanced; that is, the "right" level of quality at an appropriate and affordable level of cost. The balance is crucial.

Critical Paths

Controlling cost by use of critical paths for frequently seen, major diagnosis-related groups can be effective. Patient care must be designed in terms of appropriate lengths of stay. Financial outcomes can be evaluated from critical paths by assessing variances in length of stay and average charges per case type (Graybeal, Gheen, & McKenna, 1993). Variance analysis should focus on problems within the system that extend length of stay or drive up costs because of overutilization of resources or diagnostic testing. Adherence to a defined path supports the attempt to control system costs and prevent inappropriate utilization. Critical paths present substantial opportunity for physicians, nurses, and other health care professionals to work closely together in developing appropriate plans of care for patients. The challenges of the new health care financing systems strongly promote such collaboration.

Patient-Centered Care

Redesigned care delivery systems are changing the way that financial data are reported and analyzed in organizations. Many care delivery system redesign projects are being developed around the concept of "patient-centered care." Such models require matrix relationships. It has been shown that standard departmental budgets do not work well with patient-centered care models. New systems cannot be measured with the old tools. Such models require that greater flexibility be built into the budgeting and reporting processes. In the future, we are likely to see program-specific financial data that cross departmental lines (Solovy, 1993). This will be necessary so that teams that are not structured under one department can maintain accountability for managing costs across multiple disciplines of care and services.

Control Charts

Control charts, a CQI tool, can be used to visually display budget data. The control chart uses upper and lower control limits. The goal of the control chart is to help staff understand variances and causes of variance and to predict future performance (Solovy, 1993). By understanding the causes of budget variances, staff members will be able to come up with their own innovative ideas and strategies to control the budget, thus empowering them to manage their unit's costs. However, these financial parameters must be consistently evaluated along with quality-of-care parameters; only then is the evaluation comprehensive.

Interaction of Finance Department and Clinical Staff

Building cost management into redesign also has positive effects for the finance department. By working closely with care teams, financial staff begin to understand clinical operations and can assist care teams more fully in managing costs (Solovy, 1993). Chief financial officers are also able to make better decisions as they become part of the team and realize the need for specific resources to provide quality care.

At RWJUH, clinical care managers (nurse case managers) initially spend a significant portion of their orientation time on finance, with much of the content provided by the chief financial officer or senior financial staff. Here, they learn more fully how the organization is reimbursed and how they can better manage systems to maximize reimbursement and control costs. When planning a redesign project, nurse executives and nurse managers should encourage their financial staffs to provide financial education related to patient care for appropriate care team members.

▄CONCLUSION

John Ruskin said, "Quality is never an accident; it is always the result of intelligent effort." His words certainly ring true for nurse executives and nurse managers today. Organizations that do not provide high quality care at affordable and competitive costs simply will not survive. It is futile to undertake a delivery system redesign project without significant thought and careful planning for the integration of quality into the system. Systems are not self-maintained; they must be carefully managed. The bottom line is that the sustained success of any redesign project is proportional to the essential focus on quality and the effective management of costs.

As Paul Valéry, the French philosopher noted, "The trouble with our times is that the future is not what it used to be." Indeed it is not. But therein lies the challenge—and the unprecedented opportunity for nurse executives. We can and must provide leadership in creating new patient care delivery systems that are important for the organization, that are rewarding for nurses and other staff, but most of all, that provide patients with appropriate high-quality care. That is indeed an essential part of the new work of the contemporary nurse executive.

▄REFERENCES

Baly, M. (1991). *As Miss Nightingale said . . .* London: Scutari Press.
Barnum, B. (1991). On differentiated practice. *Nursing & Health Care, 12*(4), 171.
Bergman, R. (1993, June 20). Quantifying quality: Experts wonder what's behind numbers. *Hospitals & Health Networks*, p. 56.
Bowles, J. (1993). Reinventing healthcare: A total quality approach to improving care and lowering costs. *Fortune, 128*(1), 107–115.
Brett, J. & Tonges, M. (1990). Restructured patient care delivery: Evaluation of the ProACT™ model. *Nursing Economics, 8*(1), 36–44.
Caldwell, C. (1993). What healthcare can learn from TQM's past. *Healthcare Executive, 8*(3), 26–28.
Driever, M. (1991). Clinical interpretation and analysis of monitoring data. In P. Schroeder

(Ed.), *The encyclopedia of nursing care quality: Vol. 3. Monitoring and evaluation in nursing* (pp. 239–252). Gaithersburg: Aspen.

Finkler, S. & Kovner, C. (1993). *Financial management for nurse managers and executives.* Philadelphia: Saunders.

Fralic, M. (1992). The nurse case manager: Focus, selection, preparation, and measurement. *Journal of Nursing Administration, 22*(11), 13–14, 46.

Fralic, M., Kowalski, M., & Llewellyn, F. (1991). The staff nurse as quality monitor. *American Journal of Nursing, 91*(4), 40–42.

Graybeal, K., Gheen, M., & McKenna, B. (1993). Clinical pathway development: The Overlake model. *Nursing Management, 24*(4), 42–45.

Hackman, J. R. & Oldham, G. R. (1990). *Work redesign.* Reading, MA: Addison-Wesley.

Leebov, W. & Ersoz, C. (1991). *The health care manager's guide to continuous quality improvement.* Chicago: American Hospital.

Ritter, J., Fralic, M. F., Tonges, M. C., & McCormac, M. (1992). Redesigning nursing practice: A case management model for critical care. *Nursing Clinics of North America, 27*(1), 119–128.

Solovy, A. (1993, March 5). Champions of change. *Hospitals,* pp. 15–19.

Tonges, M. C. (1989a). Redesigning hospital nursing practice: The professionally advanced care team (ProACT™) model: Part 1. *Journal of Nursing Administration, 19*(7), 31–38.

Tonges, M. C. (1989b). Redesigning hospital nursing practice: The professionally advanced care team (ProACT™) model: Part 2. *Journal of Nursing Administration, 19*(8), 19–22.

Tonges, M. C. (1990). ProACT™: The professionally advanced care team model. In G. Mayer, M. J. Madden, & E. Lawrenz (Eds.), *Patient care delivery models* (pp. 13–35). Rockville, MD: Aspen.

Wood, R., Bailey, N., & Tilkemeier, D. Managed care: The missing link in quality improvement. *Journal of Nursing Care Quality, 6*(4), 55–65.

Zander, K. (1992). Critical pathways. In M. Melum & M. Sinioris (Eds.), *Total quality management: The health care pioneers* (pp. 305–314). Chicago: American Hospital.

Chapter 5

Evaluation of Care Delivery Redesign and Quality Outcomes

ROXANE B. SPITZER-LEHMAN   DOMINICK L. FLAREY

Health care reform, despite government intervention, has been occurring at a rapid pace over the past several years. This transformation of our nation's health care delivery system is being driven by factors originating from the external environment. The imperative to meet the demands of an ever changing, often hostile system has ushered in a myriad of strategies focused on survival and viability for health care organizations. One of the most effective strategies has been the redesign of care delivery systems.

Redesign in care delivery is rapidly evolving into a specific science with its own theoretical base of fundamental and complex principles. We are witnessing the emergence of sound methodologies for driving this process. Little has been written on redesign in health care and even less on the integration and evaluation of critical outcomes. This chapter provides a foundation for the establishment of specific methodologies related to evaluation of quality outcomes and productivity measures that can be integrated into the process of care delivery redesign.

▀ THE QUALITY AND PRODUCTIVITY IMPERATIVES IN REDESIGN

A most important imperative for redesign is the integration of quality and productivity into the process. Quality and productivity cannot be separated; rather, they must merge synergistically to produce optimal systems results. Quality and productivity come together when the primary focus is on the customers of the organization: patients, families, physicians, third-party payors, and employees. The quality imperative focuses on attaining clinical outcomes that maximize health and wellness. The productivity imperative rests on the mandate to maximize efficiencies of the system in a cost-effective way. As Lee Iacocca, president of Chrysler Corporation, said, "Quality and productivity are two sides of the same coin." Together, they provide the foundational support for delivery system redesign.

In relation to systems and role redesign, a new definition of quality

Flarey, D: REDESIGNING NURSING CARE DELIVERY: Transforming Our Future

emerges. Quality is the sum effort produced when everyone in the organization works together and shares in the responsibility to meet the needs and expectations of the organization's customers. Quality is everyone's job, from the employee who first greets customers at the registration area, to housekeepers, to professional staff, up to and including executive management.

Quality is a shared responsibility and an organizational imperative. The integration of quality into redesign becomes the process that enables achievement of the organization's Total Quality Management/Continuous Quality Improvement (TQM/CQI) initiative. When redesigning delivery systems, it is essential to incorporate the basic tenet of TQM/CQI—identifying customers' needs and expectations. Often, it may appear that the desires of some customers conflict with what other customers want; in actuality, they do not. Patients and families want attention to care needs with optimal outcomes; physicians want a user-friendly system that maximizes efficiency and supports the achievement of quality care outcomes; and payors want a highly efficient organization that moves the patient rapidly through the care delivery system while containing costs.

These customer needs blend well and impact one another in a positive way. The quality initiative in redesign must focus on such needs, and processes must be developed and managed to meet them. To effectively manage the process, it is critical that statistical measures to monitor performance and outcomes be built into redesign.

The productivity imperative in redesign is essential to the overall system's effectiveness as well as its quality mandate. Over the past decade, we have witnessed the amount of care service per patient continually rise. In other words, we are providing more and more service to patients while conceding the real mandate of providing care within a shorter time frame. Case-mix adjusted admissions, based on our current diagnosis-related groups (DRG) system, demonstrate how severely ill our patient population is. Complex clinical presentations require enormous amounts of resources to maximize clinical outcomes.

While intensity and need for services increase, hospital expenses continue to climb. In relation to the Gross National Product (GNP), health care spending can be said to be out of control. Despite this reality, over the last decade we have witnessed a consistent rise in the number of health care management positions, often at the expense of staff positions. This scenario negatively impacts productivity and mandates that we rethink our business and redesign work structures and roles to reverse this costly mistake.

Restructuring to enhance productivity while containing costs is an essential ingredient in any system redesign. Restructuring can be initiated from the top down or from the bottom up; the cadence in the process is unimportant. What is important is that form follow function and that a well-defined, thought-out, long-range plan and vision be established prior to its undertaking.

The following twenty principles, ideas, and suggestions are success strategies which will prove beneficial to those planning an organizational restructuring and delivery system redesign. They lend effectively to enhancement of quality and productivity within a redesigned system and provide a foundation on which to establish critical indicators and other criteria for evaluating the outcomes of delivery system redesign.

1. Organizational restructuring must be planned around customers. For example, if physicians are identified as a primary customer group, it may be well to have an executive level position for physician services. Clinical services must be restructured around patients. If you are not developing a patient-centered model, you are not doing real redesign.

2. Nursing administration roles must be redesigned, particularly the critical role of the nurse manager. Units can be restructured so that one nurse manager directs two or more similar units. Matrix responsibilities for nurse managers are appropriate when a system is redesigned for patient-focused care.

3. Traditional vertical departments that do not integrate well horizontally and impede the proper integration of patient services, should be restructured.

4. The role of chief nurse executive should be redesigned to become an executive position for patient care services. This nurse, the new patient care executive, should have leadership responsibilities for all nursing services as well as ancillary and primary support services. Such services may include pharmacy, respiratory therapy, physical therapy, dietary services, environmental services, patient registration, social services, and so on.

5. Restructuring should have as its primary goal the creation of a "seamless" organization in which all employees are encouraged to integrate their practices and roles around the organization's primary customers.

6. Redesign and restructuring should be focused on the organization's mission, values, history, culture, and social climate.

7. Reengineering, or redefining and redesigning work processes, should be an integral component of redesign. This involves identifying the work to be done in regard to patients and other primary customers. New work must be defined and new jobs created to match the work to the goals and objectives of system redesign.

8. Ancillary care and support services should be decentralized to the level of the patient care unit. Staff should report directly to the unit nurse manager, or reporting relationships should be designed in a matrix format.

9. New roles should be developed for multifunctional workers. When defining what tasks must be done, design should consider multiple job elements. For example, if the position of environmental staff member is decentralized to a unit level, what other elements of care and support services could be designed into the role?

10. Whenever feasible, services should be designed around the patient. This means planning for the decentralization to the unit of services such as physical therapy and electrocardiography. These decentral-

izations should be planned using a cost-benefit analysis; outcomes will vary from institution to institution.

11. Some functions and processes should be centralized. For example, a preadmission testing area, where all patient diagnostics are scheduled and effectively coordinated, will go a long way in maximizing the efficiency of a system and making it user-friendly for patients and physicians.

12. All work processes should be examined for their relevance, effectiveness, and quality imperatives. Work processes should be redesigned to achieve the goals of the project. A striking example is intravenous (IV) teams. It has been shown that IV teams are inefficient, because a significant amount of time is spent walking about the institution, and staff are generally alienated from team members when they are on the units. It has also been found that rates of IV site infection decline if primary caregivers at the bedside assume responsibility for all IV therapy.

13. Providing everyone with information is critical to a redesign and restructuring process. Everyone must know what we are measuring in terms of quality and productivity and what the measurements show. This allows all staff to participate in improving their practices to achieve greater levels of quality and productivity. More information means enhanced decisionmaking by all members of the organization.

14. Self-managed, high-performance work teams should be initiated to maximize productivity and quality outcomes. Mechanisms should be developed to evaluate and reward team performance as well as individual performance.

15. A proactive work management environment should be created. Provide employees with the resources they need to handle problems efficiently and effectively. An excellent example is when a light bulb must be replaced over a patient's bed. Requiring the staff to complete a requisition for the engineering department to replace the bulb often causes a delay of 24 hours or longer before the problem is resolved. Instead, the unit is supplied with bulbs so that the problem can be addressed immediately.

16. Redesigned systems must be physician-centered as well. Physicians are important customers of the organization, and their needs must be identified and addressed. Focusing on what physicians need to move patients through the care delivery system is vital for producing quality outcomes and efficiencies.

17. Data collection specifications must be established. This is critical to the overall total quality management process in redesign. One guiding principle is paramount: if you can measure it, you can manage it. All employees should participate in data collection and measurement. Key decisions related to these processes include a) What are you going to look at?, b) What data are you going to collect? and c) How are you going to collect it?

18. Benchmarking should be used in the overall redesign process. It is

necessary to establish what outcomes you are trying to achieve and what change processes are required to achieve them. Benchmarking can be instituted with internal data and measurements or against externally published data and outcomes.

19. Financial analysis should be built into the redesign process. This is essential for effective cost control. Financial data must be shared with everyone in the organization and used to drive effective decision making for systems redesign.

20. In a redesign/restructuring process, priority must be placed on three core elements: a) the management of quality outcomes, b) the effective management of costs, and c) an increase in overall productivity resulting in an increased ability to maximize the capacity of all resources to meet patient care and other customer needs. The above principle, while not all-inclusive, highlights key elements in the overall process of delivery system redesign. It also provides the foundation for assessing multiple outcomes, especially those related to quality, productivity, and costs. When examined critically and introduced successfully, these core elements play major roles in the transformation to an efficient and effective delivery system.

EVALUATING OUTCOMES IN REDESIGN

The evaluation of outcomes is critical to the redesign process. What to measure and evaluate are decisions that each organization must make individually. In establishing criteria for indicators, the organization must go back to its vision statements and define what outcomes it wants to achieve. Once defined, indicators and other measurements can be established, measured, and evaluated. In the authors' experience, many outcome criteria are relatively simple and may be broadly defined. What follows are suggested criteria that may be applied generically to most delivery system redesign and restructuring processes. Based on the specifics of each organization's redesign project, more particular and unique indicators can be established as well. As redesign becomes more commonplace, more detailed criteria and testable assumptions will be developed. The indications for future nursing administration research are vast.

When evaluating outcomes, criteria and indicators can be grouped into three major categories: clinical outcomes, administrative outcomes, and service outcomes. The following narrative highlights outcomes for evaluation based on these major categories.

Clinical Outcomes

Clinical outcomes focus on the evaluation of the care process as patients progress through the system. These outcomes can be very broad or very specific. Often such outcomes are assessed against defined criteria or care maps. Multiple outcomes may be evaluated, depending on the organization's objectives for quality care. The following are more generically based outcomes which may be applied across a continuum of care services.

Infection rates should be assessed and tracked for any specific trends, especially those related to nosocomial infections. The expected outcome must be a significant reduction of nosocomial infections; ideally, a zero infection rate.

Patient falls should be monitored on an ongoing basis. The redesign of care delivery should provide for more direct care by specific team members. More time at the bedside means that patients are observed more frequently, needs are taken care of in a timely manner, and assistance is more readily provided for ambulation. The expected outcome after implementation should be an absence of patient falls and concomitant injuries.

Medication administration errors should be evaluated, and an expected outcome of reduced errors should be realized. The redesigned system must focus on enhancing quality through safe practice. A significant reduction in medication errors can often be achieved after the process is evaluated and redesigned using the tenets of CQI.

Deviations or variances from defined patient care outcome maps must be evaluated. Questions that require answering are: 1) What outcomes were expected? 2) What outcomes were realized? 3) What in the system needs improvement to achieve optimal outcomes? and 4) How can these variances be consistently modified and improved over time? Analysis of variances should be an ongoing process.

Length-of-stay criteria, usually based on DRGs, must be continually evaluated after redesign. It is imperative to assess the degree to which patients exceed the established length of stay. Long lengths of stay often indicate that the system continues to lack efficiencies with which to maximize resources and move patients quickly through the care process. Impediments to achieving length-of-stay goals, such as poor discharge planning, substandard medical/nursing care, lack of family support, and poor adherence to critical paths by the professional staff, must be identified. Plans can be formulated to address such issues and correct system problems in order to achieve length-of-stay goals. Length-of-stay outcomes are excellent evaluative criteria for assessing the overall effectiveness of a redesigned care delivery system.

Administrative Outcomes

These outcomes are specifically related to the organization as a whole and the effects of the redesigned system on employees, physicians, staff, and the organization's bottom line. It is essential that these defined outcomes be measured consistently. A baseline measurement before delivery system redesign is necessary to measure the degree of impact of redesign on the organization.

Employee satisfaction is a critical outcome indicator for the success of any redesign project. A redesigned system should improve the quality of work life for employees, although this will take time. Generally, a more efficient, more effective system, driven by an intense philosophy of teamwork and patient-centered care, should achieve greater levels of employee satisfaction. If employee satisfaction has not improved to a considerable degree, the redesigned system is not effective, and an intense analysis should be done. Measures of employee satisfaction should be assessed on a regular basis. As the system matures and continues to improve, employee satisfaction should improve.

—➤ *Cost-effectiveness* of the redesigned system must be measured routinely. Cost targets must be defined early in the redesign process. Biweekly, or more frequently, financial data should be analyzed to assess the impact of redesign on overall organizational costs. If costs rise after redesign, then the model is not likely to be viable in the long term and requires intense evaluation and further redesign efforts to enhance feasibility. Many factors can interact to negate cost control, such as poor worker productivity, substandard care resulting in patient complications and increased lengths of stay, an ineffective skill mix that drives up costs, and inappropriate staff reductions resulting in enormous amounts of overtime and excessive use of agency personnel.

Analysis of *organizational culture and climate* is important to measure the success and positive impact of redesign. It is imperative that baseline assessments and reassessments be made routinely over time. A well planned, effective redesign process with continually communicated benchmarking positively impacts both the culture and the climate of the organization. The culture should grow into one of team spirit with an emphasis on patient-focused processes, a real value on education and learning, and mutual respect among staff, physicians, and management. The climate should be transformed into an environment of increased staff autonomy, encouragement and rewards for creativity and innovation, enhanced managerial support, and a real sense of cohesiveness among team members.

Recruitment efforts for physicians and employees should be evaluated. Does the redesigned system attract quality people to the organization? Has the organization developed a community reputation as a preferred place to work? Failure to achieve such outcomes indicates that the system may need to become more employee-centered. Many avenues exist for building employee-centeredness into the redesigned system. This should be included early in the planning process.

Specific employee indicators, such as incidence of sick leave, turnover rates, employee accidents, and performance measures, need to be consistently evaluated. A successfully redesigned system should reduce stressors on the staff, resulting in fewer employee health and safety problems. The new system should be attractive to employees so that costly turnovers are minimized. The new system should be user-friendly and supportive of all work roles so that employee performance improves consistently over time. Measurement and evaluation of these important indicators provide excellent indications of the degree of organizational transformation realized through the redesign process.

Service Outcomes

There are an endless number of service indicators that can be evaluated on an ongoing basis to assess outcomes of the redesigned system. The following are a few of the more simple and traditional indicators.

Patient satisfaction is the most critical indicator. There are many methods and tools available to accurately measure satisfaction. What is imperative is that such measurements be taken frequently and analyzed for developing trends or problems which can readily be corrected. Failure to listen and respond to patients' perceptions of the delivery system process will result in the ultimate failure of the organization. Data related to patient satisfaction must be regularly shared with all employees, just as clinical and financial data is. Excellent outcomes provide motivation to further improve performance; poor evaluations serve as a stimulus to rethink the system's processes and further redesign the system to achieve more optimal outcomes.

Physician satisfaction is an important service indicator. Improved levels of satisfaction can generally be achieved by involving physicians in many aspects of organizational life. When physicians are involved, they develop a sense of ownership and pride in the organization, are motivated to assist and cooperate in the change process, and gain a sense of team membership. Another strategy to enhance physician satisfaction is to keep physicians well informed throughout the redesign process. If physician satisfaction does not improve after redesign, then the new model will likely fail to achieve its defined goals.

Admissions turnaround time is an excellent service indicator to evaluate system effectiveness. A complex, bureaucratic, slow-paced system produces marked delays in this important process. Patients are sensitive to these delays and often form lasting, negative impressions of the organization based on the admissions experience. Turnaround time indicators can be effectively used as an internal benchmark against which performance can constantly be evaluated and improved.

Other important service indicators which may be considered for measurement include laboratory turnaround time, operating room utilization, ease of scheduling cases, emergency room waiting time, patients' food temperatures on delivery, turnaround times for medical record transcriptions, customer perceptions of staff friendliness and courtesy, and pharmacy turnaround times.

◼CONCLUSION

Redesign and restructuring of systems is complex. The work of redesign is a journey; it generally takes 3 to 5 years to make significant and lasting transformations. A successfully redesigned system is one that meets its defined goals and objectives and makes its visions a reality. Only by the continual measurement, evaluation, and communication of defined outcomes will the benefits of redesign be realized. Outcome evaluation is the means by which future redesign projects will be driven, culminating in the long-term process of health care system reform and transformation.

Chapter 6

Organizational Design: The Ultimate Challenge for Nursing Leadership

CAROL BOSTON

> *Revolution calls for leaders with the head, the heart,*
> *and the guts to improve the world.*
>
> —*Noel Tichy, 1993*

■ INTRODUCTION

These are unprecedented times in health care. The Clinton administration has developed a comprehensive plan for health care in the United States that calls for dramatic changes in the ways in which health care is focused, financed, accessed, and delivered. Should President Clinton's plan for health care reform ultimately be enacted into law, America will experience a social revolution in health care so profound that the impact of Medicare in the 1960s and Diagnosis-Related Groups (DRGs) in the 1980s will pale in comparison.

As is the case with any political agenda, skepticism exists as to whether the Clinton administration will be successful with efforts to have federal health care legislation reform enacted. However, national health care expenditures continue to grow at more than twice the annual inflation rate and presently represent nearly 13% of the Gross Domestic Product. Statistics soundly demonstrate the mitigating effect that rising health care costs are having on national efforts to control and decrease the steadily growing federal deficit. This sobering economic reality has already prompted congressional cutbacks in federal dollars available for health care, especially Medicare. Additionally, consumer polls consistently demonstrate decreased satisfaction with the manner in which U.S. health care is presently delivered; although notably, consumers have yet to reach consensus on which alternative to the present form of health care delivery would be the most desirable for the future.

Providers of health care across the country, anxiously monitoring federal deliberations regarding health care reform, are simultaneously taking steps to ensure organizational viability at local levels. Ever cognizant that the current health care environment is characterized by continually shrinking re-

Flarey, D: REDESIGNING NURSING CARE DELIVERY: Transforming Our Future
© 1995, J. B. Lippincott Company

sources and decreased customer satisfaction with the status quo, health care providers are challenged to ensure that their delivery systems and infrastructures are operating as effectively and as efficiently as is possible. While numerous strategies exist to meet such challenges, many organizations are determining that the very *design* of the health care organization is the single most important determinant of the organization's future success. Hence, health care organizations profit and not-for-profit, teaching and community, urban and rural, are currently examining various organizational design options that can maximize resource utilization while ensuring health care quality and effectiveness outcomes.

Not to be confused with projects that focus on the design of departments or departmental processes within an organization, the focus of organizational design projects referred to in this chapter are dedicated to fundamentally changing the entire care delivery model and its infrastructure in order to maximize organizational versus departmental efficiency and effectiveness in keeping with overall federal reform imperatives. Goals for organizations embarking on major design efforts are naturally developed unique to the organization; yet it is customary that one organizational goal for a major redesign effort includes the need to create a seamless continuum of care focused on the needs of the customer versus the needs or practices of specific functional areas or departments within health care organizations. Key factors to be considered in an organizational design effort include the organization's long-term business strategy, economic situation, customer expectations, changing payor mix, decline in inpatient utilization, case mix, and skill mix.

In health care, organizational design options tend to fall into three major categories: resizing, restructuring, and reengineering. Resizing, which typically is limited to decreasing or "downsizing" an organization's work force to support declines in inpatient volume and revenues is considered the most basic of organizational design efforts. Organizational restructuring generally requires reorganization of management structures including consolidating and eliminating positions and overall structural flattening.

Another part of restructuring is relevant department consolidation which serves to drive requisite staff eliminations that support the consolidated organization. Within recent years, considerable attention has been given to the limited ability of organizational resizing or restructuring efforts to sustain essential costs, quality, and service results over the long term (Kanter, 1990). In fact, one could question whether resizing or restructuring really constitutes true organizational redesign or merely organizational "reorganization." Resizing and restructuring may legitimately produce significant overhead savings for health care organizations in the near term. However, organizations that seek to conduct their business in the same way with fewer people typically experience increased frustration and decreased productivity among remaining employees.

While expenses are initially kept down, performance of employees, which impacts costs over the long term, suffers (Kanter, Stein, & Jick, 1992). In these situations, it is not unusual to find organizations responding to sudden but temporary increases in business volume by reinstating employees who were released during the resizing initiative.

Health care organizations need long-term, sustainable results from organizational design initiatives to ensure optimal positioning within the changing health care system. Hence, health care organizations are increasingly turning to reengineering of the entire organization as a true organizational design strategy dedicated to achieving necessary cost, quality, and service outcomes that can last. Reengineering is defined as the fundamental rethinking and radical redesign of business processes to achieve dramatic improvements in critical, contemporary measures of organizational performance, including cost, quality, service, and work life (Hammer & Champy, 1993). More simply, it means starting over . . . tossing aside old systems and traditions . . . going back to the beginning . . . in order to determine a more effective way of doing work (Hammer & Champy, 1993). For health care organizations, this means resisting the impetus to redesign pieces of the patient care delivery process within the organization (ie, the nursing care model) and instead committing to redesigning the entire process of patient care from preadmission through postdischarge, including all functions, departments, and disciplines that contribute to the overall patient care process.

To the extent that increasing numbers of health care organizations are initiating massive organizational overhauls through reengineering and not simply "tuning up" the organizational parts through resizing or restructuring, the unique leadership challenge for nurse executives in these types of projects appears unprecedented. It is acknowledged that over 50% of a hospital's operating budget represents labor costs, with a sizable portion of that percentage including direct ant indirect costs for nursing personnel. Given the financial imperatives typically tied to organizational design efforts, nursing is dramatically affected by massive organizational redesign efforts. Further, the essence of nursing, that of providing comprehensive care to individuals in order to maximize health, mandates that all aspects of nursing be considered during an organizational design initiative that seeks to integrate patient care into the organizational process. Hence, the significant impact of organizational design efforts on nurse executives and nursing warrants a careful analysis of the evolving role of the nurse executive in the world of organizational design, as well as the skill sets and leadership competencies that nurse executives need in order to be successful with organizational design. Clearly, development and demonstration of these competencies can mean the potential success of both the design project for the organization as well as the nurse executive's potential for continued success in her or his evolving role within the redesigned organization. Notably, the competencies identified within this chapter closely mirror the lists of competencies that contemporary management theorists cite as being essential for leaders of all types, regardless of any organizational design project being in progress. This begs the question as to whether contemporary health care organizations, in order to be successful over time, are constantly in a state of design, thereby necessitating leadership competencies from executives that are most responsive to this organizational design phenomenon. This question is subject for separate discussion, and will be addressed within the context of closing comments.

■ THE CHANGING ROLE

The scope of any major organizational design initiative in health care includes a careful analysis of how decisions are made throughout the organization and the management infrastructure essential to facilitating work in a radically redesigned environment. The executive team of a health care organization and the roles of all senior executives are included in this analysis in order to ensure that the senior executive roles in the redesigned organization support the new philosophies of work that are desired (eg, decision making leveraged to the point of care, self-managed work teams, etc.). Thus, the role of the nurse executive, like all other leadership roles, is subject to change in a redesigned organization.

How is the nurse executive's role changing in redesigned health care organizations? In an effort to address this question, a survey of Voluntary Hospitals of America, Inc. (VHA) hospitals was conducted in August 1992. The tables in the chapter appendix illustrate the scope of redesign occurring as of August, 1993 in VHA hospitals, reasons for redesign, as well as impact on the nurse executive's role.

This survey, while admittedly representative of one major system in this country, nevertheless provides interesting information about the nurse executive's evolving role in health care organizations that are redesigning. Notably, of the hospitals responding to the survey, 39.7% indicated that the nurse executive role was changing and 18.2% indicated it wasn't; but 42.1% did not respond to the question. The conclusion being made regarding the significant numbers of nonresponses to that question is that the design projects were not completed; hence, it was premature to indicate the change in the nurse executive's role. Of those nurse executives who indicated their role was changing because of redesign, the overwhelming majority (83.8%) indicated role expansion, thereby demanding added competencies of nurse executives for success in a redesigned environment.

■ THE COMPETENCIES

Building Shared Visions

When a health care organization commits to a true organizational design process, the organization's leadership team is challenged to develop and communicate a vision of what the redesigned organization will look like. Visions are customarily considered a picture of the organization's future, a desired future state around which the organization's people can identify with (Nadler & Tushman, 1990). Health care leaders typically have extensive experience with the visioning process. However, given the nature of organizational transformation increasingly being considered by health care organizations in design processes, the ability to build shared visions throughout the organization for an organization to look, feel and function radically different is complex.

Remember, increasing numbers of health care organizations are embarking on design efforts that seek to reengineer the very nature of how patient care is accomplished throughout the organization versus the more limited design approaches of resizing and restructuring. Hence, nurse executives challenged to provide leadership in organizational design efforts that are seeking to develop a seamless continuum of care, must work to develop a shared vision that integrates nursing practice into patient care within the desired care delivery continuum rather than isolate it. Such a vision is required both at the executive management level within the organization at which strategic decisions about organizational redesign are made as well as the staff and middle-management level. Acknowledging that most health care organizations are currently organized around specialties and disciplines instead of by core processes, the development of a shared vision for organizational design that speaks to the horizontal integration of care delivery processes versus the continuation of vertically organized departments is particularly difficult for staff and middle managers to internalize.

The need to build shared visions within the entire health care organization is obvious. The executive leadership team, including the nurse executive, can objectively identify and support a design vision that seeks to integrate care delivery processes because this approach provides organizations with untapped opportunities for efficiency and effectiveness by capturing inefficient resource utilization between departments and functions as well as within them. Nevertheless, this type of vision can be troubling to staff and middle managers educated and socialized around a discipline versus the care delivery process in its most global sense. At the executive level, the development of a shared vision for organizational design calls for the nurse executive to paint a picture that successfully integrates nursing practice into the care delivery continuum. Equally important, at the staff level, the nurse executive is challenged to ensure that staff share the vision of integrating nursing practice as the design strategy that makes sense both for the organization and for the long-term transformation of professional nursing practice in a reforming health care system that is patient-focused rather than functionally driven.

When an organization initiates a massive organizational redesign initiative, no one really knows exactly where the design is headed, what the organization will become, what will change, and how (Hammer & Champy, 1993). Because shared visions in organizational design initiatives seek to depict what the organization wants to achieve when it is done designing, shared visions can provide the entire organization with focus, direction, and powerful motivation for embracing change that will result in a positive organizational future (Kanter, 1990). During the redesign of a health care organization, the nurse executive will be faced with nursing professionals anxious about what lies ahead for the traditional and customary way in which nursing is practiced. A shared vision reflects the consensus of all stakeholders in the design process, including nursing, regarding what the organization wants to achieve when it is done designing. It will prove to be an invaluable tool for the nurse executive attempting to sustain the department's and the organization's commitment to design during the stress of the actual design process (Hammer & Champy, 1993).

Catalyzing Paradigm Shifts

The design of an entire health care organization through reengineering calls for executives who are more than just competent in managing a complex change process. The redesign of a health care organization at the level needed to demonstrate sustainable outcomes calls for executives who are catalysts for shifting the very vantage points from which people view contemporary reality. Health care leaders preparing their organizations to compete in the 21st century are challenged to shift paradigms by moving beyond current mental boundaries as well as geographic ones. Further, leaders must embrace the evolving strategic orientation of health care organizations as serving the public and community rather than maximize short-term profitability (Healthcare Forum, 1992). With the fundamental upheaval in the structure and function of health care delivery occurring during an organizational redesign process, health care executives must seek design solutions not by way of a change of action but by way of a change in overall perception (Kim, 1993).

The nurse executive's view of reality, understandably shaped by education, socialization, and experience in a health care system traditionally designed by function instead of process, can unknowingly influence an organizational design process toward continued support of vertical functionality unless the nurse executive is supportive of creating a new health care reality within the organization. This new reality for health care includes integrating departments and functions to ensure a seamless care continuum. It calls for viewing patient care as a process instead of separate events. It demands the determination of new ways to support the patient care process that make sense for the patient as opposed to the individual departments contributing to patient care within the organization.

The nurse executive leading the clinical discipline of nursing within the organization faces challenges to successfully shift this paradigm in the minds of nursing professionals, who may view the shift as detrimental to the profession of nursing. While some tasks and responsibilities traditionally accomplished by nursing professionals will be delegated to other care providers within the organization as a result of the radical design process, the design process can actually serve to transform the practice of nursing within the organization to levels historically difficult to reach. Nevertheless, abandoning tradition for new realities is a difficult task for all care providers within a health care organization, including nursing. The nurse executive needs to consistently reinforce that professional nursing is not being abandoned as much as transformed within the new realities of the redesigned health care organization. Notably, paradigm shifts for nursing in redesigned organizations, while initially perceived as radical by many, do not serve to modify that which is codified or regulated by law (ie, state nurse practice acts). In the final analysis, what is potentially "lost" in the paradigm shift are those activities assumed by nursing professionals that have always been done because of tradition, habit, or custom; thereby freeing up the nurse's time such that the scope of professional nursing practice is leveraged to the upper limits of licensure.

A Focus on Systems Thinking

In organizations, contemporary leaders are challenged to help people see the "big picture" (Senge, 1990). This calls for the elevation of employee perspectives regarding individual contributions as parts of an overall process versus isolated events. Unfortunately, individuals unable to see interrelationships between actions are confined to thinking of actions as singular events versus parts of an integrated process.

Healthcare Forum's 1992 study entitled *Bridging the Leadership Gap in Healthcare* investigated the gap between contemporary leadership competencies and those necessary to lead 21st-century organizations. Systems thinking was identified as one of six competencies critical for 21st-century leadership in health care; further, it was one of three competencies identified as being the least practiced by contemporary health care leadership. Systems thinking defies linear thinking, challenging leaders to refrain from focusing on things in a static environment and instead on things as part of an ongoing, dynamic (Senge, 1990). Notably, leaders who practice linear versus systems thinking typically implement management interventions that focus on symptomatic fixes to problems/challenges versus underlying causes (Senge, 1990).

For nurse executives assuming leadership roles in a comprehensive organizational design project, the need for the nurse executive to demonstrate as well as gain staff support for a systems approach becomes abundantly clear. When health care organizations are designed to support a seamless continuum of care that is patient-focused rather than departmentally-driven, functional specialization is abandoned for horizontal integration. For this reason, the redesign of the nursing care delivery model to the exclusion of all other organizational contributors to the patient care process represents a linear approach to organizational design. Thus, deep, sustainable results for the organization that cut across departmental lines are difficult to achieve absent a systems approach to the entire design process. Nursing care and practice is part of the patient care system; not independent of it. By focusing on the entire system and not just the domain of nursing care, the nurse executive can provide leadership to an organizational design initiative that transforms nursing practice within the desired, integrated continuum.

Systems thinking does not imply abandonment of value derived from individual components of the system. In fact, organizations seeking to shape a design that will optimally position the organization for the future are challenged to retain the value inherent in the preexisting pieces of the process, avoiding the danger of consolidating pieces of work into a process that results in the process being worth less than the sum of its parts (Kanter, 1990). Real synergy in redesigned systems can be achieved when true value of process components is retained while the foundation for creating new value for the future is laid (Kanter, 1990). The nurse executive, as part of the leadership team committed to redesigning the health care organization, is optimally positioned to ensure that nursing's essential contributions to health care are maximized in the redesigned care delivery model and organization.

Nurse executives in redesigning organizations who embrace systems thinking and are successful in assisting staff to similarly embrace this approach to the organization's patient care process are well positioned to assist staff with the role transitions typically called for in redesigned organizations. By moving away from focusing on specialized functions or departments to that of the horizontally integrated patient care system, staff roles, including those within nursing, are typically expanded to assume greater accountability for the overall patient care process and process results. In redesigned health care organizations, staff are frequently organized into various types of self-managed work teams, multidisciplinary in nature, sharing joint responsibility with team members for performing the entire patient care process, not just select process components. Job lines between team members, as appropriate, are naturally fuzzy versus clear, fostering staff appreciation for the bigger picture as a whole (Hammer & Champy, 1993). Thus, the nurse executive's skill in demonstrating a systems versus linear approach to organizational design will clearly influence the behaviors ultimately demonstrated by nursing staff expected to support a systematic versus functional approach to the patient care process.

An Enabler of Others

Successfully redesigning health care organizations to support a seamless continuum of care that is patient-focused versus departmentally driven typically includes instituting multidisciplinary work teams that are both accountable for the entire patient care process and in possession of the necessary organizational authority to make the decisions needed for total process completion. True empowerment of all employees is an unavoidable consequence of a reengineered organization (Hammer & Champy, 1993). Likewise, the organization's management structure changes from hierarchical to flat. If work and decisions about work are to be leveraged to the point at which work is delivered, then the need for a management structure dedicated to the making and checking of work decisions decreases. In reengineered organizations with work performed by teams of essentially coequal people having great autonomy, the need for managers to be supervisors becomes less essential than the need for managers to be coaches of others (Hammer & Champy, 1993).

For the nurse executive in a redesigned organization, this typically means a tremendous flattening of the department of nursing's management structure as well as potential integration of the department of nursing into a newly designed department or division of patient care services (inpatient, outpatient, or a combination thereof). Many positions within nursing administration created solely to support or oversee decision making in nursing are frequently eliminated, consistent with the desire to position as much decision making regarding patient care to the point at which patient care is delivered. Thus, the need for supervisor and director jobs in health care organizations is diminishing; strategies to consolidate units and new management positions within consolidated units are on the rise. The nurse executive's key skill in this organizational flattening process is the ability to determine what information the patient care decision makers need to make relevant decisions about patient care and what competencies these decision makers need to be effective and successful in their redesigned roles.

Jobs within redesigned organizations, although potentially fewer in number, become more complex and expansive in scope. This is true for jobs at both the staff and middle management levels. The change in roles and accountabilities of workers in redesigned organizations necessitates leaders who are skilled to influence and guide employees rather than manipulating and controlling them. In traditionally designed organizations, managers allocate work by means of design, supervision, control, and discipline. In reengineered organizations, heavily characterized by the existence of work teams focusing on processes, leaders essentially serve to support or *enable* the work of the teams, coaching teams and team members as needed. Reengineered organizations, depending on the expertise of their employees for success, need their managers to focus on the intensive, continuous development of the organization's people in order for the organization's people to demonstrate ongoing expertise with the management of the patient care process. It is short-sighted to assume that a nominal increase in training/ education of an organization's employees will be sufficient to support the radical changes in behavior and practice expected in a redesigned organization. Additionally, concepts like empowerment and accountability in a redesigned organization can sound like bureaucratic rhetoric if they aren't introduced and sustained in organizations by solid education and training efforts (Henkoff, 1993). Further, an organization with truly empowered employees can only be successful if managers believe and support their employees' acting independently to benefit both the organization and its customers (Bowen & Lawler, 1992).

A Revitalized Customer Focus

For years, leaders in health care have been pressured to ensure that all aspects of the health care organization be designed to support customer needs. In particular, the advent of continuous quality improvement programs in health care organizations during the late 1980s and early 1990s resulted in comprehensive processes to identify primary and secondary customers within health care organizations, around which select processes could be established and continuously improved.

A new day for defining customers in health care is dawning. The phrase of "patient-focused care" has evolved, from a singular approach to patient care restructuring to the prevailing theme for organizational redesign through reengineering. The move to develop a seamless continuum of care that is patient-focused and not department-driven is consistent with the strategic orientation of health care organizations evolving into the public and the community over a lifetime versus episodic treatment of illnesses as they occur. Hence, all executives in health care are challenged to evaluate recent decisions about who their true customers are. The central issue is whether the ultimate customer around whom all core processes are designed and

decisions are made in health care organizations is the actual consumer of
health care services.

For patient-focused care in a redesigned organization to be successfully
realized, the nurse executive is challenged to assist staff with supporting the
design and implementation of a care delivery model with the consumer of
health care services versus a department being the model's center. Although skill in this area appears simple, the obvious pressures that this focus
places on all core processes in health care, including those involving nursing, make this skill difficult to actually achieve. The patient-focused approach to organizational design questions all processes, first to determine
whether the process is needed for the organization's true customers (ie, the
consumers of health care) and, if needed, how the processes can best be
organized to support the customers' needs.

By using the true customer as the focus for the design process, the nurse
executive can better facilitate staff transition away from nursing care processes designed to support professional behaviors or mores and toward patient care processes designed to support the customers' needs in the broadest context. Again, this revitalized customer focus is not intended to
minimize the essential contributions of any health care discipline, including
nursing. As previously mentioned, an outcome of patient-focused redesign
is the transformation of the practice of nursing to levels historically difficult
to achieve. However, with the focus on the customer instead of the disciplines, all staff within redesigned organizations learn to achieve a balance
between concentration on their own skills and the responsiveness of working together with all disciplines for the customer's ultimate well-being.

THE ULTIMATE CHALLENGE

The role of the nurse executive in a redesigned organization is subject to
change, and the competencies that nurse executives need for continued
success in redesign processes and redesigned organizations are numerous.
The ultimate challenge for the nurse executive accepting the challenge is to
sustain the courage to participate in a leadership role in a project that turns
the organization upside down in the short term as well as the historic role of
nursing within the organization. Without question, the nurse executive is
faced with balancing the business imperative of optimally positioning the
organization in a reforming health care environment while continuing to
lead the clinical discipline of nursing. As such, the nurse executive must
confront and help others confront the traditional paradigm through which
all staff historically have viewed the way "things should be done" for radically redefining the process of patient care in a redesigned organization.

Organizational redesign is not for the fainthearted. It is for the leader in
health care who is willing to tackle the design of the entire organization in
order to ensure that the organization is both economically viable and
clearly responsive to customers' needs in a reforming health care delivery
system. The redesigned organization that supports a seamless continuum of
health care will be patient-focused versus departmentally-driven. The con-

tinuum will support care delivery that transcends the walls of individual organizations to include all organizations and entities within a defined health care network or plan. It will provide the opportunity for the transformation of nursing practice into a 21st-century health care option, with nursing's essential contributions to health care realized and maximized.

▬ REFERENCES

Bowen, D. & Lawler, E. E. (1992, Spring). The empowerment of service workers: What, why, how and when. *Sloan Management Review*, pp. 31–39.

Hammer, M. & Champy, J. (1993). *Reengineering the corporation.* New York: Harper Collins.

Healthcare Forum. (1992). *Bridging the leadership gap in healthcare.*

Henkoff, R. (1993, March). Companies that train best. *Fortune*, pp. 62–75.

Kanter, R. (1990). *When giants learn to dance.* New York: Simon & Schuster.

Kanter, R., Stein, B., & Jick, T. (1992). *The challenge of organizational change.* New York: The Free Press/MacMillan.

Kim, D. H. (1993, July/August). The leader with the beginner's mind. *Healthcare Forum Journal*, pp. 39–43.

Nadler, D. & Tushman, M. (1990, Winter). Beyond the charismatic leader: Leadership and organizational change. *California Management Review*, pp. 77–95.

Senge, P. M. (1990, Fall). The leader's new work: Building learning organizations. *Sloan Management Review*, pp. 7–23.

▬ APPENDIX 6-1.
Involvement of Institution in a System Redesign Project at VHA Hospitals

Has your institution or is your institution currently involved in a systems redesign project?

RESPONSE	PERCENT OF RESPONDENTS
Yes	73.0
No	27.0
(N = 423)	

▬ APPENDIX 6-2.
Primary Reason for Initiating the Redesign Project at VHA Hospitals

What was/is the primary reason for initiating the redesign project?

PRIMARY REASON*	PERCENT OF RESPONDENTS**
Need to reduce operating costs (213)	50.4
Other (101)	23.9
Dissatisfied customers (physicians, patients, etc.) (59)	13.9
Partnership/alliance/integration with multiple facilities (46)	10.9
Dissatisfaction of work force (44)	10.4
Substandard quality/clinical outcomes (33)	7.8
(N = 423)	

*Number in parentheses is number of respondents.
**Total is more than 100%; respondents could select more than one answer.

▬APPENDIX 6-3.
Identifier of Need/Initiator of Systems Redesign Project at VHA Hospitals
Who in the organization identified the need and initiated the systems redesign project?

POSITION*	PERCENT OF RESPONDENTS**
Nurse Executive (240)	56.7
Chief Executive Officer (154)	36.4
Chief Operating Officer (66)	15.6
Other (49)	11.6
Chief Financial Officer (45)	10.6
Governing body (34)	8.0
Medical staff (24)	5.7
(N = 423)	

*Number in parentheses is number of respondents.
**Total is more than 100%; respondents could select more than one answer.

▬APPENDIX 6-4.
Decision Makers in the Redesign Project at VHA Hospitals
Who were/are the primary decision makers in the redesign project?

POSITION*	PERCENT OF RESPONDENTS**
Nurse Executive (263)	62.2
Chief Executive Officer (173)	40.9
Nurse Manager (131)	31.0
Chief Operating Officer (96)	22.7
Other (92)	21.7
Chief Financial Officer (77)	18.2
Governing Body (41)	9.7
(N = 423)	

*Number in parentheses is number of respondents.
**Total is more than 100%; respondents could select more than one answer.

▬APPENDIX 6-5.
Nurse Executive's Role in the Redesign Project at VHA Hospitals
Which of the following best describes your role and responsibilities in the redesign project?

ROLE*	PERCENT OF RESPONDENTS**
Project leader (128)	30.3
Project team member (108)	25.5
Consultant to project (80)	18.9
Did not participate (5)	1.2
(N = 423)	

*Number in parentheses is number of respondents.

▬APPENDIX 6-6.

Core Features of Systems Redesign Project at VHA Hospitals

Which of the following best describes the core feature of your systems redesign project?

FEATURE*	PERCENT OF RESPONDENTS**
Integration/coordination of work across department lines (205)	48.5
Critical paths/protocol development (176)	41.6
Multiskilled workers (162)	38.3
Management restructure (150)	35.5
Case management (118)	27.9
Unit-based management of care (105)	24.8
Self-managed teams (73)	17.3
Other features (33)	7.8
Primary nursing (25)	5.9

$(N = 423)$

*Number in parentheses is number of respondents.
**Total is more than 100%; respondents could select more than one answer.

▬APPENDIX 6-7.

Departments Accountable to Nursing Services After Completion of Systems Redesign at VHA Hospitals

Upon completion, which support and/or operations departments were/will be accountable to nursing services?

DEPARTMENT*	PERCENT OF RESPONDENTS**
Education (114)	27.0
Social service (107)	25.3
Respiratory therapy (103)	24.3
Other department (93)	22.0
Patient transport (83)	19.6
Pharmacy (71)	16.8
Utilization review (63)	14.9
Physical therapy (62)	14.7
Hospital QA/CQI (55)	13.0
Housekeeping (55)	13.0
Matrix responsibilities (52)	12.3
Laboratory (50)	11.8
Dietary (33)	7.8
Laundry (21)	5.0
Engineering (5)	1.2

$(N = 423)$

*Number in parentheses is number of respondents.
**Total is more than 100%; respondents could select more than one answer.

▬ APPENDIX 6-8.
Transformation of Position, Roles, Responsibilities Upon Completion of Systems Redesign
Upon completion, did your position, roles, responsibilities in the organization change?

RESPONSE		PERCENT OF RESPONDENTS
Yes		39.7
Position/responsibilities were expanded	83.8	
Position/responsibilities were narrowed	4.0	
Position/responsibilities were altered	12.0	
	100.0	
No		18.2
No answer/blank		42.1
$N = 423$		

▬ APPENDIX 6-9.
Nurse Executive Position Changes with System Redesign at VHA Hospitals

CHANGE	PERCENT OF RESPONDENTS
No change; remained line	61.0
Reporting relationship changed	27.0
No change; remained staff	6.3
From line to staff	3.1
From staff to line	2.5
$(N = 159)$	

▬ APPENDIX 6-10.
Nurse Executive Position Prior to the Redesign Project at VHA Hospitals
Which of the following titles best describes your position in the organization prior to the redesign project?

POSITION	PERCENT OF RESPONDENTS
Vice President/Nursing	38.7
Vice President/Patient Care	24.5
Director of Nursing	23.5
Other	11.3
Vice President/Operations	1.7
Chief Operating Officer	0.3
$(N = 302)$	

▬ APPENDIX 6-11.
Nurse Executive Position After the Redesign Project at VHA Hospitals
Which of the following titles best describes your position (or will describe your position) in the organization after the redesign project?

POSITION	PERCENT OF RESPONDENTS
Vice President/Patient Care	40.4
Other	20.2
Director of Nursing	17.6
Vice President/Nursing	15.4
Vice President/Operations	4.4
Chief Operating Officer	1.8

(*N* = 272)

▬ APPENDIX 6-12.
Criteria Used to Evaluate Outcomes of the Redesign Project at VHA Hospitals
Which of the following best describes criteria that were/will be used to evaluate major outcomes of the redesign project?

CRITERIA*	PERCENT OF RESPONDENTS**
Reduction of costs (270)	63.8
Quality of care/clinical outcomes (262)	61.9
Customer (patient) satisfaction (259)	61.2
Staff satisfaction (247)	58.4
Customer (physician) satisfaction (244)	57.7
Other (29)	6.9

(*N* = 423)

*Number in parentheses is number of respondents.
**Total is more than 100%; respondents could select more than one answer.

Part 2
Case Studies in Redesign

Chapter 7

The "Energized" Nursing Department: Design for Change

RELLA ADAMS   MAIA BAKER   ERNESTINA BRIONES   LISA GRAY

CYNTHIA HINOJOSA-ALARCÓN   PAM WARNER

An "energized" nursing department is one exhibiting the high degree of stimulation and exchange that occurs when members of the department interact among themselves and with personnel of other departments, physicians, administrators, and board of trustees. Nursing departments of the 1990s can be described as "energized" when compared with those of the 1970s and early 1980s. In the latter era, the "nonenergized" nursing department was based on control and stability rather than freedom and change (Pratt, 1976).

Innovation 10 years ago was slow and deliberate. Even though nurses with BSNs and MSNs were taught to be role models portraying "change agents," change was difficult to promote in the clinical and administrative settings. Management of hospitals and patient care delivery remained in status quo until economics and quality of health care became the central focus. Now, regulators, reimbursement entities, and consumers demand change. Nursing professionals are innovators, and the boundaries of the new world of health care are endless. Using skills and knowledge from education and research, nursing has begun its new perspective as we move toward the 21st century.

The Nursing Department at Valley Baptist Medical Center (VBMC), Harlingen, Texas, has initiated many changes since 1989. In 1993, change is a nursing professional's prerogative. Change can occur at the patient care level or at the administrative level, through committees or as a suggestion through a continuous quality improvement (CQI) program. The avenues for the initiation of change are many and varied. The ultimate goal for nursing, as change takes place, is to benefit the patient.

This chapter highlights a few of the changes initiated by the Nursing Department at VBMC. Outcomes of change are also presented. Many of the concepts and structures represent the second or third generation of VBMC's Design for Change program.

▀RESTORATIVE CARE PATHS

As 1 of 80 hospitals in the United States selected by The Robert Wood Johnson Foundation and The Pew Charitable Trusts to participate in the grant program, "Strengthening Hospital Nursing: A Program to Improve Patient Care," VBMC entered into a new age, an age of change, whereby nursing became the foundation and impetus for innovation (Adams & Rentfro, 1991). Direction and technical assistance were provided by Shands Hospital at the University of Florida. Funds were made available to hospitals that could demonstrate innovative plans for institution-wide restructuring and redesign with nursing service as the catalyst for change. In 1989, the nursing department began to explore new opportunities to improve patient care. The result was VBMC's Design for Change program, developed and implemented as a program for analysis and enhancement of systems to continually improve patient care. The major outcomes realized from the Design for Change program include

- Development of a new case management model, the Restorative Care Path;
- Outcome-oriented services that focus on patient capabilities and restorative measures rather than on nursing tasks;
- Establishment of an associate degree nursing program on the hospital campus;
- Development and implementation of a Shared Governance Model (Nursing Department Organizational Guidelines);
- Increased awareness of fiscal responsibility in the current health care environment; and
- Implementation of a continuous quality improvement program.

One of the new opportunities and first outcomes of the Design for Change program was the Restorative Care Path (RCP). This model emphasizes patients' capabilities to promote wellness. The development of the RCP began in 1989. It has been an evolutionary process, one that has been changing and improving continuously over the past 4 years. The Care Path is a permanent part of the medical record. It details medical and nursing interventions and expected outcomes within specific time frames. Nursing interventions are based on Nursing Standards of Care correlated with Standards of Nursing Practice. The RCP replaces the temporary card system and the traditional nursing care plan (NCP). As NCPs have been eliminated, nursing standards of care have been incorporated into the RCP. This process is examined in more detail in the section titled *Standards of Care.*

The rationale for development of the RCP was to provide nurses with a tool for planning daily interventions leading to expected quality outcomes, and to ensure registered nurse accountability for overall patient care. The RCP has become a vehicle for emphasizing VBMC's nursing care philosophy: "Nursing's primary function is to restore the person to his or her highest attainable level of health." The RCP is a tool that facilitates patient care management by RNs with a focus on outcomes rather than on specific nursing tasks. It also alerts caregivers to process and outcome variances that can be monitored and evaluated both retrospectively and prospectively.

A major advantage of using RCPs is to promote and ensure professional collaboration in the delivery of care. For any case management tool to work effectively, professional collaboration must occur among nursing staff, support personnel, and physicians. The RCPs used at VBMC were developed by the nursing staff in collaboration with the other health care professionals. The RCPs span all areas of care, are unit-specific, and are based on medical diagnoses. Examples of RCPs include Myocardial Infarction, Diabetes, Laminectomy, Open Heart Surgery, Pulmonary Disease, C-Section, and Premature Infant. The RCP for Cardiogenic Shock is presented in Appendix 7-1.

This very workable tool has been adopted by the hospital and has proved instrumental in managing patient care while focusing on specific outcomes. Problems can be easily identified, and opportunities for collaboration in patient care are enhanced. RCPs focus on the delivery of quality patient care while reducing the length of stay whenever possible. If problems or variances occur, they are noted directly on the Care Path with the date and time. Information related to the variance is expounded in the variance column.

Because the process of care represents a system, the variances provide an opportunity to investigate trends and to make improvements within the specific process or the system. It is the responsibility of the Registered Nurse Clinical Manager (CM) to check each RCP for daily variances. These daily variances are monitored, and a plan of action is formulated among all the caregivers involved. The CM coordinates any changes in care and monitors the effectiveness of these changes. Variances are also monitored and trended over time. Recurrent trends are discussed, and any needed process changes are addressed. RCPs are modified according to the process changes noted. Daily variance adjustments and variance trending patterns are monitored by the CM, but solutions are arrived at from an interdisciplinary approach, including physicians. The CM coordinates the implementation of any changes with the Care Plans. Thus, a CQI event takes place.

One of the latest developments at VBMC is integrated charting. This charting format focuses on the documentation of identified variances from the RCP. Documentation is completed by an RN on a specific Nurse–Physician Progress Note. This promotes professional collaboration and communication between nursing and medicine and has been instrumental in the delivery of quality patient care. This model of interdisciplinary documentation streamlines the entire care process in the medical record. Accrediting and regulatory agencies will probably develop documentation standards in the future that use an integrated charting model.

▄STANDARDS OF CARE

To understand how standards of care at VBMC evolved, it is necessary to trace their historic evolution. In 1986, a committee was formed to develop NCPs based on major medical diagnoses. These care plans were preprinted and included a method for individualization. They were based on nursing diagnoses for each potential problem identified and included patient goals and evaluation of outcomes from nursing interventions. The care plans became the standards of care for nursing practice. With the evolution of RCPs, however, it became apparent that the NCPs were redundant, leading to duplication of information and documentation. An ad hoc committee was formed from the Nursing Practice Council with representation of staff nurses, nurse educators, and nurse managers to devise an alternative method of developing and integrating standards of care. The committee defined standards of care as broad parameters on which nursing care is based. Within the parameters are supporting standards of nursing practice. Figure 7-1 presents VBMCs major care and practice standards. The Standards of Care Manual was developed from this framework and highlights 15 standards of care.

Each standard of care encompasses several supporting standards of nursing practice based on nursing diagnoses. For example, Standard of Care V is Teaching & Learning; the supporting standards of practice include Health Maintenance Alteration and Home Management Alteration/Discharge Planning. Each supporting standard of nursing practice is clarified by a definition and includes desired outcomes, characteristics, risk/related factors, nursing interventions, and patient/family education.

RCPs were developed from the standards of care and supporting standards of practice. This facilitates consistency and department-wide understanding of the standards and ensures that they are actually built into nursing practice and the overall process of care delivery. Historically, as each nursing unit generated RCPs, unit-specific standards of care and supporting standards of practice were developed concurrently. Thus, all nomenclature and criteria are consistent. The Practice Council, which includes staff nurse membership, approves all RCPs as well as standards of care and supporting standards of practice. Standards of care and practice are dynamic and continuously evolving. They represent second and third generations of development in the overall process of change and delivery system redesign.

▆SHARED GOVERNANCE

In 1989, the Vice President for Nursing Service, the directors of nursing, and a small group of nurse managers formed a committee called the Alternative Practice Committee. The major goal of this committee was to review current nursing practice nationwide, review the literature for alternative forms of practice being tried at other institutions, and strategically consider the direction of change and innovation desired for the VBMC Nursing Department. This investigative analysis considered cost-effectiveness, patient satisfaction, nurse satisfaction as it affects nurse retention, possibility of role redesign for RNs, and creative mechanisms for effective use of resources and ancillary support personnel. The formation of the committee marked the beginning of shared governance at VBMC. In order to ensure staff nurse participation in developing innovations for patient care, a committee of staff representatives from all shifts and all levels of nursing personnel was formed on a trial unit. Orthopedics was the first trial unit for shared governance and the first unit to develop an RCP.

Valley Baptist Medical Center

STANDARDS OF NURSING CARE & STANDARDS OF NURSING PRACTICE	
STANDARD OF CARE	**SUPPORTING STANDARD(S) OF PRACTICE**
I. Nursing Process	Nursing Process: Implementation and Use of Assessment, Planning, Intervention, Evaluation
II. Safety	Injury, Potential for: Falls related to ____ (specify) Injury, Potential for: Physiologic, related to Abnormal Lab Values (specify)
III. Comfort	Comfort, Alteration In
IV. Hygiene	Self Care Deficit: Feeding, Grooming, Bathing, Toilet, Dressing, Hygiene
V. Teaching & Learning	Health Maintenance Alteration/Knowledge Deficit Home Management Alteration/Discharge Planning
VI. Psychosocial	Grieving, Dysfunctional Anxiety/Fear Coping, (In) effective Body Image Disturbance Self-Concept Disturbance Sexuality Pattern Alteration Family Process Alteration Spiritual Distress
VII. Neurologic/Cognitive	Altered Tissue Perfusion: Cerebral Altered Thought Processes
VIII. Circulation & Perfusion	Altered Tissue Perfusion: Cardiopulmonary Decreased Cardiac Output Altered Tissue Perfusion: Peripheral
IX. Ventilation	Ineffective Breathing Pattern Impaired Gas Exchange
X. Food & Fluid	Fluid Volume Excess Fluid Volume Deficit Nutrition Alteration: Less Than/More Than Body Requirements
XI. Thermoregulation	Altered Body Temperature: Hypothermia / Hyperthermia
XII. Activity & Rest	Mobility Impaired
XIII. Elimination	Bowel Elimination Alteration: Constipation/Diarrhea Urinary Elimination Alteration: Incontinence Urinary Elimination Alternation: Retention
XIV. Integumentary	Skin Integrity Alteration
XV. Infection	Potential for Infection

FIGURE 7-1   An overview of the general Standards of Care and Standards of Practice. Individual units have additional unit-specific nursing diagnoses to accompany these standards.

Unit Action Committee: The First Step Toward Shared Governance

The unit action committee is composed of elected staff and discusses clinical issues occurring on the unit with a focus on possible solutions. The nurse manager serves as facilitator. The committee comprises RNs, LVNs, nurse's aides, and secretaries, with equal representation from all shifts. As the need for collaboration is identified, ancillary support staff and physicians are invited to participate.

The committee meets routinely once a month. The representatives develop agenda items and discuss quality improvement as it affects patient care on their unit. Each representative reports committee business to the other staff members in their category of care. This structure facilitates cohesion and teamwork on the unit with a real dedication for improving patient care. Appendix 7-2 presents the working guidelines for unit action committees at VBMC. The development of shared governance at the unit level led to the eventual formation of the Joint Unit Action Committee.

Joint Unit Action Committee: The Second Step Toward Shared Governance

The chairperson of each unit action committee represents his or her nursing unit in a nursing department-wide committee known as the Joint Unit Action Committee. This committee began meeting in November 1991 and was developed to discuss clinical issues common to all nursing areas and practice specialties. It was soon realized that this committee was able to provide valuable information related to practice issues as well as resolutions to long-standing problems throughout the nursing department. The committee gained in popularity as it was consulted by nursing units considering changes in practices, policies, or procedures. Whenever a commonality of practice problems could be identified across units, recommendations for solving such problems were developed by the Joint Unit Action Committee. Guidelines for the operation of the Joint Unit Action Committee are detailed in Appendix 7-3.

This committee meets once a month. Its first major accomplishment was the review and revision of the nursing department philosophy. The revised philosophy has been the foundational element for VBMCs Design for Change program. Because it was developed with considerable staff input, it exemplifies the commitment to a model of shared governance.

Other major accomplishments of the Joint Unit Action Committee include

- Formation of the Dietary/Nurse Committee to address patient satisfaction issues;
- Formation of the Respiratory/Nurse Committee to address issues of improving service;
- Development and presentation of a Nursing Department Joint Commission In-Service program to help educate staff members about the 1993 Joint Commission on Accreditation of Health Care Organizations (JCAHO) Standards.

Council Formation: The Third Step Toward Shared Governance

After all unit action committees were in place and the Joint Unit Action Committee was meeting on a regular basis, the next phase of the shared governance model was implemented. The focus of this phase was the development and implementation of specific nursing councils. Figure 7-2 details the overall governance model and highlights the various councils.

The *Management Council* consists of the Senior Vice President of Nursing, five Directors of Nursing, five Nurse Managers, the Coordinator of Nursing Education, the Guest Relations Coordinator, the Critical Care Coordinator, and the Maternal/Child Coordinator. Five members of the Joint Unit Action Committee are also appointed. This council discusses clinical, operational, and quality improvement issues and forms CQI teams as necessary to resolve department-wide problems and redesign care processes and systems.

The *Quality Improvement Council* consists of the Director of Nursing who serves as the Hospital Quality Management Coordinator, the Coordinator of Nursing Education, Clinicians, the Infection Control Practitioner, the Critical Care Coordinator, and the Maternal/Child Coordinator. Four members of the Joint Unit Action Committee and one member of each nursing unit are also appointed. Quality issues are addressed, and unit-specific findings are reported and discussed in terms of monitoring and evaluating. Appendix 7-4 highlights the structure, roles, and responsibilities of this council.

Valley Baptist Medical Center Shared Governance Organizational Chart

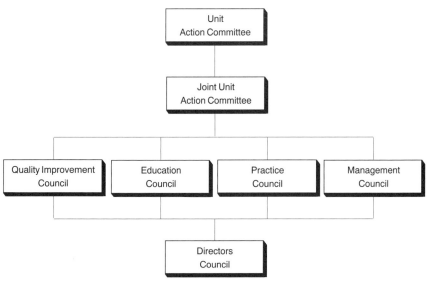

FIGURE 7-2 Organizational chart for shared governance.

The *Education Council* consists of the Coordinator of Nursing Education, Clinical Specialists, five Clinicians, two Nurse Managers, the Guest Relations Coordinator, three faculty members from the Associate Degree Nursing and Vocational Nursing programs, and the Director of Training and Development. Six members of the Joint Unit Action Committee are also appointed. This council receives information from all other councils relative to education issues and reports back to all councils through the Coordinator of Nursing Education.

The *Practice Council* consists of two Directors of Nursing, two Nurse Managers, the Coordinator of Nursing Education, and the MIS (Management of Information Services) Coordinator. Four members of the Joint Unit Action Committee are also appointed. The council monitors professional practice and clinical operations within the nursing department. It is responsible for evaluating standards of practice and standards of care and provides suggestions for innovations in nursing practice. The Practice Council also established a Policy, Procedure, and Forms Subcommittee, responsible for policy development based on practice and care standards.

The *Directors Council* was formed to discuss issues at the administrative level. Issues requiring upper management decision-making are dealt with by this council. Examples of such issues include department-wide operational and capital budget questions, analysis of the quarterly employee turnover report, risk management concerns, and quality management reports. In addition, each of the other councils submits a quarterly report to the Directors Council. This was the last council to be implemented, and it consists of the Senior Vice President of Nursing, the Directors of Nursing, the Guest Relations Coordinator, the Coordinator of Nursing Education, and the MIS Coordinator. The chairperson of the Joint Unit Action Committee and one additional member are also appointed to serve on the Directors Council. This council's duties, process, meetings, and reports meet the criteria set forth by hospital accreditation entities, particularly JCAHO.

Council Day

In order to facilitate participation of staff nurses assigned to committees and councils, preestablished meeting times are scheduled. Involved nurses are routinely given less than full patient care assignments on meeting days. Staff members of the Joint Unit Action Committee are also granted a Council Day as an added benefit. The councils focus on unit-specific quality-of-care reviews, literature searches, meeting minutes, and so on. Each council also develops its specific meeting agenda. All committees and councils are scheduled to meet on a specific day each month. This day is scheduled 1 year in advance. It is a busy day, and excellent communication flows from council to council. This established Council Day has contributed most to the success of the shared governance model, because staff nurses' attendance is scheduled and they fully participate in council activities and decision making. The benefits and outcomes of the councils far exceed the costs of scheduling staff to participate.

▬ CHAPLAIN CHARTING: INTEGRATING SPIRITUAL AND PSYCHOSOCIAL CARE

Spirituality is within the realm of nursing practice because the VBMC nursing philosophy supports holistic care. Although spirituality is addressed by both nurses and chaplains, it is not often documented. Prior to the redesign project, chaplains at VBMC were not documenting their assessments and interventions. This important element of patient care was not properly communicated. The Practice Council addressed this problem and incorporated spiritual needs as a standard of practice under the Psychosocial standard of care.

Although hospital chaplains attempt to visit every patient at least once during their hospitalization, it is the nurse who first identifies specific issues involving the spiritual needs of the patient. When this occurs, the nurse contacts pastoral services and requests a chaplain visit the patient. Initially, there was no documented evidence of follow-up that would allow the staff to assess and measure outcomes related to this intervention. A CQI committee composed of nurses and chaplains was formed to examine and redesign the process. The committee suggested that chaplains document spiritual care in the medical record. Outcomes could then be monitored, and the nursing staff could continue to plan for and provide holistic care, including care for identified spiritual needs. A Pastoral Care Consultant form was developed collaboratively between nursing and pastoral services, along with related policy and procedure.

Chaplains were given in-service training on acceptable documentation format. In assessing outcome, it has been shown that patients' spiritual needs are now being identified and incorporated into the overall plan of care. The chaplain's role has become an integral part of the multidisciplinary professional health care delivery team. Plans are now being formulated to include spiritual care in RCPs and integrated charting.

▬ EDUCATION IN ACTION

Annual mandatory in-service training programs include fire and electrical safety, hazardous waste management, universal precautions, body mechanics, and cardiopulmonary resuscitation (CPR) recertification. In the past, each employee simply viewed videos on his or her anniversary date. It was the responsibility of the Department Manager or Nurse Manager to determine the need for and arrange the viewing of videos. As the VBMC has grown, the number of employees has proportionally increased. Scheduling for mandatory in-service training sessions became difficult, and work became intensive for the managers.

An ad hoc Safety Education Committee was formed from VBMC's Safety Committee. It included nursing and ancillary representation in order to address the problem and generate alternative solutions. The committee developed the concept of setting aside one day per month to provide needed in-service training. The result was the establishment of a monthly "update day." During the month of his or her birthday, each employee is scheduled off of the unit and paid to attend the mandatory in-service training program. The nursing department further incorporated annual CPR recertification sessions as a part of the education update day. A hospital-wide computerized list of employees is generated each month and sent to managers in advance for scheduling. This process is organized and streamlined, leading to a marked increase in employee attendance and compliance with policies related to mandatory in-service training.

▄ INNOVATIONS IN CONTINUOUS QUALITY IMPROVEMENT

The progression of VBMC's quality management program toward CQI included the review and revision of the nursing philosophy. This was delegated to the Joint Unit Action Committee. The nursing department philosophy reinforces the commitment of the entire organization to quality care as well as process and system improvements. Based on this mutual commitment to quality, the groundwork was set to implement the principles of a new CQI program. The program was developed by nursing leaders and is taught, championed, structured, and rewarded by these leaders. This focus and direction empowers staff to creatively and systematically approach problems and opportunities and make improvements as identified by nursing's primary customers: patients, physicians, and coworkers.

This hospital-wide CQI program is not confined to the department of nursing but crosses departmental lines. Staff nurses become involved by serving on multidisciplinary CQI teams that study and improve processes and systems. The major accomplishments realized by this program are improved interdepartmental communication and increased decision-making authority for staff nurses, which in turn have increased job satisfaction and produced improvements in processes. Some examples are mechanisms to better meet patients' psychosocial and spiritual needs through a multidisciplinary approach, improved timeliness when responding to emergency situations (the Pronto Protocol, described later), and more timely treatment of hypoglycemic reactions (described later). Nursing practice has improved because of staff nurse empowerment and involvement in initiating change.

Customer Feedback

As part of the ongoing CQI program, nursing leaders encouraged staff to identify their customers. The nursing department then developed ways to measure satisfaction with the services it provided. The existing patient satisfaction feedback mechanism was studied and improved; it became the Valley Baptist Medical Center Report Card. This new tool is a satisfaction questionnaire given to every patient or significant other as part of the nursing discharge process, along with a detailed explanation of its importance in assisting the nursing department to improve the quality of care.

The return rate averages 50% to 60%, and trending analysis has identified many opportunities for improvement. For example, the timeliness of the admission process was identified as an opportunity for improvement. This process involved many departments, including nursing. Based on the analysis, a multidisciplinary CQI team was formed to study the admission process. Through process changes, timeliness was improved and patient feedback demonstrated increased satisfaction. The questionnaires have also provided leaders the opportunity to recognize and reward staff for high-quality care. Many patients identify "special" staff members. Those identified are rewarded with an ice cream voucher. This recognition has been well received and has served as a positive reinforcement to the overall quest for quality care and service.

Departmental Liaison Committees

Liaison committees are another methodology used to improve care through customer feedback. The Nurse–Pharmacy Liaison Committee is made up of three pharmacists, one pharmacy technician, five nursing clinical managers, and one unit secretary. If process review is recommended, a CQI team is formed from this committee to study the process and develop recommendations for improvement. This committee has been effective in improving the accuracy of medication administration records, improving the process of medication administration, and assuring the reporting and analysis of adverse drug reactions.

The Nurse–Laboratory Liaison Committee functions in a similar manner. This committee is composed of five laboratory staff members and five nursing clinical staff managers. This group has been instrumental in decreasing needle sticks through procedural changes related to the disposal of needles and other sharps, improving the timeliness of ordering and carrying out lab testing, and improving job satisfaction in both departments by promoting a better understanding of each other's roles, responsibilities, and problems.

Physician–Nurse Liaison Committee

The most innovative and collaborative quality improvement committee at VBMC is the Physician–Nurse Liaison Committee. This committee originated as a mechanism to deal with conflicts in professional relations between physicians and nurses. It has since developed into a major, multifunctional committee. The committee deals with issues of quality improvement, utilization review, risk management, and innovations in patient care. The committee has been meeting once a month for the last 4 years. Structure, roles, and responsibilities of the committee are detailed in Appendix 7-5.

The Physician–Nurse Liaison Committee functions as no other hospital committee. Quality of care and any behavior concerns between physicians and nurses or physicians and patients in the previous 30 days are addressed by the Chiefs of Staff, the Medical Director, and the Vice President of Nursing. All issues are dealt with in a timely, unbiased, concerned manner.

Inappropriate physician behavior can seriously disrupt the activities of patient care. There are multiple ramifications for nursing if this behavior is not addressed. Nursing job satisfaction may decline, and the quality and timeliness of patient care may be adversely affected. Risks of patient/family dissatisfaction culminating in legal action may also occur.

Inappropriate physician behavior is dealt with by the Physician–Nurse Liaison Committee. Most inappropriate behavior can be improved with education or addressed as a failure of the system by which patient care is delivered. If individual physician behaviors repeatedly surface during monthly meetings, physician leadership is forced to face issues they often overlooked in the past. The committee agenda and actions taken are reviewed by the Vice President of Nursing in the monthly Medical Executive Board meeting. If a particular physician's inappropriate behavior has become a trend, the Medical Executive Board must take further action. Privilege reduction is a possible recommendation.

Examples of other issues addressed through the committee include Health Care Financing Administration (HCFA) transfer denials and concerns, problems with documentation in patients' medical records, problems with emergency department on-call response, alterations of the medical record, physician–physician relations, documentation of advance directives, and implementation of integrated charting.

The Physician–Nurse Liaison Committee has intervened with physicians who have verbally abused nurses. The Chiefs of Staff visit with these physicians, and the unacceptable behavior stops. The staff nurse involved is told that this committee has taken action on the complaint. Staff nurses, therefore, feel the committee serves their purpose well in not only representing them in physician-related problems but producing results that lead to better professional relations between staff nurses and physicians. The Physician–Nurse Liaison Committee has been instrumental in empowering the nursing department.

Guest Relations Program

The Guest Relations Coordinator addresses in-house patient/family complaints regarding all aspects of care. On admission, patients are provided with an office telephone number by which to voice their concerns. All concerns are thoroughly investigated by the coordinator. Any trends identified for patient care improvement are referred to the quality improvement program. Examples of concerns that have been referred include misplaced patient valuables, visitation issues, requesting an explanation and copy of hospital bills, dislike of hospital food, delay of surgery or other scheduled procedures, and admission or discharge processes. CQI teams study the processes and develop new mechanisms to correct problems, thus increasing patient satisfaction. For example, a new process to track and document patient valuables was developed jointly by nurses and security personnel. Visitor direction maps and rule changes were initiated by another multidisciplinary CQI team. Both of these measures have enhanced patient/family satisfaction as evidenced by comments on the VBMC Report Card.

CQI Hotline

A CQI Hotline was implemented as a mechanism to gather quality improvement ideas from employees and physicians. This telephone answering machine is located in the Quality Management Coordinator's office. If an idea serves to 1) improve quality; 2) improve cost-effectiveness; 3) increase customer satisfaction; 4) improve the work environment; or 5) improve the hospital's competitive position, action is taken to investigate and implement the improved process. All suggestions are acknowledged within 24 hours of the call. A follow-up letter is sent to the caller detailing whether the idea was implemented. If the idea was not implemented, a reasonable explanation is given. There were 35 calls from staff members in the first 3 months after implementation of the CQI Hotline; 19 of the ideas met criteria and have been implemented.

Interdepartmental Quality Improvement Committees (CQI Teams)

Each nursing unit action committee serves as an intradepartmental quality improvement committee. Members are selected by their peers, and ideas for improvement are introduced to the committees.

If opportunities to improve processes are identified through patient satisfaction questionnaires, a liaison committee, the guest relations program, the CQI Hotline, or a unit action committee, a CQI team is formed to study the processes and recommend improvements. The CQI team generally consists of eight to ten staff members who are closely related to the process under study. Attempts are made to involve all departments, including physicians. The results have been very effective in promoting interdepartmental and intradepartmental teamwork, quality improvement, and communication.

Pronto Protocol

A CQI team that included physician members was effective in developing a *Pronto Protocol* (Appendix 7-6). This policy and procedure specifically empowers clinical nurses. The process was created to give nurses authority to ensure immediate, hands-on patient care by a physician during situations that previously had resulted in a delayed response of several hours or more. Examples of such situations include disagreement with a physician's orders, slow deterioration of a patient's condition with inadequate physician response, or a family problem involving a physician. The multidisciplinary team developed a protocol that outlined steps to be taken to enhance quality care in such situations. Quality concerns related to the Pronto Protocol are monitored by the Nurse–Physician Liaison Committee, and appropriate actions are taken by the Medical Staff, if necessary.

This protocol has been utilized by nurses, and each time it has been related to a lack of timely response when attempting to reach a physician for urgently needed orders. It has been effective, because patients were promptly and efficiently managed, without delay. After the Pronto Protocol has been activated, a thorough, retrospective investigation may reveal a failure of a communication tool (eg, beeper, answering service) or a more serious issue that must be resolved through physician peer review. The major advantage of the protocol is that patient care is not compromised.

Hypoglycemia Protocol
A CQI team made up of nurses, a diabetic nurse clinician, and physicians developed a hypoglycemia protocol for the nonintensive care nursing units. Improvements not only involved the development of a treatment protocol to assure timely and effective intervention, but also led to increased education for staff nurses regarding diabetic management.

Heparin Protocol
Another multidisciplinary CQI team made up of physicians, pharmacists, nurses, and laboratory personnel studied the lab monitoring process for patients on heparin therapy. A process to assure appropriate monitoring of laboratory values during heparin therapy was developed and implemented. The CQI team reported its progress to the Pharmacy and Therapeutics Committee, who will continue to monitor the process for compliance. Even though this is a physician responsibility, the multidisciplinary approach helps to enhance quality of care.

Fall Festival
Once a year, a Fall Festival is held at VBMC. This festival is educational and includes an annual update on CQI activities which occurred over the past year. It is a time to celebrate accomplishments. Employees, physicians, administrative staff, and members of the governing body attend. The Fall Festival also includes updates on Infection Control, Utilization Management, Patient Rights, and Employee Health and Human Resource activities. In 1992, 400 people attended the one-day event.

With the quality improvement support systems of customer feedback, reward and recognition for team and individual accomplishments, internal benchmarking by the nursing units, and active leadership involvement, the VBMC nursing department has made great strides in CQI.

The next step will be implementing a medical information system to assist in identifying opportunities for improvement, prioritizing those opportunities, and measuring the results of CQI activities. Another key element that will lead the way in enhancing outcome measurement is the computerization of the RCP and related variances.

■ PATIENT SELF-DETERMINATION ACT
The Patient Self-Determination Act of December 1991 mandates that all health care facilities that are Medicare- or Medicaid-funded have a mechanism of informing patients of their rights to accept or refuse medical or surgical treatment (Pennsylvania Insurance Management Company, 1993). The Act also details the right of patients to formulate advance directives and/or a durable power of attorney for health care in the event they become incapacitated.

In order to facilitate implementation of the various forms needed in different situations, a Patient Rights Decision Tree form was developed. This enhances the nursing staff's knowledge of which forms to use at a glance.

The number of consultation requests from nurses to the Guest Relations Coordinator has decreased from 25 calls per week to only seven. The nurses' role is to ask newly admitted patients whether they have implemented advance directives and whether they want their advance directives to apply to this admission. Patients are informed of their rights but not coerced to exercise them. The appropriate forms and a brochure about patients' rights are provided in Spanish or English to every patient on admission. If a patient decides to develop an advance directive, the Guest Relations Coordinator or House Supervisor is notified to assist the patient or family. Copies of the forms are provided to the patient or family.

■ NCLEX-RN SPECIAL REVIEW
Graduate nurses who fail the NCLEX-RN examination are provided an opportunity to participate in an eight-week program to prepare to retake the exam. The participant takes special written tests three times a week on various clinical subjects. If questions are answered incorrectly, the graduate nurse is given a take-home assignment in which he or she writes the correct answer with a rationale. Consequently, the student is encouraged to study and understand the answer to complete the assignment. Learning occurs when the participant must correct each wrong question and discuss it with an instructor. Fourteen graduate nurses have taken the course, with only one failure on the second NCLEX-RN exam. The remaining thirteen who participated in the program are now RNs working at VBMC.

■ CONCLUSION
Future innovations by the Nursing Department at VBMC will be directed and dedicated to quality patient outcomes. With computerization of clinical information, including critical care, nursing will be completely "paperless" within 3 years. All data are ready to be implemented in a nursing subsystem. Integrated charting and RCPs will be used throughout the patient care system. Variances from RCPs, utilization review, and risk mechanisms will be part of the overall quality management system that is currently being structured within the medical information system.

There is a commitment of resources, both financial and human, to achieve this goal. It is our mission to be patient-centered, oriented to quality, and competitive in the health care system—wherever the future takes us.

■ REFERENCES
Adams, R. & Rentfro, A. (1991). Strengthening Hospital Nursing: An approach to restructuring care delivery. *The Journal of Nursing Administration, 21*(6), 12–19.
Pennsylvania Insurance Management Company. (1993, January). The Patient Self-Determination Act: Living wills and other types of advance directives. *ECRI*, pp. 1–33.
Pratt, L. (1976). *Family structure and effective health behavior: The energized family.* Boston: Houghton Mifflin.

PATIENT NAME:_____   MR# _____

Initiated By:_____   RN Date _____   **VALLEY BAPTIST MEDICAL CENTER**

NURSING DIAGNOSES   STANDARD   PATIENT GOALS & EXPECTED OUTCOMES

CIRCULATION & PERFUSION

_____ Altered Tissue Perfusion: <u>Cardiopulmonary</u>
Initial

<u>Signs & Symptoms</u>   Patient will exhibit the following by time of transfer from unit:

Neuro:	change in mental status, i.e. restlessness confusion, disorientation, lethargy	Neuro:	Alert & Oriented
Resp..	lung congestion, dyspnea, ↑↓ resp. rate, ↓ pulse oximetry	Resp:	>12 <25 O₂Sat >94%
Cardiac:	↑↓ HR, ↑↓ BP, rhythm changes, extra heart sounds, chest pain, ↓ pulses, jugular distention, peripheral edema, weight gain	Cardiac:	HR >50<110 SBP >90 <150 CO 4-7
			SVR 900-1500 Hgb >9.0 CI 2-4
			K+ 3.5-5.5
GU:	↓ urine output	GU:	Output >20cc/h or >240cc/8 hrs
Skin:	pallor, cyanosis, diaphoresis, clammy	Skin:	Warm & dry

FOOD & FLUID

_____ (Potential) <u>Nutrition</u> Altered Less Than Body's Requirement
Initial

<u>Signs & Symptoms</u>   Patient will exhibit the following by time of transfer from unit.

Weight Loss   Eating >75% of meals.

Decrease/absence of bowel sounds, N/V, constipation   Bowel sounds; No N/V or constipation

↑↓ Glucose   Glucose >80 <150

PSYCHOSOCIAL - TEACHING & LEARNING

_____ <u>Coping</u> (In)effective: Individual/Family
Initial

<u>Signs & Symptoms</u>   Patient will exhibit the following by time of transfer from unit:

Lack of knowledge   Restate information accurately
Denial, non-compliance   Express feelings
Ineffective communication   Develop adequate communication skills
Insomnia, Oversleeping   Sleeps 4-6 hrs q night
Irritability, denial, withdrawal of family members/significant   Family will verbalize education/resource needs for coping with
(signif.)others   pt's illness.

COMFORT

_____ <u>COMFORT</u> Alteration in
Initial

<u>Signs & Symptoms</u>   Patient will exhibit the following:

Pain   Relief of chest pain 15-30 min. after medication.

                                             Relief of _____ pain 30-45 min. after
                                             medication.

                    Standard:_____

_____ Nursing DX: _____
Initial

■ **APPENDIX 7-1.** Cardiogenic Shock. RCP is initiated on admission to critical care unit. Standards of Care for the patient are listed in bold print such as Circulation and Perfusion. Supporting Standards of Practice are also shown above. Key word in Standard of Practice is underlined and used as a reference when charting in Nursing Progress Notes.

(continued)

ADMISSION DAY   Reviewed/Revised by _____ <u>RN</u> Date _____

CARDIOPULMONARY

DOCTOR'S ORDERS	NURSING ORDERS
Admission wt as soon as condition warrants.	_____ Biophysical/Psychosocial on database within 30 min of adm.
Weights q _____; record.	_____ RN Assessment on transfer adm.
On adm, BP both arms	
Vital Signs q 2-4 hrs & prn or _____	_____ Instruct pt. to turn, cough, & deep breathe.
Hemodynamics q _____	Suction prn
Notify MD of any significant arrhythmias, excessive	Assess cardiac/respiratory status q 4 h & prn
diaphoresis, hypotension, ↓↑ HR	NURSING ORDERS FOR IABP
Monitor Lab results, notify MD of abnormals.	- Document BP on & off IABP q 12 hrs at beginning of shift.
Titrate drips per orders.	- Assess pt q 4 hrs & prn & Document: mental status, cardiac status (including radial/pedal pulses & limb warmth/color), resp. status, GI (bowel sounds), GU (30cc/hr UO).
Document pulse oximeter	- Assess IABP site q 4 hrs for hematoma, bleeding, S&S of infection & Document.
ABGs prn	- Assess clear tubing for moisture/blood & Document on IABP box in flow sheet q 2 hrs & prn.
Foley catheter	- Nofity MD of any assessment abnormals.
	MONITOR IABP controls closely.
	- NEVER run on MANUAL MODE
	- Purge q 4 hrs & Document on IABP box in flow sheet (purge tubing & disc.)
	- DO NOT remove any cables from machine.
	- Check/Document catheter balloon size corresponds to disc size.
	IMMEDIATELY call Engineering after troubleshooting does not resolve alarms.

NUTRITION

DOCTOR'S ORDERS	NURSING ORDERS
	Daily weights
Diet: _____	Assess bowel sounds q 4 hrs; c/o N/V
Fluid restriction as necessary	Monitor BM's & record; if no BM, laxative of choice.
Laxative of choice	_____ Encourage pt to eat; record intake.
I & O	Assist pt to eat while femoral line(s) present.

COPING

DOCTOR'S ORDERS	NURSING ORDERS Document:
Sedatives	_____ Teach pt/signif.other of disease process, medical regimen, i.e., IABP.
If pt unable to sleep by 10 p.m., give sleeping med.	
Review Advance Directives	_____ Pt/signif. other verbalize concerns/fears of hospitalization & disease process.
	_____ Pt/signif. other offered chaplain services. Document minister visits.
	_____ Teach pt/signif.other of restricted activity.

COMFORT

DOCTOR'S ORDERS	NURSING ORDERS
For Chest Pain:	_____ Teach pt to rate degree of pain with 1-10 scale pre & post meds
Do 12 lead EKG	
NTG per protocol	Assess/document type, location & degree of pain pre & post meds.
NOTIFY Charge Nurse & MD OF CHEST PAIN	Document v.s. & other signs/symptoms.
Sof Care Mattress	Back rub/analgesics for restricted activity.
	Logroll when turning.

STANDARD:

7a-7p Initial/Signature/Credential	7p-7a Initial/Signature/Credential	7a-7p Initial/Signature/Credential	7a-7p Initial/Signature/Credential

■APPENDIX 7-1. *(continued)*

VBMC
UNIT ACTION COMMITTEE

I. MEMBERSHIP

A. Unit Action Committee shall consist of representatives from all shifts and all levels of nursing personnel on a specific unit. (Each Unit Action Committee is encouraged to have equal representation from all shifts and from all personnel [RN, LVN, NA, secretary, etc.]) The members of each Unit Action Committee shall be nominated by their peers and appointed by the Nurse Manager. The Unit Action Committee chairperson and recorder (optional) shall be nominated by the committee members and appointed by the Nurse Manager. The Nurse Manager shall serve as the committee facilitator.

B. The size of each Unit Action Committee shall be determined by the number of employees on a given unit.
1. Units with 10-20 employees shall have approximately 4-6 representatives;
2. Units with 20-40 employees shall have approximately 8-10 representatives; and
3. Units with greater than 40 employees shall have approximately 10-15 representatives.

II. DURATION OF APPOINTMENT

A. The term of appointment for each Unit Action Committee member will be 2 years.

B. The term of office for each Unit Action Committee chairperson shall be two (2) years with change over in January.

C. Any resignation of a Unit Action Committee member, chairperson or recorder that occurs during his/her term of office must be submitted in writing to the Nurse Manager. The process to replace the resigning chairperson shall follow the nomination and appointment procedure specified elsewhere in these guidelines.

III. DUTIES

A. Each Unit Action Committee shall:
1. share ideas, discuss clinical issues, and make recommendations as appropriate to the Nurse Manager.
2. give input to the Joint Unit Action Committee as appropriate.
3. promote and recommend to the Nurse Manager clinical changes to increase productivity in a positive manner; and
4. increase and encourage communication between nursing shifts in an effort to solve potential shift differences and/or conflicts.

B. Any Unit Action Committee may recommend changes in its duties by submitting any requested change in writing to the Director's Council by July 1 of each year.

IV. MEETINGS AND REPORTS

A. Each Unit Action Committee shall meet at least eight (8) times per year, shall maintain a permanent record of its findings, proceedings and actions, and shall make a report after each meeting to the Director's Council, the Senior Vice President of Nursing or designee, and the Chief Executive Officer.

B. Unit Action Committee meetings shall be on a scheduled rotation, accommodating all three (3) working shifts. Any member who is unable to attend a scheduled meeting must send a substitute from his/her shift to the meeting. The substitute shall have the same privileges as the member. Any Unit Action Committee member who has more than three (3) unexcused or excused absences shall be replaced through the process of nomination for appointment by the nursing staff.

■ **APPENDIX 7-2.** Guidelines for the operation of the Unit Action Committee.

VBMC
Joint Unit Action Committee

V.   MEMBERSHIP

Joint Unit Action Committee shall consist of the Chairpersons of all Unit Action Committees and the Coordinator of Nursing Education, who shall serve as committee facilitator. The chairperson shall be nominated by the committee members and approval and appointment shall be made by the Director's Council. All committee members shall have voting privileges.

VI.   DURATION OF APPOINTMENT

The term of appointment of each member of the Joint Unit Action Committee shall be two (2) years.

VII.   DUTIES

A.   The Joint Unit Action Committee shall:

1.   encourage communications between the units and resolve potential unit differences and/or conflicts;
2.   share ideas and discuss clinical issues;
3.   make recommendations to the Director's Council and other nursing councils and committees as appropriate regarding clinical issues; and,
4.   review the philosophy of the Department of Nursing annually and make recommendations as necessary.

B.   Joint Unit Action Committee members shall serve on Continuous Quality Improvement Teams as needs are identified.

C.   Members of other councils and committees shall report proceedings of their meetings at Joint Unit Action Committee meetings.

D.   The Joint Unit Action Committee may recommend changes in its duties by submitting any requested change in writing to the Director's Council by July 1 of each year.

VIII.   MEETINGS AND REPORTS

A.   The Joint Unit Action Committee shall meet as often as necessary but at least eight (8) times per year, shall maintain a record of its findings, proceedings, and actions, and shall make a report at least quarterly through the Coordinator of Nursing Education to the Director's Council, the Senior Vice President of Nursing or designee, and the Chief Executive Officer.

B.   Any member who is unable to attend a scheduled meeting must send a substitute from his/her Unit to that meeting. The substitute shall have all the privileges of the members.

■ **APPENDIX 7-3.** Guidelines for the operation of the Joint Unit Action Committee.

VBMC
QUALITY IMPROVEMENT COUNCIL

I. MEMBERSHIP

The Quality Improvement Council shall consist of the Director of Quality Management who shall serve as council chairperson, Nurse Managers, the Infection Control Nurse, Nurse Clinicians, the Critical Care Coordinator, the Maternal/Child Coordinator, Coordinator of Nursing Education, four (4) members of the Joint Unit Action Committee, one (1) member of each nursing unit, and the Secretary for Quality Management, who shall serve as the recorder. Additional members include the Critical Care Nurse Educator, Medical-Surgical Clinician, Enterostomal Therapy Clinician, Diabetes Nurse Clinician, and the Infection Control Nurse. All members including Joint Unit Action Committee members will have voting privileges.

II. DURATION OF APPOINTMENT

All appointments to the Quality Management Council shall be made by the Director's Council, and the term of appointment for Joint Unit Action Committee members shall be one (1) year.

III. DUTIES

A. The Quality Improvement Council shall:
    1. regularly discuss nursing clinical issues;
    2. review the quality of care provided by nursing service;
    3. prioritized opportunities to improve care;
    4. monitor and make recommendations regarding opportunities for improvements; and
    5. submit an annual quality improvement report of nursing activities to the Director's Council by July 1 of each year.

B. The Quality Improvement Council may recommend changes in its duties by submitting any requested change in writing to the Director's Council by July 1 of each year.

IV. MEETINGS AND REPORTS

A. The Quality Improvement Council shall meet as often as necessary but at least bi-monthly, shall maintain a record of its findings, proceedings, and action, and shall make a report after each meeting to the Chief Executive Officer and other nursing councils and/or committees as appropriate or desirable. Fifty percent (50%) of the members present at a meeting shall constitute a quorum.

B. Educational issues including, but not limited to, orientation and inservice shall be referred to the Education Council through the Nursing Education Coordinator. Policy and procedure issues shall be referred to the Practice Council.

■ **APPENDIX 7-4.** Quality Improvement Council enhances communication, collaboration and cooperation between all nursing units.

VBMC
PHYSICIAN-NURSE LIAISON COMMITTEE
OF THE MEDICAL BOARD

I.   Introduction

This is a revision of the prospectus of this committee, which was formed in 1989 as a means of improving collaboration between the medical and nursing staffs of Valley Baptist Medical Center.   Evidence that this committee has fulfilled its function includes development and acceptance of the "Pronto Protocol" for ensuring timely nursing and medical intervention in rapidly changing clinical situations, a decrease in the use of the medical record as a forum for physicians and nurses to critique each other, and improved understanding among physicians and nurses regarding how each group contributes to the monitoring and improvement of quality of care.

II.   Purpose

The purpose of this committee is to search for ways to improve communication and collaboration between physicians and nurses working in Valley Baptist Medical Center.   It shall fulfill this purpose by:

(a)   serving as a forum for regular and timely discussion of issues related to physician/nurse clinical practice;

(b)   seeking suggestions through physician interaction and support for innovative nursing proposals to enhance patient care;

(c)   evaluating format and content of medical records and seeking ways to improve these in order to improve the patient care process for both physicians and nurses;

(d)   analyzing instances of suboptimal communication and collaboration between physicians and nurses in a timely manner;

(e)   based upon such analysis, moving significant problems expeditiously through the quality improvement mechanism;

(f)   identifying need and opportunity for educational programs in risk management or clinical practice.

(g)   reviewing all transfer denials and concerns through written reports submitted by the House Supervisor.

The Physician-Nurse Liaison Committee will review all reports of situations involving questions concerning the transfer policies of VBMC as a part of the VBMC quality management program which is a medical peer review function.   As such the reports made to or by the Committee are privileged and confidential under Tex. Rev. Civ. Stat. Ann. art. 4495b, § 5.6 and Tex. Health & Safety Code Ann. §§ 161.031-161.033. As such the records of this committee are not subject to discovery or subpoena and are not admissible into evidence.

III.   Composition

The committee shall consist of the Senior Vice President of Nursing and the Chief of Staff as co-chairs, the Chief of Medicine, Chief of Surgery, an additional member of the Medical Board, the Director of Hospital Quality Management, and Quality Improvement Medical Advisor.

IV.   Authority

The Physician-Nurse Liaison Committee shall be a quality management and improvement committee of the hospital, whose role is to review and investigate issues and incidents related to its purpose.   It shall refer or report its findings to a committee of the Medical Staff, the Quality Management and Improvement Committee of the Medical staff, the Nursing Quality Management Committee, and/or the Chief Executive Officer, as appropriate.

■ APPENDIX 7-5.   Rules governing the Physician-Nurse Liaison Committee. This represents the second revision.

VALLEY BAPTIST MEDICAL CENTER

PRONTO PROTOCOL
(WHEN QUESTIONS ARISE INVOLVING MEDICAL CARE)

V. POLICY:

A. Statements:

If a staff member has any reason to doubt or question the care provided to any patient or believes that appropriate consultation is needed and has not been obtained, or feels that a particular physician order is not appropriate, she/he shall call this to the attention of the Nurse Manager or Charge Nurse. The Nurse Manager/Charge Nurse will discuss the concerns with the attending physician or may refer the situation to the House Supervisor. If unresolved after discussion with the attending physician, the House Supervisor will report to the Chief of the Department, wherein the practitioner has clinical privileges. The Chief of the Department may request a consultation or give medical orders. If an emergency exists, assistance may be obtained by calling the emergency department physician or by paging a Dr. 10.

The events are documented by the House Supervisor and submitted to the Senior Vice President of Nursing Service.

If the treatment in question involves administration of a medication that the nurse feels is not appropriately ordered, he/she will use the above process. The last resort may be that the physician is requested to administer the medication himself.

B. Purpose: To ensure timely and appropriate medical intervention.

VI. PROCEDURE:

A. Description: Steps to take to initiate the Pronto Protocol.

B. Steps:

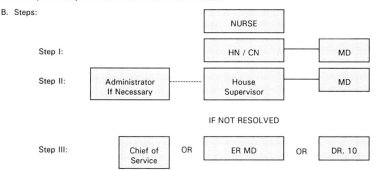

A time lapse of 15 minutes should be kept in mind, based upon seriousness of situation.

The House Supervisor shall report all Step II and Step III occurrences to the Vice President of Nursing Service.

Step II and Step III occurrences shall be reviewed by the Nurse/Physician Liaison Committee.

C. Post Procedure Observations: N/A
D. Required Documentation: N/A
E. References: N/A

■ **APPENDIX 7-6.** The House Supervisor is responsible for submitting this in writing.

Chapter 8

Third Generation Redesign: Lessons From the Field

M. LYNNE O'DAY   MARY L. FISHER

This is the story of a large urban hospital in the midwestern United States that in 1988 began a journey to restructure its systems of patient care delivery. The road had many hills, valleys, and curves which had to be traversed safely. Many lessons were learned along the way about change management. It is our desire to share that experience with you.

St. Vincent Hospital is a member of the Daughters of Charity National Health System. St. Vincent Hospital and Health Care Center, Inc., is a 1100-bed complex distributed across four sites in Indianapolis, Indiana. The system comprises a 650-bed tertiary hospital; a 150-bed stress center for mental health and chemical dependency programs; a 100-bed general hospital in Carmel, Indiana; and a 200-bed facility for the mentally retarded and physically handicapped. The initial restructuring effort began on the main campus, the 650-bed tertiary care facility.

In August 1988, St. Vincent Hospital, under the guidance of Booz-Allen and Hamilton, Inc., participated in a year-long study to determine how its hospitals could streamline their operations and allow caregivers to spend more time with patients. Out of this study evolved a new concept of patient-focused care, which St. Vincent Hospital calls Care2001.

Why restructure? Technical, highly sophisticated health care structures have become too complex. Patients, state and federal governments, health insurers, and business and industry are all demanding change. All health care providers must be ready to innovate and redesign quickly to improve the quality and efficiency of care.

Before restructuring, St. Vincent Hospital operated all of its departments as most other large modern hospitals do. Patient care revolved around centralized services. Staff spent a significant amount of time documenting, coordinating, scheduling, and transporting patients to services. Although patients at St. Vincent Hospital have consistently received high-quality clinical care, research indicated that staff spent a considerable amount of time in areas that were not related to direct patient care (Strengthening Hospital Nursing Program, 1992). It was alarming to discover that registered nurses

Flarey, D: REDESIGNING NURSING CARE DELIVERY: Transforming Our Future
© 1995, J. B. Lippincott Company

(RNs), the primary caregivers, spent less than 50% of their time on direct patient care. This statistic supported the need to find a new health care delivery system that could improve care and foster an environment for innovative change.

▄▄ PRINCIPLES

The experience at St. Vincent Hospital verifies what others have learned, that restructuring care delivery is a journey. It is a dynamic process that should be customized for each institution, patient population, and staff culture. Hopefully, the learning that occurs on this journey will spur innovation and change throughout the organization. Thus, the path is laid for making subsequent restructuring efforts more efficient and staff adjustments less disruptive. Ackoff (Strengthening Hospital Nursing Program, 1992) describes the process of interactive planning, which involves planning backward from an idealized design or from guiding principles. This participative process is continuous and holistic in that it recognizes the interdependence of units within an organization. St. Vincent Hospital developed four principles on which to base the Care2001 innovations: 1) high-quality, patient-focused care; 2) efficiency and effectiveness; 3) simplicity; and 4) an environment for innovation and change.

These principles also serve as a screening device to determine what and why additional changes should take place. Each of these principles is based on partnerships: patient and family with the physician; patient and family with St. Vincent employees and St. Vincent employees with physicians.

Patient-Focused Care

High-quality, patient-focused care is the first and fundamental guiding principle. Quality is one of the five core values of the St. Vincent organizational culture and is a key deliverable of the Care2001 program. In traditional approaches to care, many services are provided to patients at the convenience of a central department, rather than at the convenience of the patient. Additionally, many services and methods of service to patients occur to support a profession rather than patients. Patient-focused care requires a shift in operations such that processes and systems revolve around patients' needs and convenience.

Efficiency and Effectiveness

Any changes that took place for Care2001 would have to support a more efficient and more effective service. With the increasing awareness and concern about rising health care costs, St. Vincent Hospital found it imperative to deliver a service that would be more efficient in terms of time and resources. Effectiveness would be measured by quality medical outcomes and patient satisfaction.

Simplicity

Simplicity is another core value of the St. Vincent Hospital health care system, and it certainly augments efficiency. Because of the complex and highly departmentalized health care bureaucracy in acute care facilities today, system simplicity must be emphasized. In simplifying systems, we are looking at better coordination of services and, more importantly, an opportunity to eliminate unnecessary steps and processes. It is also important to delegate work among care givers more evenly and by specialization.

Environment for Innovation and Change

Peter Drucker says, "The modern hospital was essentially designed between 1900 and 1920" (Drucker, 1973, p. 784). Little change or innovation in systems and infrastructure has taken place since then. The rapidly changing external health care environment necessitates a dynamic, innovative internal environment that allows the hospital to quickly respond to the many factors affecting the delivery of patient care.

▬RESTRUCTURING PATIENT CARE

With principles in place, ways to direct future redesign efforts in a consistent manner became much clearer. Although innovation was desired, chaos was not. The principles allowed for flexibility within a framework that adhered to overall planning goals.

The Seton Unit, a general and subspecialty surgery floor, opened as the pilot redesigned unit in January 1990. This initial unit was planned using a top-down approach. As other units have evolved into the Care2001 concept, the hospital progressively has given more responsibility for redesign to unit employees. This evolution has been possible because of the influence of shared governance on staff decision-making.

Having learned a lot from working with Booz-Allen, we were better able to analyze patient requirements and implement design changes with the needs of the patient as our focus. As many services as possible had to be managed closer to the patient. The surgery population worked well for this purpose because of the way their needs clustered. This population shared needs for common laboratory tests such as electrolytes, blood urea nitrogen, creatinine, blood sugar, urinalysis, complete blood count, prothrombin time, and partial prothrombin time. The "80/20 rule" guided the selection of these tests: 20% of the tests represented approximately 80% of the volume. The tests run on the unit have differed on each Care2001 floor based on patient population needs.

Surgical patients consistently need preoperative chest x-rays and electrocardiograms (ECGs) as well as postoperative respiratory support in the form of oxygen set-ups, incentive spirometry, postural drainage, percussions, and treatments with Benylin, Mucomyst, and Albuterol. Although staff were originally cross-trained to set up and develop x-rays, the practice never evolved because of Indiana radiology licensure issues. Seton staff now have added peak flow determination to their list of respiratory skills. Such modifications continue to keep staff aware that redesign is a dynamic state that is never completed.

Impact of Physical Changes

A satellite pharmacy, mini-laboratory, and radiology room for flat plate films were included in the floor plans. The central nurses' station was eliminated, and six team mini-stations were created near each patient cluster.

With these changes, nurses were finally able to work closer to the patients as their center of activity and communication moved from the central station to these individual work areas. This physical change and the elimination of the unit secretary position supported decentralizing order entry to the team caring for the patient. Nurses became more aware of order changes and were able to more quickly intervene to meet patient needs.

The elimination of the central nurses' station provided challenges as well. Systems had to be put in place to foster unit communication, because associates rarely leave their teams during their shifts. Physicians had long been accustomed to communicating their needs to a clinical charge nurse (CCN). This was no longer possible. Not only was there no CCN, but the physicians had to find individual RNs to answer their questions about patients. The nurses were not visible in the halls because they were now in patient rooms the majority of the time. There were telephone issues as well, since the physicians' calls had to be transferred between teams with no assurance of finding the correct person the first time. Nurses were in the rooms, and there was no one readily available to answer phones. Although Care2001 was functioning well for patient care, it was vital to eliminate physicians' frustrations with the decentralized system.

Each Care2001 unit has addressed these communication issues differently. Seton prominently posts which staff work on which team. Physicians and others have been given cards with team phone numbers. On two units, the RNs now wear cellular phones that can be accessed only by physicians. For the staff, this improvement has saved many steps, because they can now answer the phone from anywhere rather than having to drop everything to run down the hall to the desk phone. The physicians have more immediate access to the nurse caring for their patients.

Nurses were supported in their practice changes by the creation of nurse server units in the patient rooms. Each nurse server consists of cabinets stocked with supplies necessary for surgical patient care, individual patient medication drawers, and a bedside computer. Nurses were able to reduce the number of trips to central linen and supply storage areas by taking advantage of the nurse servers. The bedside computer was used only for order entry. Software became the big obstacle to computerizing the nurses' documentation. These bedside computers were eliminated from subsequent Care2001 unit designs until a fully functioning system could be put in place.

The unit pharmacists began supplying unit-dose medications directly to the patients' cubicles. Pharmacy computerized the medication administration record, eliminating the need for nurses to manually record medications every 5 days. Pharmacists work closely with the care team and are readily available to consult on appropriate medication therapy with the physician and care team. They also are involved in patient education. This service positively impacts pharmacy cost by eliminating drug wastage and recommending appropriate cost-effective alternative therapies.

Seton also planned a pleasant admitting/reception area. One of the goals of the patient-focused process was to eliminate the long and unpleasant task of enduring admitting procedures in a slow, centralized unit. With Seton, patients come directly to the floor, since most are preassigned for elective surgeries. Patients who do not feel well are taken directly to their rooms, where the unit representative (UR) comes to them at a convenient time for any paperwork that must be done.

Role Redesign

The physical changes merely set the stage for the more significant redesign effort, that of role redesign (Fig. 8-1). The unit became self-contained in its staffing. Instead of cleaning services being provided by housekeeping, the unit hired a unit support assistant (USA). The USA performs traditional housekeeping duties in addition to stocking nurse servers and ordering routine supplies. Since February 1993, the USA also has been assisting with patient transportation.

A unit pharmacist serves Seton and one other unit. The pharmacist reports in a matrix structure to the clinical manager and the pharmacy director.

The UR position was created to decentralize the admitting, transfer, and discharge procedures. URs also do the chart coding and abstracting necessary for billing, precertification/recertification, and financial counseling.

The traditional titles of RN, LPN, and aide were eliminated. A single title, team care specialist (TCS) was introduced. TCSs also had their credentials identified on their name tags (eg, Nancy Nurse, RN, Team Care Specialist). They brought their clinical backgrounds to the team. The RN was still the licensed nurse and leader of the team. There were also LPN and technician TCSs.

The TCSs were selected from volunteers eager to try a new delivery system. Some technicians were licensed laboratory or radiology personnel.

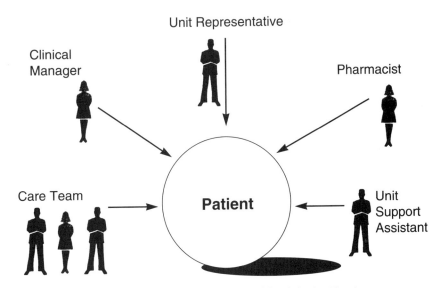

FIGURE 8-1   Pilot unit organization will consist of five job classifications.

Others had been ECG technicians, pharmacy technicians, or nurse assistants before transfer to Care2001. They were all trained in direct patient care. All TCSs underwent intensive cross-training that included phlebotomy, basic respiratory treatments, laboratory work, radiology set-ups, and ECG. The Seton education committee was established to maintain staff competencies in these areas. There is a detailed credentialing system to ensure that competencies are maintained. Because of the expense of training, the recognition that fewer people need to be trained, and the lack of efficiency in attempting to train everyone, fewer staff are now being trained in laboratory skills, and no one is now being trained in radiology.

Initially, all members of the team were considered equals. Although specific duties differed based on licensure, each team member's contributions were valuable. At first, this was translated into "no one is in charge" of the team. Teams evolved on their own. Many of the teams did not take individual patient assignments, preferring instead to work closely together to deliver care. Systems were set up to communicate what work had been completed and what remained to be done. Unfortunately, this approach took on a task orientation.

In rethinking the roles of team members, it became obvious that what was missing was a clear picture of the pivotal role of the RN. No one else on the team had the requisite understanding of patient needs; no one better understood the broad picture so as to direct the care above a technical level. Therefore, a change was made to enable the RN to direct the team in patient care. Although other TCSs had been trained to observe patients, it was the RN's responsibility to assess and plan care. A further evolvement of this RN role was the management of patients with critical pathways.

It was vital to begin developing RN leadership for the teams. A full-time educational consultant was placed on Seton to help the staff resolve some of these issues. Team building and growth in shared governance were facilitated by this informal leader (the educational consultant), who was readily accepted by the staff. The role of the professional nurse in relation to the Indiana Nurse Practice Act was clarified, and some ongoing documentation issues were resolved.

Documentation

A major strategy to streamline work that takes nurses away from patients is to eliminate duplication in charting and make it more concise and meaningful. Seton nurses spearheaded an effort to update the charting forms. The task force took more than a year to complete its work. The new forms were implemented in the Fall of 1992 on several units.

Documentation is now done by problem-oriented, focused notes based on PIE (Problem—Intervention—Evaluation) charting. If any of the patient's assessments fall within the color-coded areas on the assessment checklist, the nurse is prompted to initiate or maintain a problem note in that area. This color-coded area details patient problems requiring further assessment, planning, and ongoing evaluation. Associates assert that since they adapted to the new forms, their charting is now more concise and less time consuming.

▬MEASURES OF SUCCESS

St. Vincent Hospital has, over the years, enjoyed a high degree of satisfaction among associates, medical staff, and patients. In order to determine the success of this change process, measures of associate, physician, and patient satisfaction, quality, and cost were documented. It was the intention of the team that the patient-focused approach would enhance satisfaction, improve quality, and improve our cost position. The initial results of the patient-focused pilot unit were extremely positive. Studies indicated that quality had improved; patient, physician, and associate satisfaction had increased; an increased percentage of hours was spent on direct patient care (Fig. 8-2); and, the number of direct hours provided at the bedside had increased (Fig. 8-3).

Patients expressed, through surveys and thank-you notes, that they received more direct care from staff who showed greater concern. Patient satisfaction on the Seton unit was generally as good or higher than the hospital average. Ratings were significantly higher on overall satisfaction with the experience, the morale and teamwork of the staff, overall quality of treatment, and the caring atmosphere. Some areas, such as dietary services or the amount of time physicians spent with patients, received higher ratings compared with the hospital average even though no changes were made.

Through a survey, physicians indicated they were "satisfied" or "very satisfied" with the care given on the Seton unit (Fig. 8-4). They also appreciated the level of service relative to scheduling, medical records, pharmacy, lab, and ECG (Fig. 8-5). A full 90% rated nursing care as "better" or "much better" on the Seton unit. Perhaps the best measure of physicians' satisfaction was their expressed desire to have their patients on that unit.

Through interviews and questionnaires, the staff also rated the unit very positively. The overwhelming staff comment was that they now had greater control over their patients and what transpired in the course of delivering

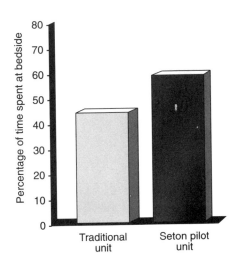

FIGURE 8-2 Percentage of time spent at bedside in traditional unit and Seton pilot unit.

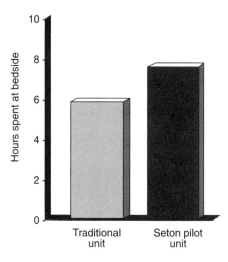

FIGURE 8-3 Hours spent at bedside in traditional unit and Seton pilot unit.

care. They also expressed satisfaction with the increased knowledge of their patients' needs and status and their expanded responsibilities, as well as the sense of belonging to a team. The RNs, particularly, noted satisfaction in having an opportunity to manage the patients' care and expressed enthusiasm regarding the physical changes to the unit. Convenient location of resources positively impacted their ability to provide care in the patients'

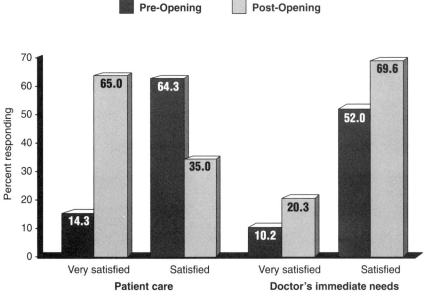

FIGURE 8-4 Physician survey responses—before and after Seton pilot unit opening showing increased satisfaction with patient care and doctor's immediate needs.

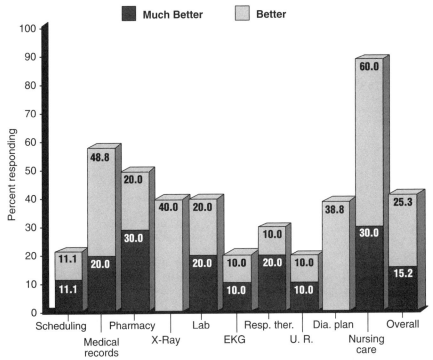

FIGURE 8-5   Physician survey responses evaluating level of service in Seton pilot unit compared with traditional unit.

rooms. LPNs were also satisfied that they could do more for their patients. Cross-trained technicians felt good about the new approach to care. They appreciated the job enrichment and the new challenges presented them. Processing of orders by the TCSs also was viewed positively. Staff could prioritize the orders and have meaningful interaction with the physician about the orders at the time they were written.

Ratings from the USAs and the URs were extremely high as well. Recognition of the positive impact of being part of a team and of their varying job responsibilities improved morale. They reported satisfaction in positively impacting the efforts of TCSs, physicians, and patients by their direct interactions. All staff saw improved timeliness in patient care as being a great bonus. The turnover for all three new job categories was very low.

The five quality indicators that were monitored (infection rates, medication error rates, intravenous administration error rate, patient falls, and skin breakdowns) had better outcomes on the Seton unit compared with a similar surgical unit. Each month, the Seton results demonstrated higher quality outcomes than those of comparable units. Staff members reported that the improvements in patient care management, problem-solving, critical thinking, and efficiency contributed to the higher quality. Interviews with staff revealed that the majority believed quality improved because caregivers had more control of the patients' care, could spend more time with their patients, and could more readily identify and treat potential complications. Patients also felt the quality of care was better on Seton. In one survey, 88% of the Seton patients rated their quality of care "better" or "much better" than expected, compared with the overall hospital average of 83%.

For the pilot unit, a financial analysis was not completed. However, the preliminary estimate indicated that there would be a reduction in the overall cost of delivering care. This was primarily seen through reductions in length of stay. There was a 17% decrease in the average length of stay for surgical patients cared for on Seton, compared with a traditional surgical unit. Also, total charges per case averaged approximately 13% less on Care2001 units compared with traditional units. These initial positive measures of success were influential in making the decision to move forward with this process throughout the hospital.

Patient, physician, and associate satisfaction, quality, and cost are continuously monitored and continue to reflect positive outcomes and trends. Patient satisfaction on the restructured units is consistently higher than on the traditional patient units. Associate satisfaction has been monitored on an annual basis through surveys. The results of these surveys reflect the enthusiasm the associates have for their work in the redesigned environment. They feel they have more control over their work and more involvement in making decisions for patients, as well as for the unit. Turnover rates and absenteeism are lower on these units than on traditional units.

Physician satisfaction has been mixed. All physicians continue to state that their patients receive better care on these units and that their patients are very satisfied with the care received on the unit. The consultants, internal medicine specialists, and family practice physicians have more difficulty practicing in this environment, because the environment is tailored to the specific patient needs of the unit. This requires flexibility on the physician's part to adapt to new surroundings and systems that may vary slightly from unit to unit. The lack of a central nursing station, charge nurse, and unit clerk, upon whom most of these physicians depended for communication and information, has been an issue that we continue to work through with the physicians. Another area of frustration for the physicians is telephone communication. Because there is not one central telephone number on each unit, there is an increase in waiting time on the phone by physicians as their calls are being processed.

As patient care units continue to thrive in the new environment, the quality indicators continue to demonstrate increasingly positive trends. The cost data has been encouraging for fiscal year 1992. The process used to evaluate the financial success was to compare similar patients of like physicians cared for on a Care2001 unit and on a traditional unit. Overall trends indicate a decreased length of stay and more efficient use of ancillary services for patients on redesigned units. The cost to the patient was less than for patients on traditional units, yet St. Vincent Hospital's contribution margin was higher, primarily because of a decrease in direct expenses per case.

By the end of fiscal year 1992, which was the financial period studied, the surgical Seton unit had been operational for 30 months, and the restructured medical unit had been operational for 14 months. It appears that the longer the unit is operational, the greater the positive outcomes (Table 8-1). With surgical patients, the decrease in gross revenue per case was 17%. This was because of the decreased number of days the patient stayed in the hospital as well as the decreased amount of services received as a result of the shorter stay. The direct expenses for these patients were down 26%, resulting in an increased contribution margin of 7%. For medical patients, the average decrease in gross revenue per case was 5%. The length of stay for these patients was higher (up 8%); however, direct expenses were down 9%. This accounted for an increase in contribution margin of 8.5%. The reasons for the trends are that

- Placing similar patients together allows the staff to become expert caregivers for that population and to tailor services to the specific needs of the patient;
- Because multiskilled (cross-trained) staff provide more patient services, they have a better knowledge of patients and their needs, allowing them to quickly identify and respond to complications and to better prioritize physician orders;
- The increased interaction among physicians and the other caregivers enhances their abilities to address patient needs; and
- With faster turnaround time for laboratory and other clinical results, the team rapidly assesses patient changes.

Involving the patients in the plan of care has also positively impacted the patients' perceptions of their illnesses and their recovery times. There has also been a decrease in positions in the ancillary departments as the work shifts to the patient care units. Departments such as housekeeping, phlebotomy, ECG, respiratory, and admitting are downsizing through attrition.

Overall reduction in management layers is another financial and organizational goal. To date, we have made minimal strides in this area.

ROADBLOCKS

There have been many roadblocks encountered along our journey. Resistance to change, both personal and professional, has challenged us at every point. Resistance is generally caused by inertia, fear of change, lack of knowledge, or inflexibility on the part of the individual. Professional territo-

TABLE 8-1   Impact on Operations—Comparison of Care2001 Unit Patients With Like Patients on a Traditional Unit

	CARE2001/6W	CARE2001/4E
Gross revenue	17% ↓	5% ↓
Deductions	38% ↓	10% ↓
Net revenue	11% ↓	3% ↓
Direct expenses	26% ↓	9% ↓
Contribution margin	7% ↑	8% ↑

rialism is something that cannot be overlooked when changing the scope of practice of a number of professional workers. Hospital policies and procedures regarding practice frequently become roadblocks to change, as do state licensure and certification laws. Poor communication can hinder any change process. There must be open, two-way communication, both vertically and horizontally in the organization. The opportunity for feedback from colleagues must be ongoing. Listening and responding to information in a timely manner becomes extremely important.

Financial constraints can also greatly reduce the success of this process. The cost of physical renovations and cross-training can be high. Overt and covert undermining and lack of support were experienced in various areas; this resulted in slowing the process and, in some cases, changing the method of achieving positive outcomes. Lack of physician involvement in the decision making process served as a roadblock. After the initial pilot project, the medical staff expressed the desire to be part of the decision-making process, as opposed to being informed of changes as they were made.

■EVOLVING ORGANIZATION

Many paradigm shifts are necessary to support the redesign process. Patient-focused care requires that the system conform to patient needs and not that patients conform to a segmented system. The end result is a lot of change that occurs relatively quickly. However, most people do seem to become accustomed to the notion that change is inevitable. Change is central to redesign because innovation is a key element to challenging old ways of operating. To the extent that an organization can actively involve its workers in change, the base for innovation broadens to include more resources.

At St. Vincent Hospital, the very way change is handled has undergone transformation. It is no longer a top-down organization, and decision making is routinely inclusive. The St. Vincent model of shared governance, called shared decision-making, has spread through the institution. This movement began in the nursing units and is now expanding to other departments.

Bringing more people into the decision-making process has proven the need to invest further in our associates. To that end, the corporation has instituted a philosophy of organizational development. Three associates have been given the title of organizational development consultant and have been assigned to head major task forces with the goal of implementing change in specified areas of the system. Task force members are educated in group dynamics and teamwork skills that cross traditional disciplinary barriers. These planning groups work to build consensus to solve fundamental issues related to patient care in their area. They are being trained to question basic premises and to work on change from a new framework. The system's core values are firmly undergirding this process.

Strategic planning has evolved at St. Vincent Hospital as well. First-line managers have become involved in strategic planning for the first time. This

Chapter 8   Third Generation Redesign: Lessons From the Field   105

process began with the entire management team retreating to rewrite the institutional vision statement. This process helped everyone center on the essential mission of the organization.

St. Vincent Hospital is reaching beyond its walls to jointly plan for the community's needs with another major health care institution. A core planning group, composed of members from both institutions, has begun to plan the roles the two institutions will play in the future. Core aims of this joint effort are to identify how future resources can be conserved and how the public can be assured access to affordable health care.

All of these massive changes associated with redesign could not take place without consideration of which organizational structures would support a more decentralized administrative model. As nursing units have developed in the patient-focused format, a layer of administrative reporting has been eliminated. In the past, a unit manager reported to a director of nursing who then reported to a vice president. Now, unit managers report directly to a vice president or to a service line manager.

Associates' roles have changed with redesign. Many nursing staff members have seen their jobs grow through cross-training into new areas and through the Coordinated Care program (St. Vincent Hospital's managed care model). To acknowledge the additional value of these services, the institution has established a compensation system to reward advanced skills and greater work flexibility. The performance appraisal system had to be restructured to reflect the real changes in work expectations under redesign. A task force has been working for more than a year to redesign the evaluation and performance compensation systems.

Another area that continues to evolve is the very nature of professional practice. Through active participation in shared decision-making, associates are creating the multidisciplinary professional practice model for the future. Unit-based councils take charge of areas that previously would have been management's purview. Quality improvement is unit-based.

Another major movement in the organization is the development of the Coordinated Care model. Coordinated Care is taking the nurses from a more technically-focused practice to a professional level of accountability for patient outcomes. The process of designing critical pathways for specific patient situations has brought the major disciplines together into a more collaborative relationship. Once nursing and medicine begin working together, instead of in parallel, a number of other benefits are achieved. The net effect is that individual nursing associates feel a greater sense of professional satisfaction in this new environment. A research study is under way to determine the payoff for patients in the Coordinated Care program. This study focuses on patient outcomes and satisfaction.

CONTINUING ISSUES

As with any fundamental change, a continuing focus is how to maintain current changes while allowing for further evolution of the model. People may, by nature, revert to previously comfortable ways of doing things. Management must constantly be alert to signs that negative breaks in the new system have begun. Here are two examples of such signs. The central laboratory set the requirement that if values for laboratory tests processed on the Care2001 units fell outside a normal range, the tests had to be repeated in the central lab. It was not until months later that it was discovered that ranges set for Care2001 unit labs were more stringent than the central lab's own repeat ranges. Another example was the discovery that the ECG department was running separate audits on errors in Care2001 unit ECGs. These reports were not sent through the regular hospital channels for quality improvement but were sent directly to cardiologists. These examples are typical of the resentment and insecurity that can develop in the redesign environment. Departments rally to protect their turf. The underlying issue is that such behavior undermines the redesign process and causes the very duplication that redesign is intended to resolve.

The task of staff development in the redesign process is endless. Not only must initial education take place in the areas of cross-training for specific clinical skills, new roles, team building, and change, but ongoing competencies must be assured.

Leadership training is another essential element central to successful redesign. As decision-making is moved lower in the organization, associates must be ready to assume a higher level of involvement in group problem-solving. A new attitude of full investment in the success of change is needed from each associate. Creative ways to provide an atmosphere in which people are willing to take the risks required for such involvement are critical. Management development is crucial to provide leaders who know how to foster trust and respect, handle conflict effectively, and get the most involvement from associates.

A patient-focused approach requires that staff skills be tailored to the needs of specific patient populations. Worker transferability becomes an issue as units become more specialized. The impact of specificity on staffing flexibility also becomes an important issue. These continuing issues provide a context for lessons learned through engaging in redesign.

▬LESSONS LEARNED

The first lesson learned through this process was the necessity of having a clear, shared vision. This vision must be communicated clearly from the top down, with enthusiasm and commitment. The specific ways to achieve the vision must be approached from the bottom up, with team involvement. The success of the pilot unit was probably the result of a top-down approach and a good dose of the "Hawthorne effect." As we moved through other units, it became apparent that change is not sustainable using a top-down approach. Feelings of ownership for the change process and the outcomes were directly attributable to the amount of involvement individuals had in the process.

Another lesson learned was the need for trust in the organization. This trust must be multidirectional: trust of the associates in the administration and trust by administration that the associates can make good decisions. If there is suspicion or uneasiness as to the depth of commitment to this process, trust wanes and the process suffers. Empowering associates, as well as the medical staff, to be involved in the change is extremely important. Working together as partners enhances the quality of the decisions that are being made as well as the timeliness of the change process. The partnership among administration, physicians, associates, and patients is paramount to success. Focusing on the patient allows professional and departmental turfs to be minimized.

Another lesson learned is to develop realistic time lines. Any change takes time. It is important not to rush the process but to move it steadily forward, overcoming obstacles along the way.

The evaluation process is another extremely important part of the overall success. How to measure the success of the change should be determined up front. This process must be specific to the change and consistent in approach. Response to the results of evaluations must occur in a timely fashion.

Communication is vital to the success of the change process. It is not possible to overcommunicate. Communication must be both horizontal and vertical. Listening is an active part of the communication process. All people, those who are directly involved in the change as well as those who may be on the periphery, should be linked in the communication process. Processing, managing the perceptions, providing opportunities for venting, face-to-face accessibility of higher authority, feedback sessions, videos, and newsletters are all ways to keep people informed of the process.

Customizing and tailoring the process to the individual unit is extremely important. This includes assessing the readiness of the associates and physicians for the change as well as carefully studying the patient population to be served. Supporting the units after they have undergone the initial change process is also integral to the long-term success and sustainability of the change.

Another lesson learned is the necessity for changing in response to evaluation results and supporting innovation after the initial conversion to patient-focused care. Individuals from previously converted units have a major impact in mentoring staff in the planning phase of the unit. Frequent praise and celebrations also are extremely important. The successes are many, but in this process of massive change, taking the time to celebrate and praise frequently gets overlooked. As the organization evolves, our vision for the future becomes even clearer.

▬ VISION

Systems thinking and embracing change in an innovative environment, one in which managers, associates, and physicians work together to create a patient-centered system, is the vision for the future. Decreased department definition and increased matrix organization, in which groups of partners from across the organization work together for a common outcome, will become more commonplace. This fosters increased commitment of the workers to the organization. There will be a decrease in the number of departments, an increase in multiskilled workers, and a significant change in management's role as the associates embrace their new roles. This will result in decreased layers of management in the organization. To support a partnership team system, there must be changes in the methods of compensation and evaluation. An enhanced career development model that supports clinical competency, role definitions, teamwork, and leadership must be developed. An automated medical record with better information systems supporting these changes is also something envisioned for the future.

This is an exciting journey that we embarked upon in 1988. Along this road we have been faced with numerous challenges, opportunities, and successes. There will be many additional opportunities awaiting us as we continue to strive to provide a better system for patient-focused care in the acute care environment. We are fortunate to be able to expend time, energy, and resources for such a worthwhile experience.

▬REFERENCES

Drucker, P. F. (1973). *Management.* New York: Harper & Row.
Strengthening Hospital Nursing Program, National Program Office. (1992). *Strengthening Hospital Nursing: A program to improve patient care.* St. Petersburg, FL: Robert Wood Johnson/Pew Charitable Trust..

Chapter 9

Differentiated Practice: The Evolution of a Professional Practice Model for Integrated Client Care Services

JOELLEN KOERNER   LINDA BUNKERS   S. JO GIBSON

RICHARD JONES   BECKY NELSON   KALEEN SANTEMA

As the health care world mirrors the chaos of profound changes occurring in today's world, nursing is called on to respond in new and relevant ways to the changing needs of the society it serves. Leading, shaping, and support- ing the change of a corporate nursing practice is a great opportunity as well as an awesome responsibility. To be clear and consistent in this effort re- quires that the model and the process be built on a sound theoretical foun- dation.

Chaos theory (Briggs & Peat, 1989) has shown that turbulence, irregular- ity, and unpredictability are everywhere and that they operate under laws of their own rather than randomly. The laws of chaos are found in many pat- terns that support life, patterns such as human heartbeat and human thought, clouds, the structure of galaxies, the creation of a poem, the spread of a forest fire, and the evolution of life itself. As order falls apart into chaos, a new order moving closer toward wholeness emerges. Thus, it is the work of leaders to support individual, group, and societal movement through chaos in a way that brings harmony and wholeness to the universe.

Within health care organizations and professions, the old paradigm viewed the system as a well-oiled machine. Cybernetic principles applied to the work and the worker. Much as in the functioning of a thermostat, man- agement would establish a set point for behaviors, actions, and outcomes. If individual, group, or organizational performance fell below or rose above the mark, corrective actions were mobilized to once again return to homeo- stasis. The model was appropriate at the beginning of the industrial revolu- tion but is woefully lacking in this rapidly changing postindustrial era. It allowed no room for critical thinking or integration of inevitable change, always maintaining conformity and one uniform standard of achievement and production.

A more functional model today is that of the learning organization, with the individual and group viewed as a whole brain. This systems view asserts that life is a dynamic web of interrelated events, with no one part being more fundamental than any other. According to physicist, chemist, and Nobel laureate Ilya Prigogine (Prigogine & Stengers, 1984), a living organism is a self-organizing system, which means that its order is not imposed by the environment but is established by the system itself. In other words, self-organizing systems exhibit a certain degree of autonomy. This does not mean that the system is isolated from the environment. The system interacts with it continually, but the interaction does not determine its organization; it is self-organizing. Prigogine demonstrated that living, self-organizing systems not only have the tendency to maintain themselves in a state of dynamic balance, but also can transcend themselves, reaching out creatively beyond their boundaries to generate new structures and new forms of organization. The organism may undergo the process of transformation and self-transcendence, involving stages of crisis and transition, and achieve an entirely new state of balance.

Gregory Bateson (1979) looked for patterns beneath patterns, and for processes beneath structure. His concept of mind is essential to self-organization. He defined mental process as the dynamics of self-organization, which means that the organizing activity of a living system is mental activity, and all of its interactions with its environment are mental in nature. Mind and self-organization are different aspects of the same phenomenon, the phenomenon of life: mind is the essence of being alive.

It was the firm belief of nursing leadership at Sioux Valley Hospital (SVH) that the profession was composed of intelligent individuals who, if properly supported, could create and design a care delivery system that would better organize their work. So the work of redesign began, with the structure, process, and outcomes held within the hands, hearts, and minds of the entire practice.

■ BASIC COMPONENTS OF A PROFESSIONAL PRACTICE MODEL

Extensive review of the literature, numerous conversations with nursing leaders around the country, multiple brainstorming sessions in various staff committees, and the expert guidance of nursing consultants and a nursing theorist led to the development of a professional practice model which embodied four key components: 1) differentiated nursing practice—a form of internal case management; 2) shared governance—a form of shared decision-making; 3) collaborative practice—a model for interdisciplinary planning and dialogue; and 4) case management—a care delivery system for clients beyond the walls of the hospital.

Differentiated Nursing Practice

Differentiated nursing practice is a philosophy that focuses on the structuring of roles and functions of nurses according to education, experience, and competence (National Commission on Nursing Implementation Project, 1989). It establishes that the domain of professional nursing is broad, with multiple roles and responsibilities of varying degree and complexity. It assumes that nurses with different types of educational preparation, expertise, and background bring different competencies to the workplace (Primm, 1987). It seeks to assure that the work of nursing is carried out by the most appropriate nurse in the most appropriate fashion. Comprehensive, cost-effective care is provided by the collective discipline of nursing through the integration of those services across the continuum of care into a synergistic whole.

The nursing practice at SVH established three distinct career roles for the staff: 1) associate nurse—whose responsibility was for the shift of service, with a strong focus on physiologic stabilization and comfort of the client; 2) primary nurse—whose responsibility extended from admission to discharge, with a strong focus on integration of medical and nursing orders, client education, and a well-prepared and timely discharge; and 3) clinical nurse specialist (CNS)—whose focus was for the illness episode across the lifespan, expanding beyond the walls of the institution into multiple health care arenas with a strong focus on case management and client advocacy. Specific job descriptions, evaluation tools, and salary scales were developed for each role. Entry into the primary nurse role was granted to staff through a choice and competency program, whereas the CNS position required a master's degree (Koerner, 1990; Koerner, 1991a; Koerner, 1992; Pitts-Wilhelm, Nicolai, & Koerner, 1991).

Shared Governance

Shared governance is a decision-making and management model whereby the staff manage their clinical practices at the unit level while coordinating corporate issues and standardizing practice issues at a house-wide level (Koerner, 1991b). Each unit has four councils (which include other disciplines as appropriate) that represent the four components of shared governance in relation to the clinical delivery of client care on the unit:

- The *practice council* establishes standards of care and manages issues that emerge in relation to maintaining those standards;
- The *education council* educates staff to maintain standards, coordinates unit-based cardiopulmonary resuscitation recertification, and manages the educational budget for the unit;
- The *management council* manages the activities of the unit, including self-scheduling, hiring and termination of staff, and management of capital equipment budgets, that ensure availability of resources to meet the established standards; and
- The *quality assurance/research council* evaluates and measures care to assure maintenance of standards of practice, performs research studies for the practice, and performs joint studies with physicians and other provider groups.

Four similar house-wide councils (which are unique to nursing) exist to integrate the work of the practice and coordinate nursing's work with the rest of the organization. Nurses joining SVH are credentialed into the practice and evaluated through a peer review process annually.

Collaborative Practice

Collaborative practice occurs between nursing and the medical community in various medical staff committees as well as ad hoc task forces that meet on specific issues. Various liaison committees such as nursing/pharmacy and nursing/laboratory meet monthly to examine issues of mutual concern and design futuristic strategies that enhance the work of all practitioners. As the organization is moving into client-focused care with multiskilled technicians introduced to the units of service, interdisciplinary teams are emerging to facilitate planning and implementation of care in broader fashion.

Case Management

Case management has been identified as a model of care delivery that serves the needs of the client across the continuum of care (Cohen & Cesta, 1993; Ethridge & Lamb, 1989). The concept and its development are used as the exemplar for the final two stages of model development at the unit level (see *Stages III & IV—Development and Implementation*).

▀THE PROCESS OF REDESIGN

The context surrounding change is a dynamic force that shapes and instructs the work of an organization responding to it. The work of redesign for the nursing practice at SVH began in the late 1980s during a severe national nursing shortage. Professional nursing in the state of South Dakota was challenged with the governor's decision to open six schools of licensed practical nursing as an answer to providing adequate nursing personnel for the state. A Statewide Project for Nursing and Nursing Education was launched to demonstrate that the old paradigm, "a nurse is a nurse," was inadequate for the complexity inherent in contemporary health care. The model of differentiated nursing practice was selected to demonstrate the unique characteristics and contributions of associate degree and baccalaureate nurses in a restructured health care setting. A steering committee was established for this statewide project, Dr. Peggy Primm was hired as the consultant to the project, and the work of redesign began (Koerner, Bunkers, Nelson, & Santema, 1989).

The design project at SVH went through four distinct phases to reach full implementation. The first two phases, *Assessment* and *Design*, were focused on macro-planning activities, while the later two phases, *Development* and *Implementation*, focused more on unit-specific micro-applications of the model.

Stage I—Assessment

During the initial phases of redesign, establishing a clear baseline regarding the total organization, the environment, and the work of professional nursing is essential. It identifies strengths and weaknesses in the current system, which creates a pathway for redesign.

The corporate organization was the first focus for assessment. Administrative interest in and support for a change in client care delivery was foundational to the success of such an undertaking. Corporate structures for communication and decision-making had to be strong to support a radical restructuring of the care delivery system for clients, because increasing client acuity coupled with a decreasing length of stay was taxing all care providers within the hospital. Cost and quality impact of a new care delivery model had to be considered and shared with executive management as the purpose and objectives of redesign were sold to the administration.

Simultaneously, the same issues were addressed within the department of client services as nursing administration examined the readiness of nursing for such a venture. Critical issues discussed first by the administrative team with nurse managers, and then with the full nursing practice, included questions such as the following:

1. What is our primary objective in client care delivery?
2. How are we currently meeting this objective?
3. What is our current definition of health and nursing?
4. What is contemporary nursing practice if a "nurse is not a nurse is not a nurse"?
5. Does our current philosophy support these beliefs?
6. Which are the elements of our care delivery system that work well, and which elements are problematic?
7. Which support structures (ie, documentation, quality assurance, staff development, management support, communication, and decision-making) work well and which are problematic?
8. What is the current status of client, physician, and staff satisfaction?
9. What are the current working relationships between nursing and other clinical and support service departments?
10. What is nursing's relationship to the community as the pattern of chronic illness and early discharge continues to evolve?

Baseline data was acquired through the use of various research tools, focus group discussions, and networking with other hospitals and health care agencies involved in the statewide project. Careful analysis of all the data revealed a corporate readiness to move forward with the project.

The role of nursing administration in such a venture is to create a compelling vision for change, to broker information to the various publics within the organization and beyond it, and to support the evolution of consensus among the various stakeholders by clarifying and unifying perceptions and expectations that eventually merge into a common vision (Koerner, 1989). Using data, information, and stories geared to each specific group's concerns and expertise is a taxing and exhilarating political opportunity for nursing leaders involved in work of this magnitude.

Stage II—Design of the Model

Establishing a prototype is exacting work which takes considerable time and energy, calling on one's greatest creativity. This is a very critical stage of the process, for the model that evolves sets the direction for the entire practice. The design must evolve from the lived experience of the staff if it is to be relevant and successful. An invitation was extended to the entire nursing practice, with a stipulation that a positive vote of 85% must occur for the unit's inclusion as a pilot project unit. This level of commitment is imperative if the project is to succeed.

The practice at SVH discovered that several elements are essential to the success of a project of this magnitude.

1. A *committee charter* is a document that defines the goals and objectives of the project, committee composition, length of time individuals are expected to devote to the project, responsibilities of committee members, and what the organization will contribute (ie, 2 paid hours of meeting time each month, with an expectation that committee members will contribute an equal amount of time in preparation for those meetings).
2. A *steering committee* is a group of individuals who give leadership to the entire project. It should include staff and management from each unit participating in the design of the model, support service personnel, and administrative representatives who can communicate on an ongoing basis between the corporate and practice sides of the issues, keeping each group informed of progress.
3. *Group norms* are an established list of process and decision-making issues that give form to the group's work, identifying the accountability of each member to the group and the project (ie, how many meetings can be missed, whether the meetings are to be open or closed, voting or consensus as the mode of decision-making, etc.).
4. *Assumptions* are a shared list of common understandings. The group must give a common definition to their work, identifying the assumptions that underlie it. It creates a shared set of beliefs that give guidance to the work and unify the vision for all.
5. *Unit-based committees* mirror the steering committee in composition and function. These groups generate ideas and outcomes which then are coordinated and integrated by the steering committee.

Design is a circular process. The ideas are generated and given to demonstration units for testing and evaluation. Feedback brought back to the steering committee is evaluated, modifications are made, and the process is repeated until mutually satisfying experiences are occurring on all units in the pilot project.

Communication is another key to success. Activities of the project must be communicated to the entire practice, especially to those not involved directly. Much fear, suspicion, and misrepresentation can be eliminated with clear and timely communication. A communication book was placed on each nursing unit, containing the materials and minutes of activities occurring on the pilot units, so that the entire practice had access to the same data. All meetings were open, and agendas were posted so that staff members could choose to visit a meeting if a particular agenda item held special interest for them. Periodic presentations by the pilot units were made for the entire practice as well. A similar level of dialogue was occurring simultaneously with executive management, to keep the corporate side informed. A key rule in work design is "No surprises!"

After the prototype has been developed and positive outcomes shown, it is ready for micro-level application at the unit level. The developmental phase finds each unit tailoring the model to fit its unique situation. Implementation then occurs as each unit is ready to adapt its world to the practice-wide prototype.

Stages III and IV—Development and Implementation

After a model prototype has been developed, it is moved to the micro-level, the unit of service. Based on the theoretical framework of a learning organization with the capacity for self-organization, local autonomy and discretion was given each unit based on several integrating factors. Standards of practice and standards of care were used as the unifying and integrating focus for professional nursing practice throughout the organization. Guiding principles were established for each component of the professional practice model that had to be maintained, but their application at the unit level could be designed to address and honor the uniqueness of that unit. For example, the four components of shared governance had to be present on each unit. Some of the smaller units combined practice and education, along with management and quality assurance, creating two rather than four councils. Thus, all components of shared governance were present and functioning on each unit irrespective of the number of councils.

Development and implementation is a circular, ongoing process. Housewide councils communicate and coordinate the experimentation that occurs at the local unit level; the local unit is where true redesign occurs. Each project is defined so a shared belief is present throughout the practice. Clearly defined and measurable goals are established to guide and direct the process at the unit level and unify a practice-wide outcome. Finally, the work is always labeled "work in progress," as each innovation leads to another new discovery. A slogan that permeates the practice is, "Change is the norm, stability an illusion." Each piece of work is challenged with an intent to improve; thus, the creative process is dynamic and never ending.

INTEGRATED CLINICAL PATHWAYS. The development of case management began with the design of pathways. An integrated clinical pathway (ICP) is defined as an interdisciplinary plan of care used in managing the client's care through an acute episode of illness. It is a tool used to case-manage client populations by medical diagnosis or surgical procedure in the acute care setting. ICPs map or outline care on a time line and are specific to a physician or physician group. Various time lines are used, including

- Day-by-day—for surgical and less complex medical diagnoses in which care is routine and predictable;
- Steps or stages—for stages of labor in vaginal deliveries and for more complex medical diagnoses such as premature neonate (stage by gestational age) and cardiovascular accident (crisis/diagnostic, stabilization, rehabilitation, and preparation for discharge);
- Presenting signs and symptoms—for emergency room clients and clients coming from rural facilities; and
- Across other settings—includes physician's office visits before admission and home health or long-term care follow-up after discharge.

SVH established four goals that served as the impetus for the development and implementation of ICPs: 1) control length of stay and cost without jeopardizing quality of client care; 2) promote interdisciplinary collaboration; 3) streamline the documentation system; and 4) encourage active client/family participation in the plan of care.

The planning process for ICP began in January 1992 with the establishment of a nursing task force with two representatives (one primary and one associate nurse) from each unit. Others, including a CNS, quality review manager, nurse researcher, and computer expert, served as consultants to the task force. A project director coordinated the implementation and evaluation phases of the program. To begin, each unit targeted its top two diagnoses by volume or loss. The unit-based practice councils were actively involved in developing their respective units' pathways. The task force communicated a monthly update to the house-wide practice council.

Obtaining physician support is a prerequisite to achieving the identified goals. Various strategies on how to approach physicians are outlined in Display 9-1. Physicians also need to have their fears allayed that ICPs could serve as affirmative defense legally. On the east coast, where litigation is prevalent, physicians who have protocols/pathways are actually winning legal battles. As managed care and cost constraints become more prevalent, physicians will be required to have their treatment plans outlined. Over the course of a year, SVH involved 125 physicians in the development and implementation of the pathways.

The vision of establishing an ICP as the comprehensive plan of care required an intensive review of the entire documentation system. The goals for documentation that resulted were as follows.

DISPLAY 9-1   *How to Approach Physicians with Clinical Pathways*

Approach influential physicians who are interested in high-quality, cost-effective care.

Emphasize that pathways are guidelines, *not* standing orders.

Individualize for each physician or physician group to reflect personal practice patterns and avoid the charge of "cookbook medicine."

Delineate how pathways enhance the quality of care:

1. Clearly defines the physician's expectations.
2. Valuable orientation tool for nurses, students, residents, physicians covering for one another, other disciplines, and patients/families.
3. Details for the patient/family education required.
4. Sequences interventions predictably and in a timely manner to achieve an appropriate length of stay with expected patient outcomes.
5. Improves continuity and enhances communication for patients who transfer across nursing units.

Emphasize that tracking data through variance analyses facilitates changes of identified inefficiencies in hospital systems.

1. Streamline documentation from a nursing as well as an interdisciplinary perspective, eliminating all unnecessary and duplicate forms.
2. Establish interdisciplinary progress notes.
3. Ensure accessibility of interdisciplinary documentation forms.
4. Ensure readily retrievable data for
   a. Communication between health care teams.
   b. Legal documentation.
   c. Reimbursement purposes.
   d. Trending for continuous quality improvement (CQI).
5. Develop standards of care and standard operating procedures to support the documentation system.

Integrating charting by exception and focus charting are being demonstrated as viable options. Since nursing diagnoses, interventions, teaching, and client outcomes are part of the clinical pathway, the pathway becomes the standard of care. Focus notes are written only if the client is unable to achieve an identified outcome on the pathway or if there is a critical change in the client's assessment.

The Kardex, which communicates valuable information including individualized client care needs but is not part of the permanent record, has been largely eliminated. The clinical pathway now incorporates the valuable Kardex information that used to be discarded at discharge.

The acuity system was also merged with the clinical pathways. Clients who are on pathways and following the course as planned are easily tabulated into the computerized acuity system.

Active participation in the plan of care by the client and family is readily achieved by reviewing the information on the clinical pathway and individualizing special needs. The pathway clearly defines the expectations and provides the mental preparation necessary for clients to achieve a timely discharge and recovery. Since the clinical pathway contains abbreviations and acronyms in medical terminology, it is necessary for a nurse to explain most of the entries. For this reason, a version of the pathways titled "Client Pathway to Recovery" has been developed for clients.

With shortening lengths of stay and little time to outline a detailed plan of care for each client, clinical pathways offer a preplanned format so the care can be individualized and tailored to address unique client needs. In terms of role delineation, the associate nurse can deliver the care and/or modify it on a shift-to-shift basis. It is the primary nurse's responsibility to screen clients who have complex discharge, planning, education, and psychosocial needs and to manage the care from admission to discharge on the unit. Primary nurses also track the exceptions to the clinical pathways, which are variances that are analyzed to resolve system issues and barriers to recovery.

The outcomes of clinical pathways, in terms of decreasing length of stay and hospitalization charges, can be found on Figure 9-1. There has been no increase in complications or readmissions. An improvement in targeted quality indicators relative to each specific pathway has been noted. Other favorable outcomes have included client and family satisfaction from the

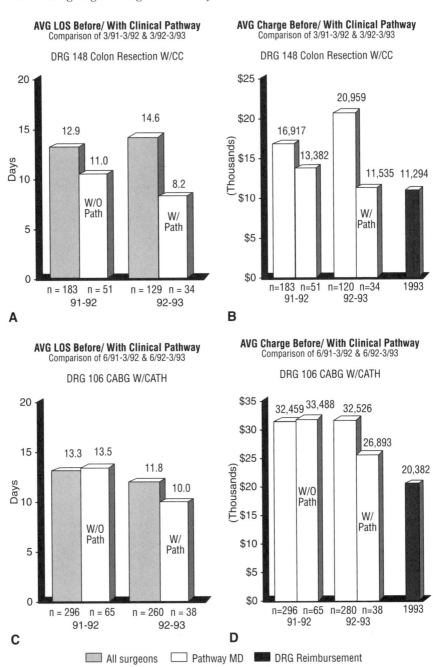

FIGURE 9-1   Clinical pathway outcomes on length of stay and hospital changes.

perspective of being actively involved in their care and knowing the expectations. Physician satisfaction has been enhanced, because clinical pathways maximize time efficiency by facilitating client rounds and necessary orders for the day. Nurse satisfaction has increased because the ICPs help nurses decrease charting time, enhance comfort in caring for unfamiliar client populations, and anticipate necessary orders.

The supportive clinical information system provided by ICPs is an essential component of an integrated care delivery system. Bringing clinical sophistication to the scene without the physician or CNS always having to be present is a most rewarding benefit.

Future plans for ICPs include continuing the pathway into the home care setting by providing the clinical expertise of an acute care primary nurse for follow-up (Maturen, 1993). This will provide the physician with the confidence necessary to discharge clients at an earlier time with the appropriate follow-up detailed in a clinical pathway format that includes nursing interventions, teaching, and client outcomes. Further work needs to be done with the interdisciplinary teams in relation to documenting on the pathway and on the progress notes. Documenting on one form would provide less duplication of documentation and effort. A valid point to be negotiated is which discipline will establish ownership of the tasks. This is being addressed as two client-focused care units evolve, being unveiled in September 1993. Computerization of pathways, integration of automated variance tracking, the CQI process, and computerized documentation also need to be pursued. In order to reduce hospital costs and respect the diagnosis-related groups, research must be conducted with ICPs to identify the variables that influence cost in a particular client population (Nugent, 1992).

CLINICAL NURSE SPECIALIST AS CASE MANAGER.   Case management was the most recent component of the model to be developed. Recognizing that certain clients have comprehensive health care needs beyond acute, episodic hospital care, the SVH Center for Case Management was created to address the needs of these select clients. This unique program was established in response to concern about chronic medical conditions causing multiple readmissions, the decrease in reimbursement, shorter hospital stays, and the need to coordinate services in the hospital with other programs across the health care continuum.

The nursing practice at SVH was fortunate to have the examples of pioneers in the field, including the Tucson Carondelet St. Mary's model and the model of St. Joseph's in Wichita (Rogers, Riordan, & Swindle, 1991; Ethridge & Lamb, 1989). Designing case management to meet the needs of our unique institution and clients proved to be the challenge.

The first hurdle to overcome was that of barriers and which division would establish ownership for case management. Since the health care system is too complex for any one individual to comprehend, it was crucial that all disciplines and departments understand their respective valuable and distinctive contributions to make case management a success. A corporate diagram was designed to calm this turf issue debate (Fig. 9-2). The design

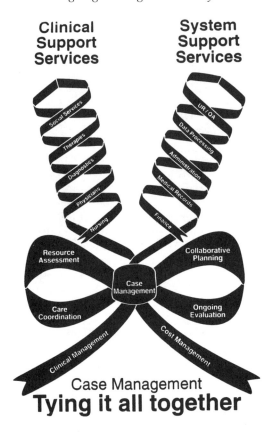

Clinical Support Services

System Support Services

Case Management
Tying it all together

FIGURE 9-2 Case management corporate diagram.

team recognized that pulling together all of the resources was the only way to accurately portray the financial and clinical picture fully.

In the early developmental stages, it became evident that dialogue and networking had to occur within the organization as well as in the community outside the main campus. A house-wide case management task force, led by the vice president for client services, was established to address the need for a seamless, integrated system across all health care settings. Areas in which collaboration and possibly partnering were needed included home health, rehabilitation, long-term care, ambulatory care, rural health, and prevention and wellness.

The program began as a demonstration project under the guidance of Dr. Margaret Murphy, Research Consultant, and Connie Burgess, Catastrophic Illness and Reimbursement Consultant. The CNSs were designated as case managers for the demonstration project, linking with clients who met at least two of the following criteria:

- Chronic illness or high-risk pregnancy;
- History of frequent admissions or utilization of emergency services;
- Fixed financial resources, causing financial risk for the hospital;

- Inadequate caregiver support, or lives alone;
- Cognitive or developmental deficit; and
- Decreasing coping capacity or emotional support needs.

These criteria were used for all clients across the life span.

The role of the CNS as case manager was to assess, monitor, and mutually plan and coordinate health care services to respond to the individual needs of these complex clients and families. Since high-quality, cost-effective, coordinated, and continuous health care was the ultimate goal, it was imperative that interdisciplinary and interagency collaboration transpire. This eliminated duplication of time, services, and dollars.

A conceptual framework was designed to depict client flow and augment referrals from primary nurses (Fig. 9-3). Ideally, clients are identified during a hospital stay or emergency visit so that the CNS can be introduced and have direct face-to-face contact during the crisis period. After clients have returned to the comfort and privacy of their own home environment and the crisis of acute hospitalization is over, it is difficult for them to under-

**Sioux Valley Hospital Center for Case Management
Conceptual Framework**

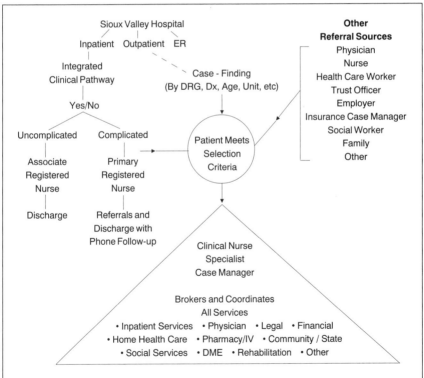

FIGURE 9-3 Conceptual framework for case management.

stand the benefits of case management. The critical time period to introduce case management and begin establishing a rapport with the client and family is toward the end of an acute care stay or shortly after discharge. Nurse case management referrals were developed to facilitate timely referrals while the clients were still hospitalized. Other referral sources include physicians, social workers, other nurses and health care workers, trust officers, employees, insurance case managers, and families.

Building on the existing shared governance model, and to expedite the structure and process for case management at SVH, the 16 CNSs evolved as a group practice with the four councils. Executive management consisted of the chairs from each council, a nursing administrator, the director for home health and hospice, and the vice president of client services. The director of the Center for Case Management, a CNS, coordinated all case management efforts with the chair of the CNS management council.

A total of 28 clients were included in the demonstration study. Demographic data is summarized in Table 9-1. Coordination of the entire spectrum of these case-managed clients proved beneficial. Using the 28 clients as their own control, a considerable impact was made in decreasing length of stay by 33% and charges by 62%. The overall net financial impact was $477,445, a 75% decrease in loss for the managed clients (Table 9-2). The constant presence of a CNS provided the clinical expertise and relationship with clients and families to broker and coordinate services in all health care settings. Providing this vital link optimized quality care, decreased fragmentation, and promoted the appropriate use of health care dollars for these clients and families with complex needs.

The CNS focus of case management with these clients was wellness, health restoration, and health maintenance, emphasizing the importance of empowering clients to maximize self-care capabilities or achieve a dignified death. Enhanced client perception and satisfaction with care has evolved for several reasons:

- Having a consistent person (the CNS) coordinate care;
- Having a nurse and an advocate to contact at any time;
- Actively participating in care; and
- Being informed and knowledgeable about the disease process, progression, and options for care.

Other clinical outcomes being studied with case-managed clients include functional abilities through activities of daily living (ADL) and instrumental activities of daily living (IADL) scores. Caregiver strain scores, which identify changes in perception of stress and coping ability, are also being addressed.

Comments made by physicians of case-managed clients have been favorable. Physicians have realized greater time efficiency, since these clients essentially have a plan in place if readmitted. Phone calls, especially during the night from desperate family members, and inappropriate phone calls to physicians have diminished. This has been facilitated by routine, more frequent contacts during the day, initiated by either the CNS or the client or family.

TABLE 9-1   Demographic Data for Case-Managed Patients (Study = 28 Patients)

Patient Age	
Range	18 mos–82 yrs
Age 0–18	14%
Age 19–61	29%
Age 62+	57%
Gender	
Male	36%
Female	64%
Ethnicity	
White	96%
Native American	4%
Other	0%
Payor	
Medicaid	29%
SVH Blue Cross/Blue Shield	4%
Private insurance	7%
Medicare	60%
Self	0%
Selection Criteria for Case Management	
Fixed financial reimbursement	90%
Chronic illness	82%
Frequent admissions/ER visits	68%
Lives alone/Inadequate support	46%
Emotional/Coping deficit	46%
Cognitive/Developmental deficit	25%
Referral Source	
CNS case manager find	42%
Primary nurse	39%
Physician	14%
Other	4%

From a nursing perspective in general, and a CNS perspective specifically, case management offers the privilege to participate in clients' lives in an autonomous way that nurses have been taught and anticipated but never actualized in their practice. Case management provides an opportunity to practice all of the role components of a CNS as defined by the American Nurses Association: expert clinician, educator, consultant, researcher, and administrative/change agent. This is a timely program to integrate as nurses are being challenged to identify their unique role and contribution to clients in a restructured health care system.

The future of case management at SVH requires integration of all corporate components of the concept. Batey (1983) has observed that social integration requires three components: unifying vision, shared decision-making, and local autonomy. A coordinating committee has been established to provide these elements to the organizational efforts toward case management. The working definition of case management adopted by the

TABLE 9-2 CNS Case Management Fiscal Summary 4½ Month Study Period (Study = 28 Patients)

PARAMETER	BEFORE CNS CASE MGMT*	WITH CNS CASE MGMT	PERCENT OF VARIANCE TOTAL
Total Admissions			
Inpatient	46	30	35
Outpatient	17	10	41
Emergency room	9	27†	300†
Inpatient Days			
Total days	346	229	34
Intensive care days	67	27	60
Mean LOS per patient	12.3	8.2	33
Financial			
Total charges	$815,895	$311,384	62
Mean charges per patient	$29,139	$11,121	62
Range of charges	$926–$290,253	$0–$73,049	
Total reimbursement	$178,383	$161,509	10
Percent of charge reimbursed	22	52	30
Mean CNS hours/Pt/Mo	0	2.6 hrs	
Range of CNS hours	0	1–42 hrs	
Estimated CNS cost	0	$10,192	
Cost per patient	0	$364	
Net Financial Impact	$–637,512	$–160,067	75

*Previous 12 months divided by 2.6
†41% of reported ER admissions were from one patient.

group is, "an integrated health management network in which care is coordinated over the continuum for individuals or groups." If a fluid, seamless environment with continuous flow is to evolve, the three components of case management that require integration are acute care, outclient/community care, and prevention/health maintenance (Fig. 9-4). Group work is now focused on developing a corporate as well as individual health management packages, along with processes that assure timely and efficient delivery of them.

Other future work includes further studies with case management clients (Lamb, 1992) and a focus on outcomes. Additionally, the CQI process will be incorporated and a fee structure established. Marketing the role of case management to the public will be carried out, along with an aggressive political action plan to assure proper legislative and regulatory support for advanced practice nursing within the state.

Case management, implemented internally through ICPs and differentiated practice roles and externally through the CNS, offers a methodology to address the majority of clients' health care needs (Fig. 9-5). Boundaries may appear blurry, but overlap is necessary at all levels of differentiated practice to avoid fragmentation and prevent clients' slipping through the cracks.

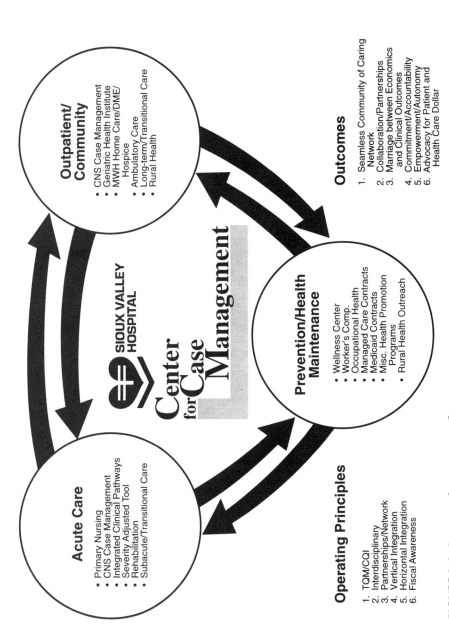

Outpatient/Community
- CNS Case Management
- Geriatric Health Institute
- MWH Home Care/DME/Hospice
- Ambulatory Care
- Long-term/Transitional Care
- Rural Health

SIOUX VALLEY HOSPITAL

Center for Case Management

Acute Care
- Primary Nursing
- CNS Case Management
- Integrated Clinical Pathways
- Severity Adjusted Tool
- Rehabilitation
- Subacute/Transitional Care

Prevention/Health Maintenance
- Wellness Center
- Worker's Comp.
- Occupational Health
- Managed Care Contracts
- Medicaid Contracts
- Misc. Health Promotion Programs
- Rural Health Outreach

Operating Principles
1. TQM/CQI
2. Interdisciplinary
3. Partnerships/Network
4. Vertical Integration
5. Horizontal Integration
6. Fiscal Awareness

Outcomes
1. Seamless Community of Caring Network
2. Collaboration/Partnerships
3. Marriage between Economics and Clinical Outcomes
4. Commitment/Accountability
5. Empowerment/Autonomy
6. Advocacy for Patient and Health Care Dollar

FIGURE 9-4 Integrated components for case management.

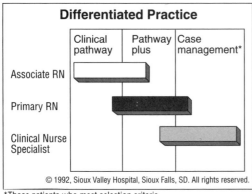

*Those patients who meet selection criteria.

FIGURE 9-5 Levels of differentiated practice.

■ SUMMARY

The work of design is a complicated process that releases much energy and creativity as well as some fear and anxiety within all participants. It is imperative for the organization to demonstrate a readiness for the work, and to supply the participants with resources and materials to use in the design of a new reality. The organization must support the innovation and testing through inevitable multiple false starts in its journey toward creating a nourishing environment that provides timely and accurate communication and in turn fosters trust. Failures must be viewed as an essential step in discovery by celebrating the individuals who take the risks of a pioneer.

Management at the corporate and unit levels must be kept one step ahead of the staff so that true and supportive leadership can be provided toward a common vision for the entire practice. And finally, whatever amount of time is required to achieve the outcomes desired must be given. Unit-based cultures require different time lines and varying approaches to a common goal, each valid and sustaining for that particular unit. By celebrating our diversity and honoring our common work, nursing can create care delivery models appropriate for a restructured health care system for the 21st century. In fact, we are the only group that can.

■ REFERENCES

Bateson, G. (1979). *Mind and nature.* New York: Ballentine.

Batey, M. (1983). Structural consideration for the social integration of nursing. In K. E. Barnard (Ed.), *Structure to outcome: Making it work* (pp. 1–11). Kansas City, MO: American Academy of Nursing.

Briggs, J. & Peat, F. D. (1989). *Turbulent mirror: An illustrated guide to chaos theory and the science of wholeness.* New York: Harper & Row.

Cohen, E. L. & Cesta, T. G. (1993). *Nursing case management: From concept to evaluation.* St Louis, MO: Mosby.

Ethridge, P. & Lamb, G. (1989). Professional nursing case management improves quality, access and costs. *Nursing Management, 20*(3), 30–35.

Koerner, J. (1989). Implications of differentiated practice models for nurse executives. *Aspen's Advisor for Nurse Executives, 4*(12) pp. 1, 6–8.

Koerner, J., Bunkers, L., Nelson, B., & Santema, K. (1989). Implementing differentiated practice: The Sioux Valley Hospital experience. *Journal of Nursing Administration, 19* (2), 13–22.

Koerner, J. (1990). The relevance of differentiated practice in today's environment. In C. Boston (Ed.), *Current issues and perspectives on differentiated practice.* Chicago, IL: American Organization of Nurse Executives. (AHA Catalog No. 154830).

Koerner, J. (1991a). Building on shared governance: The Sioux Valley Hospital experience. In I. Goertzen (Ed.), *Differentiating nursing practice: Into the 21st century.* Kansas City, MO: American Academy of Nursing.

Koerner, J. (1991b). Integrating differentiated practice into shared governance. In T. P. O'Grady (Ed.), *Implementing shared governance.* Hanover, MD: Mosby Year Book.

Koerner, J. (1992). Differentiated practice: The evolution of professional nursing. *Journal of Professional Nursing, 8*(6), 335–341.

Lamb, G. S. (1992). Conceptual and methodological issues in nurse case management research. *Advances in Nursing Science, 15*(2), 16–24.

Maturen, V. (1993). New critical pathways expand case management to the home. *Hospital Case Management, 1*(5), 96–99.

National Commission on Nursing Implementation Project. (1989). *Nursing practice patterns: Differentiating practice.* Milwaukee, WI; Author.

Nugent, K. E. (1992). The clinical nurse specialist as case manager in a collaborative practice model: Bridging the gap between quality and cost of care. *Clinical Nurse Specialist, 6*(2), 106–111.

Pitts-Wilhelm, P., Nicolai, C., & Koerner, J. (1991). Differentiating nursing practice to improve service outcomes. *Nursing Management, 22*(12), 22–26.

Prigogine, I. & Stengers, I. (1984). *Order out of chaos: Man's new dialogue with nature.* New York: Bantam.

Primm, P. (1987). Differentiating practice for ADN and BSN prepared nurses. *Journal of Professional Nursing, 3*(4), 218–225.

Rogers, M., Riordan, J., & Swindle, D. (1991). Community-based nursing case management pays off. *Nursing Management, 22*(3), 30–34.

Chapter 10

Collaborative Management: Nursing Administration Component in an Integrated Delivery System

RHONDA ANDERSON   CHERYL B. STETLER

The Strengthening Hospital Nursing program, as described in Chapter 3, "is about collaboration and commitment...about finding new ways—the best ways—of getting the work done" (Strengthening Hospital Nursing, 1992, p. 1). Hartford Hospital was one of the recipients of grants for this program from The Robert Wood Johnson Foundation and The Pew Charitable Trusts (RWJ/Pew grants). Collaboration and organization-wide commitment are two key elements in its restructuring program. Patient-centered redesign (PCR), as the grant came to be called, focused from its inception on the *overall* delivery system; nursing was neither the subject nor the primary focus. This deliberate approach was intended to convey the message that *all* departments and disciplines were to be involved because all played a role in improving patient care. It recognized the fact that a hospital is an integrated network of people and systems. Neither nursing nor any other single department or profession can alone create the type of change envisioned for Hartford Hospital, that is, "creation of an innovative, patient-centered, hospital-wide delivery system that continuously improves quality and utilizes resources cost-effectively" (Patient-Centered Redesign, Internal Publication, Hartford Hospital, 1990).

Despite this institutional, collaborative approach to implementation of the Strengthening Hospital Nursing grant, changes within the nursing department were expected to be significant. At the half-way point of this five-year project, this expectation is becoming reality. This chapter describes expected and unexpected grant-generated changes specifically related to nursing administration, with particular emphasis on the impact of a collaborative management structure. It explores factors, such as patient-centeredness and organizational commitment, required to move such a traditional system, and uses the conceptual framework of "re-energizing a mature organization" (Beatty & Ulrich, 1991) to further demonstrate strategies that facilitate achievement of an integrated delivery system.

 Flarey, D: REDESIGNING NURSING CARE DELIVERY: Transforming Our Future

▬ ENVIRONMENT AND CULTURE OF HARTFORD HOSPITAL

Hartford Hospital is a 139-year-old urban medical teaching center with 850 beds; 752 physicians; 6,000 employees; 39,500 patient discharges and 200,000 emergency and outpatient visits per year. It has a research program and an active facilities development program. Hartford can be considered a mature organization that, according to Beatty and Ulrich (1991), "has based its success on security and stability." In the unstable, challenging environment of the 1990s and beyond, such an organization must "respond to changes in a manner that will revitalize its structure and its competitive edge" (Beatty & Ulrich, 1991, p. 16).

Before the grant, this mature organization was characterized as a typical, "paternalistic" hospital driven by a medical model. Its culture, based on an internal survey, was seen as highly centralized, traditional, and staff-centered, with unilateral decision-making, more competition than collaboration, and departments and services that functioned in isolation rather than as parts of an integrated system.

The department of nursing, an inherent part of the overall organization, could basically be characterized in the same manner. This department was also mature, stable, and successful. It was highly centralized, and functioned like other vertical systems, in a fair degree of isolation. Collaboration was certainly valued, and efforts had been made to formally implement a collaborative practice model (Koerner & Armstrong, 1983). Administratively, the chief executive officer (CEO) and president had also taken steps to make the vice president of nursing an integral member of the executive team (eg, moved her office to the administrative suite and appointed her to the corporate planning steering committee). Managerial relations between nurse managers and their medical counterparts, however, were more cooperative than truly collaborative. The essential ingredient of collegiality, defined as "readiness to be mutually helpful as well as readiness to communicate constructively in order to accomplish the goals of the group or organization" (Reeder, 1983, p. 502), was not well established. Relations between nurse managers and other traditional clinical and nonclinical departments were variable. Some were cooperative, but others were characterized by ongoing conflict. The overall state of affairs was best described by two barriers to the delivery of care identified in the Hospital's initial RWJ/Pew grant application: 1) hospital-wide systems which were not designed to support the optimal delivery of patient-centered, cost-effective care; and 2) poor delineation of authority, accountability, coordination, and activity among health care providers.

▬ PATIENT-CENTERED REDESIGN PROGRAM

"A fundamental change in the U.S. hospital—from a discipline-driven, departmentalized institution to a patient-driven, unified one" (Strengthening Hospital Nursing, 1992)—this is the purpose of the Strengthening Hospital Nursing grant and of Hartford Hospital's vision-related project. To implement this vision, objectives were set to redesign collaborative practice, redesign information systems, and redesign organizational systems. The latter objective is the focus of this chapter and included redesign at the tactical (nursing unit), operational (service or department), and strategic (hospital-wide) levels. Multiple innovations related to practice, management, systems, and roles were implemented as part of each level of redesign; but a central, integrating innovation was the creation of *horizontal, collaborative management*.

The initial structure that set collaborative management into action was termed a *triad*. Triads are a type of collaborative management team (CMT). This organizational innovation established a formal relationship whereby targeted individuals (ie, the director of nursing, clinical chief, and administrative vice president for a specific service) were given collective responsibility for delivery of patient-centered, cost-effective care to a common population of patients. It recognized the inherent interconnectedness of these individuals, their departments and services in meeting the needs of patients across a continuum of care and within the overall system of care delivery.

By early 1992, six triads had been formed as part of the PCR program in the following clinical services: obstetrics/gynecology, medicine/cardiology, pediatrics, general surgery, psychiatry, and emergency medical services/trauma. Two so-called "subtriads" had also been formed, one in the labor and delivery suite with the head nurse, the assistant head nurse, an obstetrician, and an anesthesiologist, and another in the emergency center with the medical director, administrative director (a nurse), and head nurse. Over time, a supertriad evolved and included the CEO/president, the vice president for medical affairs (a physician), and the vice president for patient operations. The last, an administrative clinician role, was newly formed by the CEO/president to modify the hospital's organizational structure consistent with the PCR program and was filled by a nurse, the primary author of this chapter. This top executive CMT provides leadership, general direction, and oversight for the organization's ongoing programs and services.

Another central, integrating strategy in the PCR program was a set of core concepts: 1) patient-centeredness, 2) collaboration, 3) participation, and 4) outcomes. Display 10-1 provides definitions of these concepts, widely disseminated within Hartford Hospital, that are used to guide the behavior of triads and others throughout the organization.

Implementation and Overall Impact of Triads
Each of the six triads received an orientation to the core concepts of PCR as well as expectations for collaborative management. Each was expected to establish a set of service goals that included PCR innovations, such as implementation of health care teams, clinical critical paths, multiskilled employees, and targeted system changes. Goals were to be approved by the supertriad, which provided a visible form of organizational commitment and involvement. This executive CMT would also evaluate the triads' collective performance on an annual basis. Individually, triad members would continue to report and be accountable along traditional lines. For example, all of the nursing directors would report to the vice president of patient operations for the quality of nursing care in their individual division.

The exact manner in which triads began to implement collaborative

---

DISPLAY 10-1   Core Concepts of Patient-Centered Redesign as Described in Internal Communications

1. *Patient-Centeredness:* We have a hospital because patients need care. Patients are our most important customers. This is true to *everyone* in the Hospital, whether on a patient unit, in a clinical department, or in areas such as finance or engineering that affect caregivers and/or affect patients' overall experience at Hartford Hospital. In essence, everything done at Hartford Hospital is a patient-related event.
2. *Collaboration:* In order to meet the needs of our patients, we must first work together as a team, meeting each others' needs. Collaboration is essential, because neither delivery of care nor flow of goods, services, money, or patients through our system can be accomplished by isolated individuals or departments.
3. *Participation:* Given that patient care is the business of everyone in the Hospital, everyone is responsible for helping to create patient-centered redesign. This means keeping yourself informed of related activities, being open to change, and relentlessly wanting to continuously improve everything we do for whomever we do it.
4. *Outcomes:* In order to continuously improve quality and ensure the efficient and effective use of resources throughout Hartford Hospital, we must "manage by fact." Expected results must be clearly identified, data collected, progress measured, and the next steps toward continuous improvement taken. This approach applies to clinical practice, management of our delivery system, management of all aspects of daily operations, and personnel management.

---

management varied, in part because of the individuals involved and the nature of the clinical services. Some established service rounds, in which triad members went to their patient units to obtain information from staff on delivery needs; others did not. All, however, established a new meeting structure in which the three individuals routinely worked on their goals and clinical service business. Because the focus of this chapter is nursing administration, a more in-depth background is not provided (Stetler & Charns, in press).

In the fall of 1992, in-depth interviews were conducted with all triad members and other key stakeholders. One theme that emerged was a feeling that this collaborative focus was of value and qualitatively different from previous relationships. A written 1992 survey of 108 representative stakeholders, including 11 of 14 triad members, indicated that triads were beginning to have a discernible, positive impact on how departments and services approached their work. (Data were usually obtained during routine meetings, and lack of 100% response from triad members was not seen as significant.) Specifically:

The mean *level of triad impact* as perceived by the total sample was 3.69 on a 7-point Likert scale. At the time of the survey, a number of department heads were not yet formally integrated into PCR; as this structure has evolved, the figure would now be greater.

The level of impact as perceived by triad members themselves was, as expected, higher, at a mean of 4.55.

The mean *characteristic of the triads' impact* as perceived by the total group was 4.38 indicating their impact was positive on the 7-point negative-positive Likert scale.

The characteristic of this impact perceived by triad members themselves was also positive, at a mean of 4.40.

For triads, the increased time and workload initially required of each member to conduct collaborative business, as well as the slow movement of decentralization of authority to triads, likely kept the latter score from being higher.

Overall, there was a statistically significant change in perceptions of the organization's culture, with a shift to characteristics defined as consistent with the PCR program. For example, the Hospital was now seen as more patient- than staff-centered and more internally collaborative than competitive.

Interview comments were consistent with this quantitative data, as indicated by the following statements:

- "There is really a different attitude institutionally . . . Our mission was always to provide the optimum level of care, but . . . our organization was never really structured to do that . . . PCR is helping us to do that with . . . more collaboration" (physician, not in a triad).
- "I really see the integration between the nursing, the management, and the physician perspective as a very effective and constructive thing and in a way, it's so obvious that it needs to happen, it surprises me the way that it's taken a grant to kind of put it together" (vice president, not in a triad).
- What has changed is "the collaborative point of view...people are buying into it, I think . . . they're beginning to feel certain of its empowerment to be involved in the decision making process" (physician, in a triad).
- "I think the biggest change has been the working together of administration and nursing and physician. I found that quite frankly rather than it being a situation where I was almost always putting out fires of one sort or another administratively, that meeting on a regular basis and knowing what's going on in the department and having the opportunity to discuss it regularly . . . have made it a much more prospective process rather than reactive process. And from the point of view of time, . . . the use of my time is more efficient" (vice president, in a triad).

▬ NURSING ADMINISTRATION WITHIN PATIENT-CENTERED REDESIGN

As previously indicated, at the time the Strengthening Hospital Nursing grant was received, the department of nursing was a stable, mature organization. It had a long history of strong nursing leadership and a structure familiar to many similar organizations. Specifically, it had five clinical nursing directors at the department head level, each with responsibility for a cluster of units. Some of these clusters, or services, were historically more homogeneous than others. Each director had several head nurses reporting directly to her, and there were ongoing efforts to flatten the organization by assigning assistant directors to staff functions within individual services.

A strong, centralized office controlled activities such as quality assurance, budgeting, the float pool, equipment purchase, and personnel management and negotiated for nursing as one of many centralized, vertical systems. Nursing was thus seen as one homogeneous entity and, given its sheer size, a strong department that some felt was primarily concerned about itself. Power and control were invested in several associates of the vice president of nursing, who were recognized decision-makers. This gave nursing a seat at the decision making table but did not actualize the element of decision making closest to the patient. Even though some thought nursing was a powerful department, staff nurses and head nurses felt they did not have a direct voice in clinical or operational decisions.

Despite the title of the national grant, the PCR program was explicitly not about strengthening nursing but rather about improving patient care. The PCR program staff, the grant steering committee, and the department of nursing were careful to minimize the focus on nursing in order to reinforce the fact that this was an institutional project. Members of these groups understood that a patient-focused *vision* was the critical element, and the only way to achieve this system-oriented vision was to involve everyone. On the other hand, to improve patient care and impact resource utilization, it was recognized that those directly responsible for patient-centered, cost-effective care—the triads—had to play pivotal roles in a redesigned delivery system. In turn, they had to have the support of both clinical and nonclinical departments to achieve expected outcomes. Over time, this concept evolved into an understanding that support departments were suppliers for intermediate customers, who were the ones directly linked to patient care delivery; this latter role was particularly true for the triads. The role of nursing administration in this equation is highlighted throughout the remainder of this chapter, along with factors that have influenced related changes. This includes movement toward decentralization, a general PCR program expectation that is having a clear impact within the department of nursing.

Nursing as Part of a Collaborative Management Team: The Director Level

In the previously cited survey, nursing directors perceived the level and nature of impact of triads slightly more positively than did triad members as a whole. Their mean score for impact was 4.80, and for characteristic of impact, 4.60. Content of in-depth interviews on the concept of Strengthening Hospital Nursing, conducted in the spring of 1993, reaffirmed these positive perceptions regarding CMTs (Stetler & Anderson, in press). All of the directors believed that nursing administration had been strengthened through the PCR program, although some felt more strongly than others about progress. Directors, unexpectedly, also found that their meaning of "strengthening" had changed. A few examples illustrate this point:

"What I learned out of the grant process is that it actually works a whole lot better and quicker when it's a total approach. When all the areas around you are also looking at strengthening and changing . . . and when people start to think the same way, then that strengthens everybody."

"When you [the interviewer] came in and I looked at what the interview was going to be about, I thought, "strengthening hospital nursing," I truly don't see it as nursing, it's more like it's providing better patient care."

The Strengthening Hospital Nursing interviews suggest that part of the reason for these positive reactions was that nursing directors had acquired more influence—not for nursing, but rather for patient care and for moving the system. Directors were now recognized as pivotal stakeholders in the delivery process, in part because of the referent power they had acquired by:

- Being directly associated with powerful individuals (ie, the clinical chief and the vice president);
- Being the member of a new paradigm group that was perceived to be, and indeed was, invested with authority; and
- Removal of a layer of authority in the nursing department and empowerment as leaders and decision makers in the nursing structure.

In terms of the second and third points, if a nursing director called a department "on behalf of the triad," she was likely to receive a customer-oriented response. This was often not the case before the restructuring project. A case in point can be cited: a director had tried through multiple requests and attempts to have a long-standing equipment problem resolved, to no avail. Upon making unit rounds, the triad heard of the issue, called on various vertical departments, and within a short period of time a patient-centered solution was found. Another nursing director stated, "You could be equally assertive in the two different systems and get now what you . . . couldn't get before . . . . You've got the backing of and support of the other individuals as opposed to being divided." As PCR evolves (eg, as customer-supplier relationships between CMTs and vertical supporting systems are formalized), this influence as a member of a CMT will grow.

Another example of empowerment through enhanced, meaningful involvement is seen in the contrast between the old and new paradigm of capital budgeting. In the past, nursing directors felt they had virtually no input because the process was primarily controlled through the central nursing office. The department of nursing, as a traditional vertical system, had one list submitted to cover approximately 40 units. In the new paradigm of triads, the director participates as an equal partner in development of a patient-centered, service-based capital budget submitted by the triad (Stetler, Fagan, Hanson, Biancamano, & Curry, 1994).

Another area in which director influence was strengthened is within the triad service itself. Two of the directors noted increased access to seats of influence, such as medical department meetings, in which they now enjoy a more explicit role. Three of the five directors explicitly spoke of enhanced collaborative relations and a concomitant increase in shared problemsolving among CMT members. One change noted by a nursing director was:

> *Before the triad there used to be head-to-head conflict and we would do battle . . . and come up with totally different alternatives as a solution to the problem. . . . That has evolved over time to more collaborative relationships in decision-making and then to changing it to [identify] whose decision it really is, and the decision . . . [is being] made much better these days.*

With other examples of empowerment, the directors spoke about now being able to make decisions, make better decisions, solve problems, and, in general, move the system. With this ability to improve patient care, in reality all members of the triad were strengthened.

Nursing as Part of a Collaborative Management Team: Other Levels
In the first 2 years of PCR, considerable emphasis was placed on development of the new collaborative management structure at the upper levels. Only a few head nurses or assistant directors were immersed in PCR, although the next phase of development will drive this aspect of change. Two of these head nurses, in subtriads, and five assistant directors involved in some type of collaborative management relationship were interviewed regarding the concept of Strengthening Hospital Nursing. Page constraints prohibit an in-depth review and analysis; however, a book in preparation provides more detail (Stetler & Charns, in press).

Overall, the response of these nurse managers echoed that of the directors. In general, they believed nursing administration had been strengthened in the overall process, but not yet to the hoped-for extent. Excerpted comments speak to the perceived strengthening at the directors' and their own position levels. These comments focus on the power of the new triad paradigm, a patient-centered focus, and the move to decentralization:

> *"For many years there was a lot of problem regarding patient management . . . , it was a real source of frustration and it did, I think, cause a rift between Physicians and Nurses and it was like the traditional 'no, it's your responsibility . . . so it's your problem; (now with PCR) we looked at the issue and it was . . .' these patients need to have these procedures done, what is the best way we can expedite getting these procedures done for this patient' " [assistant director]*

> *"Nursing is now in the loop . . . now there's a structure . . . and it's acceptable to try to solve the problem and it's not nursing against medicine . . . it was like 'we've got a problem . . . and we need to solve it'. . . . and it wasn't nursing just being resistant and not wanting to take these patients" [head nurse].*

■ FACTORS THAT INFLUENCED THE CHANGING NURSING ROLE

Factors that influenced the strengthening of nursing administration at Hartford Hospital are many and complex. Beatty and Ulrich (1991), however, describe four principles which they believe are key to the success of organizational renewal efforts such as PCR. As applied to this mature department of nursing, these principles provide a framework for describing specific strategies which have contributed to the shift from an old to a new culture. An overview of these renewal principles is provided, followed by sample strategies.

1. *Instilling customer perspective and focusing on customer demands.* This requires a willingness to honestly self-assess current paradigms and behaviors and to involve and listen to the customer. In particular, for hospitals, that means the patient and the patient's family.
2. *Increasing capacity for change.* Mature organizations must reset their "internal clocks" or norms for the speed with which decisions are made and work-related movements occur. To enhance their ability to change, organizations should focus on
   a. *Alignment,* or the extent to which organizational components such as structure, policies, procedures, systems, and roles are all focused on shared goals. Such alignment facilitates integration, creates congruence among multiple organizational activities, and results in positive reinforcement of desired behavior.
   b. *Symbiosis,* or the extent to which an institution is able to remove both internal and external barriers or "toll gates." Internally, self-contained vertical systems or turf-oriented departments can create such boundaries, as can layers of hierarchy.
   c. *Reflexiveness,* which refers to whether or not the institution is a *learning* organization. Renewal can come from "reflecting on past activities and learning from them."
3. *Altering management activities within the organization.* There are two categories of management activities: hardware, or organizational strategy, structures, and systems, and software, or employee behavior and mindset. Beatty and Ulrich's principles are not mutually exclusive, and it is evident that such renewal activities overlap with customer mindsets and alignment. Because hardware and software are integrally related, renewal must obviously include both. The former can involve visioning, restructuring, and other innovative strategies. The latter requires attention to the organization's culture and policies.
4. *Creating empowered employees who act as leaders at all levels of the organization.* Individuals need such aspects of empowerment as accountability, responsibility, control, and influence over related factors if work performance is to be optimal. Work performance in turn must be focused on a vision and values that are clearly communicated and understood. Leaders throughout the organization must possess appropriate competencies, which are frequently described by the term transformational leadership (eg, "walking the talk" and ensuring

one's behavior reinforces, rewards, and recognizes the new visions and values).

▬APPLICATION OF RENEWAL PRINCIPLES
TO CHANGES IN NURSING ADMINISTRATION
Customer Perspective

Four of the five nursing directors noted "patient-centeredness" in their descriptions of growing empowerment. For example:

> *I felt that we simply were not going to any longer not question, in a very fundamental way and at a high level, things that impacted negatively on patient care ... [After] getting the key players together ... there seemed to be a high level of defensiveness on the part of some; when we approached it as a problem solving patient flow issue, it turned around entirely.*

In the survey on culture, conducted several months before the Strengthening Hospital Nursing interviews, directors had noted a dramatic shift in the organization's level of patient-centeredness, from a low mean of 1.80 (on a 7-point Likert scale) before PCR to a rating of 4.60 after its initiation. (A post–then method was used whereby respondents concurrently compare the level of an item for two points in time.) This increased focus on patient-centeredness presumably reflects a growing change in behavior among both directors and their peers, as indicated by reports of an increased ability to influence decision-making and problem resolution.

Increasing the Capacity for Change

PCR is also concerned about the second principle of renewal, increasing the capacity for change. In terms of alignment, a special committee was established to create ongoing change within the vertical department of nursing. Nursing administration now routinely incorporates PCR and related changes into all facets of operations. Other methods for reinforcing change include integration of PCR goals with annual department goals and with goals of directors and head nurses.

Symbiosis was enhanced through the mandated association of triad members and by inclusion of staff in important forums. For example, nursing directors, for the first time, were included in the annual meeting of the board and medical staff, and head nurses now participate in department-head forums in which there is ongoing communication with the supertriad.

Steps to make Hartford Hospital, and the department of nursing, a learning organization have included use of consultative sessions for directors on self-assessment as well as periodic surveys and interviews to encourage reflection on what has happened, why, and what should happen next.

Management Activities

Managerial restructuring was a major element in Hartford Hospital's organizational renewal and the resultant strengthening of nursing. Shifting the paradigms or old cultural beliefs was equally important. Within Beatty and Ulrich's (1991) framework, inclusion of nursing directors in triads and other nurse managers in subtriads reflects both significant hardware and software changes. Likewise, the role of vice president of patient operations altered management activities and traditions throughout the organization and hastened the rate of change. This individual, as the nurse executive, initiated decentralization within the department of nursing by flattening the traditional hierarchical structure. This change, consistent with principles of PCR, realigned and restructured decision making and authority closer to the patient; for example, the head nurse role now incorporates human resource and fiscal management accountability. Along with changes in the director role, the need for an accountant and an associate responsible for departmental supplies and equipment was eliminated.

The nursing directors, as line accountable managers, are now charged with development of policy and procedures (in collaboration with staff), credentialing, and department leadership activities, including description of a vision for professional practice. Two traditional associate positions with decision-making responsibilities relative to policies, procedures, and operations have been eliminated. Management of departmental business has been shifted to the directors, and overall activities are managed within a forum of decision-makers (eg, head nurses and directors). The outcomes of this restructuring are that head nurses now have accountability for decision making at the unit level, and staff and personnel in other departments respond to head nurses and directors according to their new leadership role. The structural outcome is a more streamlined, decentralized department with fewer nursing administration associates.

Empowered Employees
Decentralization and restructuring efforts have provided nurse managers with a real opportunity to lead the department in making the PCR vision a reality. Staff nurse empowerment should obviously follow.

In these newly empowered roles, nurse managers have identified new skills and competencies which they believe are needed to effectively operate in a CMT. Financial knowledge is one identified competency; others include refined assertiveness skills, "public championing," and negotiation/communication skills.

■ SUMMARY
An integrated management and delivery system is the cornerstone of future success in a reformed health care system. One cannot, however, just say the system will be integrated, or dictate collaboration. Core concepts that build a firm foundation for integration must be put into operation. At Hartford Hospital, such concepts center on collaboration, organizational commitment, and our primary customers, the patients. A cross-discipline structure has been built to support decision-making closest to the patient, with teams of individuals who are given accountability to effectively and efficiently manage the outcomes of patients' care. In order to continue its success, a highly centralized, autonomous nursing department had to become less hierarchi-

cal and integrated into a new, collaborative, organization-wide management and delivery system. The evolution and success of these efforts across the institution are exciting. The change process is continuous, and much learning and change are yet to be accomplished; still, nursing administration is successfully collaborating to benefit both professional nursing practice and the quality of patient care.

Acknowledgment is given to the jointly sponsored grant from The Robert Wood Johnson Foundation and The Pew Charitable Trusts, "Strengthening Hospital Nursing: A Program to Improve Patient Care," and to the National Program Office. Their support helped make implementation of collaborative management a reality.

■ REFERENCES

Beatty, R. W. & Ulrich, D. O. (1991, Summer). Re-energizing the mature organization. *Organizational Dynamics*, pp. 16–30.
Koerner, B. & Armstrong, D. (1983). Collaborative practice at Hartford Hospital. *Nursing Administration Quarterly, 7*, 72–81.
Reeder, S. (1983). Collegial staff relations and assertiveness in nurses: Do they make any difference in patient care? In N. Chaska (Ed.), *The profession of nursing: A time to speak* (pp. 500–514). New York: McGraw-Hill.
Stetler, C. & Anderson, R. (in press). Strengthening hospital nursing: What does it mean? In C. Stetler & M. Charns (Eds.), *Collaboration in health care: Hartford Hospital's journey in changing management and practice.* Chicago: American Hospital Association.
Stetler, C. & Charns, M. (in press). *Collaboration in health care: Hartford Hospital's journey in changing management and practice.* Chicago: American Hospital Association.
Stetler, C., Fagan, J., Hanson, M., Biancamano, J., & Curry, S. (1994, October 2). Patient-centered redesign: More collaborative, clinical input into capital budget decisions. *International Journal of Technology Assessment in Health Care.*
Strengthening Hospital Nursing Program, National Program Office. (1992). *Strengthening Hospital Nursing: A program to improve patient care.* St. Petersburg, FL: The Robert Wood Johnson Foundation and The Pew Charitable Trusts.

Chapter 11

Workplace Redesign at Mercy Medical Center, San Diego: Care 2000

JOLENE TORNABENI   VICKI DEBACA

Change creates an uncertain environment and leads to concern and fear of the unknown. People are usually comfortable where they are, and they often resist change; however, change may be mandated by the external environment. The authors discuss the changing health care environment and its effect on Mercy Medical Center, San Diego, California. The process of redesigning patient care delivery to meet these challenges is presented.

▬ THE CHANGING HEALTH CARE ENVIRONMENT
Changes in the health care environment during the last decade impacted Mercy Medical Center and most health care organizations across the country. Capitated payments resulted in decreasing health care reimbursements and began driving the transformation of organizations to maintain financial viability. The message was clear: organizations had to change their business operations if they were to survive.

Because labor costs consume the largest portion of hospital operating expenses, staff reductions and downsizing of the typical hierarchial administrative structure have been the popular mechanisms of cost savings. By 1986, Mercy Medical Center had experienced several years of declining revenue and reimbursements, resulting in the need to reduce its work force. This reduction eliminated 180 positions. Turnover in senior management positions provided a real opportunity to redesign and restructure at the executive level. A new executive role was strategically designed which combined a traditional nurse administrator position with a clinical services administrator role. This provided an opportunity to restructure reporting relationships.

▬ RESTRUCTURING FOR INNOVATION
The newly created role was that of vice president, hospital operations, having administrative responsibility for nursing, laboratory, radiology, pharmacy, cardiology, respiratory, rehabilitative, and psychiatric services.

Flarey, D: REDESIGNING NURSING CARE DELIVERY: Transforming Our Future
© 1995, J. B. Lippincott Company

The role was designed so that all direct patient care services are under one executive. The former structure often resulted in poor interdepartmental relations and barriers which negatively impacted patient care. The old structure was a traditional, vertical hierarchy which segregated the components of care delivery under various executive domains. Interdepartmental problems were frequent and were caused by a lack of cooperation between departments, a poor understanding of the roles and responsibilities of each department, and a real sense of departmental infallibility and turf protection.

Structuring all professional direct patient care services under one executive's leadership laid the foundation for the development of a patient-focused, collaborative care model. Patient needs became the priority over departmental needs. Work began to transform the culture into one of a team spirit driven by a commonality of partnership in professional practice. The recent implementation of a decision-making model of shared governance provided a strong foundation for staff responsibility and accountability in working together to make decisions at the unit. The culture and climate slowly evolved into one in which staff empowerment was valued and nurtured.

Benefits of the redesigned executive position and structure were evident almost immediately. Communication among department directors who reported to the same executive was enhanced. Long-standing, interdepartmental problems were discussed and more readily resolved. Increased cooperation, collaboration, and problem-solving between disciplines were apparent. The management team was transformed, and soon vision statements were written that focused on a radical redesign of processes and systems by which the delivery of patient care would be enhanced in a quality and cost-effective way.

Through a long developmental process, department directors moved from a problem-oriented focus to a management model based on goals achievement. The directors' major goals were to improve the delivery of patient care, enhance the quality of services, and transform the practice environment to one of patient-centeredness. The role modeling of these behaviors by department directors directly affected how the staff interacted with one another. Their ability to succeed in problem resolution and effective collaborative practice was due in large part to the redesigned structure that minimized the segregation of departments. This change in culture and organizational climate laid the foundation for advancing a new organizational philosophy.

■THE MOVE TO REDESIGN

Over a three-year period, so much progress was made in changing attitudes and work relations that the organization began to consider extending the benefits of this model of collaborative relations to other areas of the organizational structure. Driving this decision was the continued decline in reimbursements, making it even more imperative for the organization to design new and better ways of doing business while maintaining quality patient care and customer satisfaction.

Restructuring the way care is delivered and redesigning it around patients rather than the needs of the organization was thought to be a somewhat radical change but necessary to ensure Mercy Medical Center's growth and success. Such a change had to involve the entire organization, and would probably generate resistance and fear. Also, the organization did not have the expertise or experience to implement this type of project. Despite these restraining forces, the organization made a commitment to begin Care 2000, a patient-focused redesign project.

A decision was made to employ health care consultants to assist with the evaluation and early implementation phases of the project. The redesign planners felt, based on their previous experiences, that consultants would be able to provide a framework for the types of data to collect, recommend information sources, and quickly perform an analysis without a long start-up period. Another advantage was that consultants could view processes from an unbiased perspective, since they would not be caught up in the internal politics and power struggles of the organization.

The criteria for selection of a consultant were based on experience in the area of restructuring, willingness to work with the hospital staff, and costs. The firm of Booz-Allen and Hamilton was invited to provide an organizational assessment at Mercy Medical Center. The analysis took place over a two-month period from November 1990 to January 1991. The goal was to collect data that would provide a baseline assessment of the organization's current systems of care delivery. The entire organization actively participated, to some degree, in the initial assessment. The consultants identified the types of information to collect. These suggestions were reviewed by key personnel, and a customized needs assessment was developed. The internal staff assisted with collecting and interpreting the data.

The analysis provided a new perspective on many of the traditional procedures and structures and pointed out the complexities and inefficiencies in many of the processes and systems of the organization. This comprehensive assessment included analysis in the following areas: work processes and work flows, documentation, job descriptions and caregiver qualifications, patient interactions, time spent scheduling and transporting patients, and administrative structures.

Work Processes and Work Flow
With the assistance of the consultants, key hospital staff identified two common procedures for analysis: chest x-ray and chemistry panels. The typical process flow for a chest x-ray at Mercy Medical Center consisted of 64 steps, from the physician's writing the order to placement of results on the medical record. Of these, 57 steps were required to move things or people, record information, and coordinate the process. Only 7 steps involved direct patient care related to performance of the chest x-ray. Common problems with the chest x-ray procedure included lengthy waits for elevators, unavailability of the patient for transport, lengthy waits in the radiology depart-

ment before the procedure, waiting for a transporter to return the patient to the unit, and charting results in the patient's medical record. Analysis of the process flow for a chemistry panel was similar. Forty-two steps were required to perform the procedure; only 6 steps involved technical skills to perform the blood draw and analysis. The other steps involved transporting and delivering the specimen, processing paperwork, and distributing results.

Work sampling surveys were also done to determine the amount of time patient care staff spent in each of five categories of care: transportation, direct patient care, documentation, coordination of care, and idle time. The results of work sampling indicated that only 36% of time was spent in providing direct patient care. The complexity of work processes, highly specialized job activities, and the time spent coordinating and transporting patients to services left little time for direct patient care.

Complexity in Documentation

Documentation of the complex processes involved in patient care had become increasingly burdensome. Several studies have found that documentation can take from 39% to 60% of nurses' time (Childs, 1990; Weber, 1991). At Mercy Medical Center, studies demonstrated that documentation accounted for 30% of the caregivers' time. Part of the reason for this prolonged time was the need to chart similar information in several places and the reliance on a predominately paper record.

Narrow Job Descriptions and Limited Qualifications

In recent years, the trend in health care has been to increase specialization of services (Borzo, 1992). This specialization has become increasingly evident in the work provided by hospital staff. For example, electrocardiograms (ECGs) are usually taken by a limited number of centrally located personnel. In order to obtain an ECG for a patient, numerous steps are required for scheduling and coordination beforehand. Phlebotomy is another example of service specialization. Most institutions have created categories of workers to draw blood even though registered nurses, already on the unit, are licensed and skilled in phlebotomy and intravenous therapy.

Increased specialization and centralization of services has resulted in an increase in the number of caregivers seen by patients. It has been estimated that during a normal hospital stay patients have contact with 50 to 60 employees (Cassidy, 1992). At Mercy Medical Center, the typical number of employees interacting with a patient during a 3.2-day stay was 54.

Scheduling and Transporting Patients

Because the hospital was designed around centralized services, much time was spent coordinating services through the central department, arranging for transportation of patients to the central department, waiting for the procedure, returning the patient to the unit, and distributing test results to the medical record. Owing to the complexity of this system, some clerical positions existed solely for the purpose of controlling and monitoring these processes.

The design of services in centralized departments, often far from patient care areas, resulted in additional time required to transport patients to scheduled procedures. In one study sample of elevator response time, it took more than 5 minutes to transport patients from the 10th floor to the main radiology suite. Transportation of supplies and material also increased waiting time.

Administrative Structures
The organizational analysis demonstrated that work processes within the organization were very complex. The organization was structured vertically, with many small, specialized units comprised of staff who were limited in their skill and ability to do more than one or two major tasks. This resulted in increased lag time in the overall delivery of care. The system was costly and nonproductive. Work was very fragmented, because systems and processes had been created to benefit departments rather than patients. The organization was designed vertically, but patients moved horizontally in the care delivery system. This information on how the organization was structured and how work was carried out through multiple low-value tasks clearly demonstrated how inefficiently the work was done. This understanding was critical for the staff to comprehend in order to accept the need for change. Staff response was overwhelmingly positive. With staff support, the organization made a commitment to undertake the Care 2000 redesign project. The three major goals of patient-focused redesign were 1) to continuously improve the quality of patient care, 2) to enhance the services provided to the patient, and 3) to provide services in a cost-effective manner.

■GENERATING SUPPORT
It was critical to assure top-down support for a change of this magnitude. This was not simply a project but rather a complete transformation in how work within the organization would be processed. High visibility, support for change, and clear expectations were essential. In order to ensure the success of the project, a considerable investment of senior management's time was required to gather support from critical groups.

Members of senior administration and department directors approached physicians who were leaders, innovative thinkers, and most likely to support the change. Select physicians were invited to make site visits to the few hospitals that had restructured and redesigned. These physicians quickly identified the benefits of the project and later served as strong advocates for the project. This core group of physicians effectively sold the project idea to the general medical staff.

Support from the board of directors was essential for obtaining resources to fund the project. Presentations were made through a series of meetings to explain the intent and the scope of the project. Discussion of the assessment data, objectives of the Care 2000 redesign project, the time line for implementation, resources needed, and expected results of the restructuring and redesign were presented. The governing body wanted to understand the need for restructuring and the expected outcomes. Key to gaining board support was the unitary voice of senior administration and support from the physicians.

The board was overwhelmed by the physicians' commitment to the project. As a result, the board empowered senior management to proceed. Financial, clinical, and service outcomes were clearly articulated and shared with the board. Senior management committed to sharing the results on a routine basis with the board.

REDESIGNING CARE DELIVERY

In November 1991, implementation of the patient-focused program began with two demonstration units, one surgical and one medical. Using the findings of the needs assessment, and in conjunction with Booz-Allen and Hamilton, Mercy Medical Center adopted five operating principles to serve as a guide for its restructuring process: 1) streamline and simplify documentation requirements; 2) place services closer to the patient; 3) broaden caregiver qualifications and skills; 4) simplify processes; and 5) aggregate patients with similar care needs.

Physical remodeling of the demonstration units included physical changes and environmental enhancements, integration of ancillary services on the patient care unit, and staff education. It has been strongly recommended that organizations undertaking a restructuring project pay attention to involvement of the staff as the restructuring process proceeds (Henderson & Williams, 1991). In order to include extensive involvement of the staff, multidisciplinary committees were established to plan and implement various stages of the restructure and redesign. Guided by a core steering group, committees were formed to address each of the identified anticipated needs (facilities, equipment, documentation, human resources, communication, etc.).

Physical Changes

Assessment data was used to identify the high-volume services used on each of the two pilot units. Each unit was remodeled to allow for the space and equipment needs of these services. For the surgical unit, which provides a large number of orthopedic services, a substantial amount of square footage was allocated for rehabilitation services, such as physical and occupational therapy. Although plans originally included accommodations for a permanent x-ray room, prohibitive costs, regulations, and lower than anticipated volumes caused this idea to be abandoned in favor of using portable equipment for the majority of procedures.

Each patient care room was designed to include a patient server. The patient server accommodates a bedside computer terminal, locked medication drawer, and the majority of supplies necessary to provide daily care. This eliminated the need for an area in which to store central service items. In keeping with the idea that each unit is in essence a mini-hospital or separate operating unit, the entryway to the patient unit was remodeled to include a reception desk and work area for activities related to admission and discharge, such as insurance documentation, financial advisement, and performance of medical record activities. All preadmission testing is now done in this admission area.

Services

One of the key principles of redesign is to identify services frequently used by patients and to restructure those services from central departments to the patient care units (Borzo, 1992). The type of high-volume services differed on each of the two demonstration units. The central core of each unit was redesigned to accommodate the needed ancillary services. Besides the need for physical therapy on the surgical unit, the high usage of medications and intravenous drug therapy led to the incorporation of a satellite pharmacy.

On the medical unit, two high-volume services were respiratory therapy and laboratory services. To meet these needs, a laboratory was staffed and equipped, and a respiratory care area was added to house the commonly needed equipment and supplies.

Personnel

In addition to redesigning the physical environment, work restructuring also occurred. Employees have now become "partners" in delivering patient care. Four new partner roles have been defined. Clinical partners are licensed professionals, such as registered nurses, pharmacists, and medical technologists. Technical partners are staff who have had previous patient care experience, such as radiology technicians, pharmacy technicians, licensed vocational nurses, and nursing assistants. Administrative partners are those who play key roles in the admissions and medical record functions. They include admissions representatives, financial advisors, medical records coders, and nursing secretaries. Service partners provide support services for the overall functioning of the unit. Service partners include environmental service technicians, food service helpers, transporters, laboratory assistants, and central service technicians.

Direct patient care is provided by a care pair. One member of the care pair is always a registered nurse who has the responsibility to coordinate and oversee the entire plan of patient care. The other member of the care pair may be another clinical partner or a technical partner. Assignments are made in order to assure that the services required by the patient population are met by the skill mix of the care pair. Care pairs provide care for five to nine patients and work together as a team, having the same scheduled working days.

Cross-training

Cross-training is an essential component of restructuring. It reduces fragmentation caused by highly specialized service providers and eliminates departmental barriers (Brider, 1992; Cassidy, 1992). The goal of cross-training is to increase the number of multiskilled personnel in the patient care area. By increasing the scope of job duties, caregivers are able to address patient needs without long waits or other delays. In addition, having multiskilled providers decreases the number of patient contacts over the course of hospitalization.

Organizational analysis identified waiting time for services to be provided as a major concern of patients. Because of extreme job specialization, only certain workers had the knowledge or skills necessary to provide certain services, such as passing patient food trays, ambulating patients, or drawing blood. Finding the right provider to perform the needed task frequently caused delays in service.

The education committee, consisting of representatives from all departments and led by two clinical nurse specialists, developed an extensive training program for all partners. One component of preparation consisted of providing service partners and administrative partners training in basic patient care skills. This substantially increased the number of providers who were able to assist patients with simple needs, such as ambulation and meal service, and to provide basic care and comfort measures. Skill blocks consisting of specialized training to increase the scope of a partner's skills were also developed. For example, training in respiratory therapy techniques and phlebotomy was provided to licensed nurses; technical partners were cross-trained to provide select respiratory and ECG services; and pharmacists now assist with medication administration, such as the first dose of antibiotics, and other patient care services.

Reassignment of ancillary staff to the units necessitated a change in traditional reporting relationships. Guided by a philosophy of increasing teamwork and breaking down the traditional barriers created by the department hierarchy, all partners working on a patient care unit now report to the director of the unit. Such a structure has increased the responsibility and accountability of each person to the team and keeps them centered on the patient. Through a matrix reporting system, these employees continue to maintain ties to their specific disciplines. Such ties are important for maintaining competency, keeping abreast of new techniques and technology, and maintaining quality controls.

■ IMPLICATIONS FOR NURSING

In a traditional setting, the only staff members whose work revolves around the patient are nurses. In a restructured environment, nurses are able to provide an enhanced level of care. Redesign of the physical environment allows more time to be given to direct patient care activities rather than spending it obtaining supplies and coordinating procedures. Reassignment of other disciplines to the patient care unit creates a team approach to care and increases the number of resources readily available to assist with patient needs. The availability of additional staff members increases the nurses' ability to deliver comprehensive care by coordinating and delegating tasks to other cross-trained team members and assuring that quality patient care is provided in a cost-efficient manner. Having all services centered on the patient suddenly has everyone focused on the same mission—the care of

patients. Having all staff located on the patient unit provides a real opportunity for all disciplines to acquire a better appreciation of one another's
skills, abilities, and contributions to the delivery of quality patient care.

▬REALIZING OUTCOMES
The three major goals of our patient-focused redesign were 1) to continuously improve the quality of patient care, 2) to enhance services provided to
the patient, and 3) to provide services in a cost effective manner.

Quality
The Care 2000 redesign project was expected to have a major impact on
several key indicators of the quality of care provided to patients. One concern voiced during the course of cross-training and the broadening of caregiver skills was the need to ensure competency of the staff. This objective is
being met by ongoing staff evaluations such as retraining, skill-a-thons, and
annual skill appraisals. Indirect measures of the quality of care, such as mor-
tality, infection rates, and number of unexpected complications, have decreased or remained the same.

Other indicators, such as patient length of stay (LOS) and incidence of
medication errors, show improvement from preimplementation rates and
are superior to those of comparable units. On one restructured unit, the
patient fall rate has decreased from 6 per 1000 patient-days to less than 3
per 1,000 as a result of the increase in the amount of time spent in direct
patient care. A decrease in the pneumonia rate, from .41 to .20 per 100
discharged patients, is attributed to having additional cross-trained employees reinforcing preventive respiratory treatments on a more consistent
basis. Monitors of cross-trained procedures have shown no increase in laboratory errors and no decrease in the quality of chest x-rays or ECG's performed on the unit.

Service
Evaluation of the service component of Care 2000 includes both subjective
and objective monitors. The impact of restructuring on direct patient care
was an increase in time spent by registered nurses providing care. Direct
care time increased from 30% to 41%. The incorporation of ancillary services on the unit also decreased the amount of time nurses spent in coordinating and transporting patients. A reduction from 26.3% to 22% was realized. Continued improvement in systems and technology is anticipated to
decrease this component even further.

The work of the decentralized ancillary services has also been streamlined. Before restructuring, chemistry panel results required 42 steps and
required, on the average, 121 minutes to complete. This same process now
requires 26 steps and can be accomplished in 57 minutes.

Improvement has been seen in the amount of time required for patient
admissions to the unit. With decentralization of the admitting process to the
units, emergency admission time has fallen from 13 minutes to less than 2

minutes. Routine admission time, once almost 12 minutes, has decreased to 2 minutes. Decentralized admitting personnel are more flexible and available to provide admission services on the unit or in patients' rooms.

Subjective evaluation of service is also important. Patient satisfaction surveys on the restructured units have scored the highest gains ever experienced in the institution, and a positive trend continues. Physician satisfaction surveys have also demonstrated an increase in physicians' perception of the quality of care provided to their patients as well as the availability and competency of caregivers to assist them (Jones, DeBaca, Tornabeni, & Yarbrough, in press).

Caregiver surveys, both before and after implementation, were designed to provide information about staff perception of the restructuring. Overall responses showed support of the changes. Significant improvements were seen in interdepartmental and intradepartmental functioning, work group effectiveness, and the level of satisfaction in providing patient care (Jones, DeBaca, Tornabeni, & Yarbrough, in press). Staff satisfaction has also resulted in decreased turnover.

Cost
The evaluation of cost savings, already complex in the hospital environment, will take longer to complete. Not all anticipated cost savings have been realized in the initial steps of restructuring. Since only a small volume of work has been transferred out of the central department, with only two units restructured, there is still a need to retain the basic infrastructure. Cost savings are expected to be more pronounced as two additional units are restructured. This will allow for a more significant decrease in centralized department activities. Our initial, tangible cost savings were realized from work restructuring and process improvements. A reduction in the work force of 28 full-time equivalent positions was possible. This reduction was accomplished primarily through turnover, retirement, transfer, and cross-training of personnel.

Costs were also impacted through a decrease in LOS. The LOS for our three high-volume diagnoses on the surgical unit has been reduced by one day. This reduction is attributable to the availability of specialty services, such as physical therapy, on the unit; decreases in the waiting time for test results, allowing physicians to make quicker decisions about patient progress; and improved effectiveness of the caregiver staff.

Ancillary costs have also been reduced. Continued monitoring and stocking of supplies directly to patient rooms has resulted in fewer delays in patient care and fewer emergency or stat charges. Lost charges have diminished substantially. Availability of professionals, such as the pharmacist, on the unit has resulted in closer monitoring of patient medication regimes and more communication with physicians, thus preventing problems. Pharmacists provide more recommendations for less expensive therapies and are able to troubleshoot problems and prevent complications.

Other cost savings, not quantified at this time, have resulted from decreased personnel turnover, improved patient outcomes (eg, reduced falls), elimination of process steps, elimination of duplicate infrastructures and ancillary services, reduction of management and supervisory staff, and more efficient utilization of personnel.

▬CONCLUSION

Restructuring is now complete on four inpatient units, and plans are being formulated for two additional units and outpatient services. Evaluation of the project has been overwhelmingly positive. Every level of the organization, from the board of directors down, believes that the objectives of improving quality and service while maintaining cost objectives have been met. Patient, physician, and staff satisfaction have increased. Complex processes have been streamlined. Care has been improved, and waiting time, patient transportation time, and staff down time have been reduced. Work sampling analysis shows that more time by the staff is now spent in providing direct patient care.

Although change is not always welcome, it often provides the impetus to examine the way processes and systems operate. The challenge to create new systems has led to improvements in both the processes and outcomes of patient care through a patient-focused redesign. Continued implementation and refinement of patient-focused care at Mercy Medical Center will allow us to remain at the forefront of the health care reform movement. The Mercy mission rings true even a century later: providing quality care to those we serve—the patients!

▬REFERENCES

Brider, P. (1992). The move to patient focused care. *American Journal of Nursing, 92,* 26–33.
Borzo, G. (1992). Patient-focused hospitals begin reporting good results. *Health Care Strategic Management, 10,* 17–22.
Cassidy, J. (1992). Patient focused delivery promises to reshape hospitals. *Health Progress, 73,* 20–24.
Childs, B. W. (1990). Bedside terminals: One of the answers to the nursing shortage. *Health Informatics, 7,* 37.
Henderson, J. M. & Williams, J. (1991). Ten steps for restructuring patient care. *Health Care Forum Journal, 36,* 50–54.
Jones, K., DeBaca, V., Tornabeni, J., & Yarbrough, M. (in press). Implementation and evaluation of patient-centered care. In K. Kelly, (Ed.), *Series on nursing administration.* St. Louis: Mosby Year Book.
Weber, D. (1991). Six models of patient focused care. *Healthcare Forum Journal, 34,* 23–28.

Chapter 12

STARs: Interdisciplinary Care Across the Continuum

SUSAN L. BECK   CHERYL L. KINNEAR

Patients encountering today's health care system often meet with chaos. As they tell their story over and over again, they often ask, "Doesn't anyone around here talk to each other?" The typical patient interacts with numerous and often inconsistent caregivers who do not appear to provide care based on a sound and comprehensive plan. Much of this disorder results from how the people who provide patient care are organized. Hospitals are traditionally structured into departments specific to the specialized work which they perform (eg, nursing, physical therapy). Although such traditional hierarchical bureaucracies are effective in organizing the operations of the hospital's individual departments, they are not the most effective model for the organization of the primary product, patient care.

This chapter describes an alternative approach to patient care delivery which has been developed and implemented at the University Hospital (UH), a 392-bed teaching hospital that is part of the University of Utah Health Sciences Center in Salt Lake City. Service Teams with Appropriate Resources (STARs) is a model that restructures more than nursing care. The model is interdisciplinary to the core and is designed to provide superior, quality, cost-effective care across the episode of illness and spectrum of health care delivery.

▬ THE MODEL

STARs is a system of organizing care to cross the boundaries of geography and time. Each STAR is a consistent, stable team of caregivers working together to plan, coordinate, and implement care to achieve desired outcomes. Each interdisciplinary STAR is uniquely designed to best meet the needs of a specific group of patients from the time of their initial contact with the system to the period beyond discharge. The key characteristics are presented in Display 12-1. Team membership is customized to the service needs of the patient group, with the intent of improving resource utilization, as staff composition and mix are matched to patient needs.

DISPLAY 12-1 *Characteristics of Each STAR*

- Structured around a specific patient population (eg, by age, diagnosis)
- Sites of service identified (eg, patient care units, clinics, home care)
- Consists of a customized team of core members assigned from each site of service
- Consultative and supportive team members identified
- Patient care coordinator manages care across the continuum
- Involves interdisciplinary collaboration in planning, implementing, and evaluating each patient's plan of care
- Provides for STAR accountability for quality and cost of service

---

A new key nursing role in the model is the STAR patient care coordinator (PCC). This role provides an opportunity for the professional nurse to manage the care of a group of patients across the continuum and to facilitate the work of an interdisciplinary team. The PCC acts as a liaison between the patient and family, hospital services, and the community.

It is important to distinguish the STAR model from two common nursing care delivery systems: team nursing and nursing case management. Since the STAR is an interdisciplinary, system-wide team and not a unit-based nursing team, the STAR model differs significantly from team nursing. Although there are certain similarities between the role of the PCC and that of a case manager, the STAR includes not only a PCC who is managing the care across traditional boundaries but a team of caregivers who work collaboratively to provide and improve patient care.

For example, within the neuroscience service, a neuro-oncology STAR was developed to care for patients with brain and spinal cord tumors. The core team members, those who care for all patients assigned to the STAR, include the neurosurgeon, neuro-oncologist, a social worker, a pharmacist, physical, occupational, and speech therapists, and a clinical dietician. Physicians are instrumental STAR members; their care of patients improves through collaboration with a consistent team of caregivers. Nursing personnel include registered nurses (RNs) and assistive personnel in the neuroscience unit and two ambulatory clinics. A nursing liaison has been appointed from home care service. The neuro-oncology administrative secretary is also an important core team member. The STAR PCC manages the care of neuro-oncology patients from the time of their entry into the system for diagnosis, throughout their cancer treatment, and often through the palliative management of the patient and support of the family preceding death. Consultative members (eg, radiation oncologist, clinical nurse specialists) and supportive STAR members (eg, nurse managers) are also used.

Perhaps the most powerful characteristic of the STAR model, however, is that the team develops responsibility and accountability for both the quality and cost of patient care. Quality improvement becomes patient-centered and interdisciplinary. Cost control becomes part of the business of clinicians. The objectives of the STAR model are outlined in Display 12-2.

▬ THE PLANNING PROCESS

The STARs model is one of three programs that resulted from a strategic planning initiative supported by a grant from The Robert Wood Johnson Foundation and The Pew Charitable Trusts as part of a national initiative, "Strengthening Hospital Nursing: A Program to Improve Patient Care." The background and framework for this program have been described elsewhere (Taft & Stearns, 1991; Donaho & Kohles, 1992; see Chapter 3). The purpose of the strategic planning process at UH was to redesign patient services to provide superior-quality, cost-effective care across the continuum of service and to improve the supply and utilization of professional resources. The three innovative programs that resulted from this planning endeavor, and which comprise UH's *Program to Improve Patient Care*, were subsequently funded as part of the five-year implementation phase of the national Strengthening Hospital Nursing program.

The planning process was structured as a hospital-wide effort using an

---

DISPLAY 12-2   *Objectives of STARs*

To improve the quality of care by:

1. Improving communication and collaboration across disciplines and throughout the continuum of care
2. Shifting accountability for establishing standards and monitoring quality to the multidisciplinary team of caregivers
3. Improving continuity of care through a multidisciplinary plan of care and better coordinated services provided by a team of consistent caregivers

To provide more cost-effective care by:

1. Efficiently using professional and nonprofessional resources
2. Shifting accountability for establishing standards (diagnostic tests, length of stay, etc.) and monitoring costs of care to the interdisciplinary team of direct caregivers
3. Improving recovery of unreimbursed costs

To increase work satisfaction and staff retention by:

1. Increasing autonomy, empowerment, and participation in decision-making
2. Providing clinically-based advancement options for nurses
3. Increasing personal satisfaction and sense of achievement in work performance

Copyright 1990, University of Utah Hospital, *Program to Improve Patient Care.*

approach grounded in the notion of identifying, involving, and managing stakeholders—those individuals, groups, or organizations that have a stake in what the organization does (Emshoff, 1980; Fottler et al., 1989). Stakeholders in both new and existing groups actively participated in the planning (Beck, Hartigan, & Belsey, 1993). A new group, the strategic planning team (SPT), included internal stakeholders who crossed the hospital organization vertically from top to bottom and horizontally across the continuum of care. The SPT was trained and supported in the work of overall strategic planning. A systematic approach to communicating with existing groups was used throughout the planning process.

The SPT used an interactive planning model developed by Ackoff (1981). Interactive planning encompasses designing and inventing ways to bring about a desirable future. Interactive planning uses a systems approach based on the fundamental interdependence of a hospital's organizational structure. The newly developed stakeholder structure provided a framework for a participative planning process at UH. Stakeholders learned and applied an idealized design process to create a vision of what could be and then "plan backwards" to realize the vision.

The vision of the STAR emerged from the interactive planning process. A task force was established to extend the level of stakeholder involvement to include more disciplines and staff. The group, led by a member of the SPT who was a nurse manager from the surgery clinic, expanded and refined the vision. A critical component of the design was that stakeholders in each service area would be involved in creating and customizing STARs to fit their respective patient populations. Neuroscience and rehabilitation services were selected as the first two areas for implementation. These services were selected as demonstration areas for several reasons:

1. They involve complex, interdisciplinary care.
2. Rehabilitation already employed a team orientation to care.
3. Patients in these units typically were transferred to different units during a hospital stay, and these areas therefore provided a view of the potential problems of interfacing between different services.
4. Patients in these services often required outpatient follow-up, and thus they could represent the continuum of care.
5. The potential existed for physician, nursing, and administrative leadership.

Two planning teams, consisting of major stakeholders from each service, convened to review historical data (diagnosis-related groups, length of stay, census, demographic characteristics, acuity, common patient needs, frequently used resources, etc.), and divide the patient population into the groups that formed the basis of organizing STARs. The planning teams identified patient populations, sites of services, and core (consistent), consultative (occasional), and supportive members for four patient groups: neuro-oncology, spinal cord injury, traumatic brain injury, and cerebrovascular accident/amputee. Project staff then met with each department to discuss how specific staff would be assigned to the appropriate STAR.

The design of the role and position description for the PCC was a critical aspect of developing the STAR model. The position description and title for the new role went through multiple iterations with input from the STARs planning teams, nursing management, human resources, and the steering committee for the entire project. A valuable lesson was the importance of selecting the right name for a new role. Working titles included patient services manager, lead nurse, and finally, patient care coordinator. Negative implications of language came to the surface as stakeholders experimented with titles and their acronyms.

The generic responsibilities of the PCC were finally completed and approved for pilot testing. In developing these responsibilities, comparisons were made to existing roles and job responsibilities. Certain aspects of the roles of the primary nurse (eg, comprehensive intake assessment), clinic nurses, and the assistant nurse manager (eg, staff orientation) were included in the new role. The original intent was that the assistant nurse manager role would be eliminated and the responsibilities would be shared by the PCC and a newly created position, that of administrative assistant. The STAR model also provided the flexibility for each STAR to customize the role of the PCC to its needs. Responsibilities unique to each STAR (eg, monitoring patient progress on cancer treatment protocols) were identified.

Important decisions in developing the position were related to the necessary qualifications, resources, reporting relations, and hiring process. Job requirements for PCC include a bachelor's degree in nursing, 2 years of nursing experience in a clinically-related area, excellent interpersonal skills, and skills in leadership, team relationships, communication, and organization. Although it was recognized that a nurse with an advanced practice degree would be better prepared for the position, it was decided to make this a "preferred" qualification because of the shortage of masters-prepared nurses in the geographical area. Four vacant full-time equivalent positions within the nursing practice department were reallocated to fund the demonstration without requesting additional resources. Salary was recommended by the human resources compensation committee and was comparable to that of an assistant nurse manager. Detailed planning for required resources such as office space, files, and pagers is recommended; lack of attention to this task led to frustrations for the PCCs and an unnecessary barrier to implementing their role. The PCC reported to a unit-based nurse manager in the short term. The open hiring process was coordinated by this nurse manager, who arranged interviews for applicants with staff and assigned STAR members. After four PCCs were hired and team members were assigned, the process of implementing the STAR model began.

▬IMPLEMENTATION

The first step of implementation was to convene the members of each STAR. One-day retreats were organized for each of the four STARs and included core, consultative, and supportive members. The goals of the retreats were

- to provide an opportunity for STAR members to become acquainted;
- to establish a common vision of the STAR concept;

- to identify what would constitute success for the STAR and what individual member contributions were necessary for success;
- to identify the roles of individual members with regard to patient care and the STAR;
- to begin to establish the norms of the STAR; and
- to establish communication methods for the STAR.

The retreats were organized by the project staff and supported by a consultant specializing in organizational change. Support from management was solicited in order to assure that STAR members were able to attend.

At the retreat, an overview was presented describing the purpose, characteristics, and objectives of the STAR. Discussions related to roles in patient care revealed some overlap and duplication in the areas of patient advocacy, problem identification, and discharge planning. STAR members identified team roles as an important area for development. Various members described how they could coordinate resources and provide information and expertise to the STAR. All members agreed that each individual should have responsibility for identifying "glitches" in the system and should bring them to the STAR for discussion and problem-solving. Members acknowledged that building the STAR would be a developmental process and asked each other to take the development of the STAR seriously, be committed, continue in their efforts, and not let the process "fizzle out." An initial plan for STAR communication was agreed on; it was designed to provide for discussion, information sharing, problem-solving, and feedback.

Development of the Patient Care Coordinator

The orientation and development plan for the STAR PCCs was organized into phases to allow for flexibility and customization of the orientation according to the individual's previous experience and background. The theories and skills addressed in the phases were aligned with anticipated developmental milestones of the STAR. Specific content areas included in the curriculum are presented in Table 12-1. Activities to achieve the objectives varied from classroom educational sessions to observational experiences with STAR members. Established departmental orientation sessions were used when available. The PCCs found observational experiences and discussions with STAR members very helpful. Real-life critical incidents were used to apply knowledge related to interdependence, communication, and team building during weekly meetings.

To support a new role such as the STAR PCC, it is important to structure activities for application of new knowledge and skills and for close interaction with other STAR members. One must avoid assumptions about basic skills. Supporting the development of skills related to mediation, project management, organization, and leadership was identified as critical. The PCCs required a clear understanding of the organizational structure of the hospital and information about the political history of hospital departmental relationships. In retrospect, PCCs stressed the importance of education related to change theory and group dynamics. Because of the evolving nature of the role, the process of educating the PCCs is ongoing.

TABLE 12-1   **Orientation/Development Curriculum for STAR Patient Care Coordinators**

PHASE	CONTENT AREAS
I. Hospital orientation	University hospital Nursing practice department Ambulatory care services Ancillary departments Organizational structure Communication systems
II. STAR orientation	STAR concept Role in the change process Sites of care STAR member roles
III. Leadership development and team building	Interdependence Group dynamics/communication Setting goals Roles Conflict management Power Team assessment Planned change
IV. Quality improvement	Continuous quality improvement Foundation skills Meeting management skills Team leadership skills Process improvement skills
V. Cost improvement	Third party payors Managed care Cost monitoring Analyzing cost data Developing strategies

Excerpted from *STAR Patient Care Coordinator Orientation/Development Plan,* University of Utah Hospital, 1993.

Team Roles

Over the first year, role overlap and role conflicts between STAR members began to emerge. Project staff supported the STARs to manage conflicts through team meetings and through focused discussions among the specific individuals involved. Approaches such as responsibility charting (Gilmore, 1979) and nominal group technique (Delbeq, Van de Ven, & Gustafson, 1975) were used to clarify and negotiate roles. Frequent evaluation, by the individuals involved, of role decisions and members' compliance with those decisions helped to refine and assure their understanding.

Especially difficult areas included the PCC's role in relation to those of primary nurses and ambulatory care nurses in the clinic, the role of the physician's secretary within the STAR, and the roles of various STAR members (home care nurse, social worker, clinic nurse) in managing the patient after discharge. Communication of patient information necessary for STAR members to function in their agreed roles was identified as essential and proved to be an ongoing challenge. The STAR members and project staff learned over time that detailed and rigid definitions of roles, a "my job/your job" line of thinking, can erode the kind of role flexibility required to realistically care for a group of patients as a team. Trust between members must be established, with the goal of sharing responsibilities in a flexible way that is based on the situation at hand as well as on individual team members' talents and desires.

Formative Evaluation and Redesign

Because of the dynamic nature of teams, STAR members were encouraged to approach their initial efforts with the expectation of ongoing redesign and fine-tuning. Indeed, formative evaluation throughout the first year of implementation resulted in significant changes to the original design. Constant attention to the original vision helped to assure that adjustments were made in the process to attain this vision.

Revisions in the design ranged from shifts in STAR membership and roles to major changes in the continuum of care. For example, some core members of the neuro-oncology STAR were redefined as consultative members based on limited involvement, over time, in the patient caseload. The responsibilities of the PCC were clarified as the role developed and team roles were negotiated. The scope of responsibilities was narrowed as it became evident that the job was too overwhelming. Examples of current responsibilities of the PCC are illustrated in Table 12-2. The continuum of care for three of the demonstration STARs, those originally based in rehabilitation, was extended to include the prehospitalization and acute phases of care. Changes to the design were also driven by external factors, such as shifts in treatment modalities to ambulatory care. Ultimately, the customized nature of the STARs will provide a structure that enables a well-developed team to respond quickly to internal and external forces.

▬PROGRAM EVALUATION

Evaluation plans are centered on the impact of the STARs on patient outcomes, quality and cost of care, and staff satisfaction. Extensive baseline data were gathered on the variables listed in Table 12-3. As the program progressed, it became evident that documentation of successes required gathering qualitative as well as quantitative data. Case studies and process-related stories provided a rich source of information that was incorporated into program evaluation.

Certain aspects of the STARs proved to make data retrieval extremely challenging. Because of the existing functional, departmental culture at UH, it was difficult to obtain cost data related to the full continuum of care from preadmission to postdischarge. The potential of each STAR to have multiple physician members in different services (eg, neurosurgery, neuro-

TABLE 12-2   Examples of Current Patient Care Coordinator Responsibilities

RESPONSIBILITIES TO PATIENTS AND FAMILIES	PERFORMANCE CRITERIA
Educates the patient and family regarding the STAR and how to use the hospital system. Provides or arranges for additional patient education or reinforcement as needed.	Patients and families demonstrate an ability to identify team members and differentiate roles of key members on the team. Patient and family demonstrate appropriate use of the hospital system as evidenced by examples such as seeking care at the appropriate entry point (eg, clinic, emergency room, etc.), utilization of hospital resources, etc.
Monitors the interdisciplinary plan of care across the continuum of care while continually identifying and accessing appropriate resources necessary to meet patients' needs.	Patients' and families' needs are identified and addressed by the appropriate team member as evidenced by documented outcomes on the interdisciplinary plan of care.

RESPONSIBILITIES TO THE STAR	PERFORMANCE CRITERIA
Collaborates with STAR members to establish regular communications to ensure the dissemination of the patient's plan of care. This includes initiation of patient care conferences as needed or as determined by STAR members.	Regular communication occurs between STAR members and consultative members to develop and document an interdisciplinary plan of care. STAR members have access to the interdisciplinary plan.
Ensures and/or organizes the development, implementation, and review of STAR-specific standards of care, the STAR interdisciplinary continuous quality improvement program, group peer review, and a system of monitoring and influencing cost of care.	PCC leadership and coordination efforts result in STAR continuous quality improvement efforts being developed, implemented, and revised as necessary. Quality improvement efforts reflect health care service redesign that improves or maintains quality, promotes holistic care and provider options, reduces health care costs, and helps to meet patients' expectations.

Excerpted from *STAR Patient Care Coordinator Position Description and Evaluation,* University of Utah Hospital, 1993.

oncology, and rehabilitation), required developing complex data retrieval programs. Limited hospital personnel resources to assist with data retrieval and report preparation can make this type of evaluation a very time-intensive task. Early involvement of information systems administration and staff is critical to a successful evaluation.

Early indications show a positive impact of the STAR model on team member relationships, communication, and quality of care, as reported by

TABLE 12-3   STARs Program Evaluation: Examples of Specific Variables and Tools*

VARIABLES	TOOLS
Quality of care	Patient satisfaction survey Patient-centered phone survey[†] QM monitors Functional status indicators
Cost of care	Cost per patient per day Readmissions within 30 days Use of resources (lab, diagnostics) Emergency room visits
PCC job analysis	Work sampling Case load
Staff satisfaction	Work satisfaction survey[‡] Interviews
Indicators of success	Telephone survey of STAR members Patient focus groups

*Table adapted from University Hospital, *Program to Improve Patient Care,* 1992. Phase II of a Five Year Implementation Proposal, unpublished document submitted to Strengthening Hospital Nursing: A Program to Improve Patient Care, Salt Lake City, Utah, University Hospital.
[†]Patient-Centered Care Telephone Survey, Picker/Commonwealth Patient-Centered Care Program, Boston, Mass.
[‡]Stamps, P. L. & Piedmonte, E. B. (1986). Nurses and work satisfaction: An index for measurement. Ann Arbor, Michigan: Health Administration Press.

STAR members. In a recent interview of STAR members, one individual stated, "The STAR has made the interdisciplinary team more aware of each other and willing to work as a team." Another commented, "People have more equal responsibilities to initiate solutions to problems." The PCC is seen as "another person to support patient care when the primary RN is not available." At the initial retreats, many of the individuals involved in the care of the patient had never met face-to face, did not know how to contact each other, or were not aware of the various talents and services available. These same members now meet on a regular basis to plan together the care of the patient.

Quality and cost of care have been improved by smoother transitions before admission, between units, and during discharge. As described by one member, the STAR works to "address the needs of the patient earlier and address those needs that could be neglected if there was no STAR." The role of the PCC was credited as "coordinating the care across units, which decreased the patient's length of stay." Patients were "made aware of different costs of equipment and encouraged to participate in planning their care and the cost associated with the equipment." STAR members also reported that "discharge has been better facilitated and the admission process has been sped up" and that the "STAR program helped to increase communication within the interdisciplinary team for better patient care."

Problem areas continue to exist, and other areas are targeted for continued development and improvement including team communication systems, STAR member access to information, and role clarification. As one STAR member put it, "miscommunication and overlap of jobs" can result in worse coordination. Formal training related to monitoring and improving quality and cost is just beginning. Communicating the concept of STARs to others not directly involved is an ever present challenge. Continued evaluation and revision will be an ongoing process.

▬CONCLUSION

The development and implementation of interdisciplinary teams that cross the continuum, as described here, requires careful planning, support, and ongoing evaluation. The STARs represent a step beyond restructuring nursing care; the focus is patient care. Nursing can go beyond the confines of its discipline, and nurses can lead the future of patient care delivery as key players within an organized, patient-centered team of interdependent care providers.

University Hospital's Program to Improve Patient Care at the University of Utah in Salt Lake City is supported by a grant from The Robert Wood Johnson Foundation and The Pew Charitable Trusts with technical assistance provided by the national program, Strengthening Hospital Nursing: A Program to Improve Patient Care at St. Anthony's Hospital in St. Petersburg, Florida.

The authors would like to acknowledge Jackie A. Smith, Miriam O. Young, Mimi Y. Liu, and Judith Jensen for their review and critique of this manuscript. This work would not have been possible without the energy, creativity, and vision of all of the stakeholders at University Hospital. We especially want to recognize the pioneering efforts of the patient care coordinators: Martha Bray, Tracy Harris, Michelle Leiter, and Adele Shelley. Special thanks to project co-directors Evelyn G. Hartigan, Associate Administrator, Patient Care Services, and Dale Gunnell, Chief Operating Officer.

▬REFERENCES

Ackoff, R. L. (1981). *Creating the corporate future.* New York: John Wiley.

Beck, S. L., Hartigan, E. G., & Belsey, G. W. (1993). *Application of an interactive planning model to improve patient care.* Unpublished manuscript. University Hospital, Salt Lake City.

Delbeq, A. L., Van de Ven, A. H., & Gustafson, D. H. (1975). *Group techniques and program planning: A guide to nominal group technique and Delphi process.* Glenview, IL: Scott Foresman.

Donaho, B. A. & Kohles, M. K. (1992). *Gaining momentum: A progress report.* St. Petersburg, FL: Strengthening Hospital Nursing Program.

Emshoff, J. R. (1980). *Managerial breakthroughs: Action techniques for strategic change.* New York: AMACOM.

Fottler, M. D., Blair, J. D., Whitehead, C. J., Laus, M. D., & Savage, G. T. (1989). Assessing key stakeholders: Who matters to hospitals and why? *Hospital & Health Services Administration, 34*(4), 525–546.

Gilmore, T. (1979). Managing collaborative relationships in complex organizations. *Administration of Social Work, 3*(2).

Taft, S. H. & Stearns, J. E. (1991). Organizational change toward a nursing agenda: A framework for the Strengthening Hospital Nursing Program. *Journal of Nursing Administration, 21*(2), 12–21.

Chapter 13

ProACT™ for Pediatrics: Work Redesign and Nursing Case Management

NANCY SHENDELL-FALIK

The Professionally Advanced Care Team (ProACT™) model was developed in 1988 at Robert Wood Johnson University Hospital (RWJUH) in New Brunswick, New Jersey. This patient care delivery model encompasses nursing case management within a restructured work environment. The initial impetus for an alternative practice model was the nursing shortage. The gap between nursing supply and nursing demand provided a unique opportunity to redesign systems to more efficiently and effectively use the professional nurse. Today, the compelling force for expansion and evolution of the model is no longer a nursing shortage but rather the high unit cost per nurse and the need to maximize patient throughput in the acute care setting. It is imperative that the finite human and financial resources of the hospital be managed proactively to ensure high-quality patient care in the most cost-effective manner.

The philosophical and institutional requirement for a new practice model guided our strategic thinking and provided a framework for the development of a new approach to the delivery of patient care (Ritter et al., 1992). It was determined that the model would have the following key characteristics:

- High in quality;
- Patient-centered;
- Supportive of nurses and other staff;
- Satisfying to staff;
- Physician friendly;
- Institutionally integrated;
- Compatible with our case mix, volume, and intensity;
- Based on the uniqueness of each patient care area;
- Based on evaluation research;
- Use integrated multidisciplinary care teams; and
- Supportive of institutional objectives.

Flarey, D: REDESIGNING NURSING CARE DELIVERY: Transforming Our Future

Evaluation research was conducted to measure the effects of ProACT™ on a busy medical-surgical unit, analyzing quality of care, cost of care, and patient and staff satisfaction. The initial study, reported by Brett and Tonges (1990), yielded very favorable results. Those outcomes, in combination with an increasing acuity, increasing volume, and a changing case mix, prompted the implementation of ProACT™ in the Children's Center in March 1992. The Children's Center comprises three distinct units: pediatrics, adolescent, and pediatric intensive care, which contain 24, 16, and 7 beds, respectively. In addition, these units are part of a joint designation as a Specialty Acute Care Children's Hospital of Central New Jersey. The Children's Center comprises 47 of RWJUH's 416 beds. RWJUH is an academic medical center and the core teaching hospital of the University of Medicine and Dentistry of New Jersey–Robert Wood Johnson Medical School.

WHY REDESIGN?

Work redesign projects begin with assessing whether reconfiguring the patient care process is the proper way to address particular situations (Tonges, 1992). The shortage of professional nurses and other health care workers was a situation which initially drove such action.

At RWJUH, a steering committee was formed and became the catalyst for shaping the future of patient care delivery. The interdepartmental teamwork and strong vision led to the development of unit work groups to restructure the work environment and redesign roles.

The unit work group conducted work analysis in each of the Children's Center units. The work analysis questions, which were considered vital to the work design process, were

- What work is being done?
- Is each task or activity necessary? Appropriate?
- If it is, who is doing it?
- Who could or should be doing it?

The answers to these questions demonstrated that nurses spent significant time on non-nursing functions and that the system in place was not optimal for children and their families. Opportunities to maximize resources, enhance continuity, and personalize care were evident.

DESCRIPTION OF THE MODEL

The ProACT™ model has four key distinguishing features:

- Delineation of two distinct roles for registered nurses—the primary nurse and the clinical care manager (CCM);
- Creation of the CCM role, combining high-quality clinical management with aggressive financial responsibilities (this is the nurse case manager role);
- Supervised use of assistive personnel in the delivery of direct nursing care; and

- Expansion of clinical and nonclinical support services at the unit level to relieve nursing staff of inappropriate tasks and improve the quality of service experienced by the patient and family.

Professional Nursing Roles

In the ProACT™ model, there are two professional nursing roles: nurse case manager and primary nurse. "Nurse case management is defined as a care delivery system which organizes patient care by specific case types and focuses on the achievement of outcomes within appropriate time frames and resources" (Zander, 1990, p. 1). At RWJUH, the nurse case manager is unit-based and referred to as the CCM. The CCM manages the hospital stay for a caseload of patients to ensure that outcomes are achieved within an established time frame using appropriate resources.

The CCM manages a caseload of patients by using clinical care protocols. The clinical care protocol provides a guideline for what the average patient with a particular diagnosis will experience during hospitalization. It defines predictable and critical targets which must be met in order to adhere to the expected hospital length of stay. Protocols are developed for specific diagnosis-related groups. The first protocols developed were those for the most frequent admission diagnosis for each of the Children's Center units developed. High-cost, high-volume, and high-risk criteria were considered in subsequent protocol development. Protocols outline expected outcomes within particular time frames and were developed in collaboration with physicians and other health team members.

On admission of the patient to the hospital, the CCM initiates the protocol with the patient's physician and facilitates the patient's progress in achieving the identified goals. The case manager works actively with the child and family to coordinate all services. This includes assessing the need for services, validating knowledge and understanding, scheduling complex diagnostic tests, mobilizing resources, promoting communication between all members of the health team, and early identification of problems.

Potential or actual problems in meeting outcomes are identified as variances. After they are identified, the CCM takes appropriate action to correct variances in patient care. For example, the CCM carefully evaluates any child involved in a multiple trauma to ensure that placement for posthospitalization rehabilitation does not become a negative variance. A variance analysis is completed for each patient at discharge that identifies and explains deviations from the expected plan. This provides a means to track system patterns and trends which are problematic in facilitating the achievement of necessary outcomes. After careful analysis, the case manager may articulate a need to reexamine and revise systems to streamline patient care delivery and enhance coordination of care. "Nurse case managers have a broad vision of patient care needs, especially as they relate to desired outcomes" (Bower, 1992, p. 16).

A good working relationship between the primary nurse and the CCM is essential. Case management respects and values the primary nurse–patient relationship. ProACT™ is an approach that reinforces the importance of the primary nurse to assure excellence in patient care. The CCM strives to maximize the nurse's ability to remain at the bedside to assess, plan, and evaluate nursing care for a primary group of patients. The primary nurse and CCM often consult and work collaboratively to troubleshoot any problems identified. The primary nurse assumes responsibility for direct patient care and delegates appropriately to support personnel. The primary nurse in the Children's Center works 12-hour shifts, 3 days per week. The CCM works 5 days per week and also participates in an on-call schedule. This schedule fosters the delivery of high-quality, coordinated patient care and minimizes fragmentation.

The American Nurses Association recommends that the minimum preparation for a nurse case manager is a baccalaureate degree in nursing with three years of appropriate clinical experience (Bower, 1992). In accordance with this standard, RWJUH requires a baccalaureate degree in nursing, although a master's degree is preferred. Two years of relevant clinical experience with a minimum of 1 year at the institution is also preferred.

New Unlicensed Multifunctional Roles

There are four new multifunctional roles which comprise the unlicensed support personnel in the ProACT™ model in the Children's Center. These are the support service host, pharmacy technician, clinical services technician (CST), and critical care technician (CCT).

The first new multifunctional role is that of support service host. This role combines traditional functions of housekeeping, dietary services, and central stores with a number of tasks previously performed by nursing personnel. These tasks include making unoccupied beds, preparing patients for meals, and distributing linens and water. The support service host monitors the unit's level of supplies and patient care equipment daily. The support service host also assists in cleaning toys in the Child Life Center. With the introduction of this new support service host role, the nursing assistant has been relieved of making unoccupied beds, restocking supplies, and cleaning functions and is able to perform more direct patient care activities as delegated by the nurse. The nursing assistant is now able to routinely perform specific gravity measurements, vital sign monitoring, intake and output, as well as direct services related to a patient's hygienic needs. Call lights are answered more promptly, and the unit is less cluttered because the nursing assistant performs frequent environmental rounds. During these rounds, the nursing assistant is also instructed to check crib and bed side rails and the appropriateness of toys, which enhances the safety of the pediatric unit. The reshaping of the nursing assistant role has been made possible by the development of a support service host role. Both roles support the provision of ancillary services at the unit level for maximum support of patients and nurses.

The second multifunctional support role is that of pharmacy technician. The pharmacy technician, under the supervision of a registered pharmacist, assumes responsibility for all medication-related work except actual administration. The pharmacy technician prepares medications, intravenous solutions, and medicated drips and organizes them based on each individual's medication schedule. The technician also attaches, flushes, labels, and changes intravenous tubing. The medications are then delivered to the central medication room on the pediatric and adolescent units and to each bedside supply cart in the pediatric intensive care unit. In all three units, the pharmacy technician reorders unit stock and emergency medications and counts narcotics at the change of shift with a registered nurse. Pharmacy technicians perform these functions on the day shift in the Children's Center. The pharmacy technicians are high school graduates who have successfully completed a training program by the pharmacy staff at RWJUH.

Another multiskilled worker, the CST, was introduced to the model, building on the pharmacy technician role. This specialized worker performs the tasks of phlebotomy and electrocardiography (ECG) in addition to pharmacy functions. The CST responsibilities are further redefined to meet the specific needs of the unit or service. In the Children's Center, the responsibilities are primarily pharmacy and phlebotomy because of the infrequent need for ECGs for this patient population. The CST performs all peripheral blood work in addition to all functions of the pharmacy technician. This assures the nurse that stat blood work and drug levels (ie, peak and trough levels) can be accomplished in a timely manner without multiple calls to the laboratory or physician. Individuals who fulfill the CST role have prior experience as phlebotomists or pharmacy technicians. During the evening shift, a CST is scheduled to perform these functions.

The CCT, who functions solely in the pediatric intensive care unit, is the most sophisticated assistive personnel role. This position was developed in the ProACT™ Model for Critical Care (Ritter & Tonges, 1991). The CCT is the most highly skilled multifunctional worker. The CCT performs a variety of tasks that were previously performed by critical care nurses but can safely be delegated to properly trained and supervised support personnel.

CCTs are usually students with some knowledge of health care. These include individuals enrolled in nursing or medical school or paramedic and emergency medical technician courses. These types of programs are offered in the immediate vicinity, which facilitates recruitment of qualified applicants for the hospital. In addition, the university teaching environment provides a rich learning experience, which is very attractive to prospective employees. As designed in the ProACT™ Model for Critical Care, the core of the CCT's job is task-oriented functions which are performed routinely throughout the shift. Some of the highlights of the CCT's role in the pediatric intensive care unit include

- Taking routine vital signs;
- Performing unit-based laboratory tests, such as nasogastric aspirate and stool guaiacs;
- Obtaining finger-stick blood glucose levels;
- Assisting with cardiopulmonary resuscitation;
- Performing emergency equipment checks; and
- Setting up the critical care bedside for admission.

Individualized unit worksheets have been developed to facilitate patient care delivery and improve efficiency. Although primary nurses receive intershift reports, the CCT is beginning to perform their routine functions. After the primary nurse has received a comprehensive report, he or she is able to specify tasks for the CCT based on each child's individual needs. The presence of the support service host, pharmacy technician, CST, and CCT have enabled the primary nurse to concentrate on the delivery of direct patient care, thus fostering a stronger nurse–patient relationship. In the Children's Center, nurses now spend more quality time with children and their families, and support personnel are available to assume other functions, such as obtaining necessary supplies, ensuring medications are available for administration, and completing labwork. The development of various multiskilled workers, which expands clinical and nonclinical support at the unit level, has provided new opportunities to facilitate professional nursing practice.

Environmental Redesign

In analyzing the work of each unit, it was determined that the critical care areas would benefit from environmental redesign as part of the restructured delivery system. Four elements were centralized in the traditional system and have become decentralized with ProACT™ in the pediatric intensive care unit. These new changes are the supply system, pharmaceutical system, phone system, and narcotic key system.

Supplies are now stocked in a multidrawer cart, similar to a crash cart, located at each child's bedside. This cart is filled with a 24-hour supply of items needed to meet a patient's daily needs. The cart is restocked daily by the support service host.

The second system that is now decentralized is pharmaceuticals. Pharmacy supplies are located in the first drawer of the bedside cart, which is locked. The pharmacy technician delivers a 24-hour supply of medications, intravenous solutions, and tubing to this drawer daily. This drawer also contains extra needles, syringes, sterile saline and water, heparin lock flush, tincture of benzoin, Tearisol and Lacri-Lube, which are often used. With this system, primary nurses are better able to remain at the bedside and deliver patient care.

Phones have been installed at each child's bed space for use by the health care team; therefore, a nurse can call a physician or ancillary department without leaving the patient's bedside. This enables the nurse to continually monitor a critically ill child without creating gaps by running to a central area to use the phone. This phone system is considered a great asset by the staff.

Lastly, a set of narcotic supply keys is distributed to each primary nurse at the beginning of the shift. This saves valuable time in determining who has the keys to access the narcotic cabinet. At the change of shift, a key count is performed during the narcotic count to verify all sets of keys have been returned. The narcotic key system has been very successful and has now been expanded to the pediatric and adolescent units.

The impetus for changing the supply, pharmaceutical, phone, and narcotic key systems in the pediatric intensive care unit was to maximize the primary nurse's time at the bedside and enhance quality patient care. In restructuring the delivery of patient care, it is important to consider all possibilities and create the design that fits the work environment.

Cost

Every hospital is continually challenged to be creative in the delivery of high-quality patient care while working in environments with tremendous cost constraints. The need to become more cost-effective with changing reimbursement patterns and health care reform is certainly evident. ProACT™ is designed to be budget neutral. Without incremental cost, the unit's budget after implementing the model in the Children's Center was equal to the budget before implementation. This was a necessary prerequisite for administrative approval and a key strategy for successful implementation.

ProACT™ increased the number of total full-time equivalent positions within the Children's Center. This is because of a decrease in the number of registered nurses providing direct care and an increase in the number of multifunctional support workers. This change in staff mix was facilitated by shifting role responsibilities and fully maximizing every position within the model. The case manager role on the pediatric unit was financed in two ways. First, the assistant head nurse role on the day shift was eliminated. Secondly, the changing mix of employees and nurse-to-patient ratios made additional dollars available to support a second nurse case manager in the pediatric unit. In this way, salary costs remained budget neutral.

It is apparent that the nurse case manager can achieve significant cost savings through effectively using resources, minimizing fragmentation, and increasing patient throughput in the hospital setting. "The CCM's role in minimizing cost and maximizing revenue, while enhancing quality of care, is an extremely important component of the model" (Tonges, 1989a, p. 38). With the trend toward competitive managed care environments, a restructured model must have a patient focus that maximizes efficiency, enhances revenue, demonstrates desired outcomes, and ensures quality care.

▄ EVALUATION

Evaluation research with a preevaluation and postevaluation design was used to determine the effects of ProACT™ on work environment, patient satisfaction, staff satisfaction, quality of care, cost of care, and utilization of hospital resources.

In each of the three units, the following variables were measured 1 to 2 months before implementation of ProACT™ and 6 to 8 months after implementation: acuity, average daily census, workload, occupancy rate, labor costs per patient-day, nonproductive costs per patient-day, average nonsalary costs per patient-day, patient satisfaction, nurse job satisfaction, physician satisfaction, incidents, infections, length of stay, revenue, turnover, and sick time (Table 13-1).

Each of the cost and quality variables was monitored over time to evaluate trends. Data are analyzed to determine positive effects and areas that

TABLE 13-1 Evaluation Process

OBJECTIVE	VARIABLE
To devise and institute a restructured work design in the hospital setting.	Work environment
To create rewarding roles for caregivers.	Staff satisfaction: Physician Nurse Ancillary
To ensure optional quality patient care.	Quality care: Number of infections and incidents Nursing process Nursing outcome Patient satisfaction
To maintain cost effectiveness while reducing the length of stay.	Length of stay Labor cost per patient-day Nonproductive cost per patient-day Average nonsalary cost per patient-day Turnover Sick time
To efficiently use hospital resources	Nursing care hours per patient-day Workload (census × acuity) Occupancy rate

need improvement. Figures 13–1 and 13–2, for example, illustrate positive outcomes for satisfaction and cost. Clear graphic representations are used to provide rapid and thorough evaluation of complex data.

Head nurses, directors, and members of the senior nursing management group intervene as necessary if areas of improvement are identified. Evaluation of this nature provides valuable information to determine if the model is meeting its stated objectives. Findings provide direction and guide modifications and future enhancements of the ProACT™ model.

MODEL MAINTENANCE

In the development of a new patient care delivery system, it is imperative to create a mechanism that supports and facilitates complex changes. During the planning phase for implementation of ProACT™ in the Children's Center, several support structures were put into place. First, each team, comprised of nursing, support service, and pharmacy staff on the pediatric, adolescent, and pediatric intensive care units, met weekly with the head nurse. The purpose of these meetings was to integrate all roles into one high-performance team. The director of management systems attended the meetings and served as an unbiased observer and recorder. He produced minutes of the meeting using a format that identified accomplishments and clarified activities and issues for resolution by support service, pharmacy,

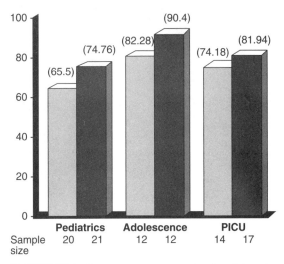

FIGURE 13-1   Survey responses evaluating job satisfaction before and after implementation of the Pro-ACT™ model. Possible score range was 23–115. PICU, Pediatric Intensive Care Unit.

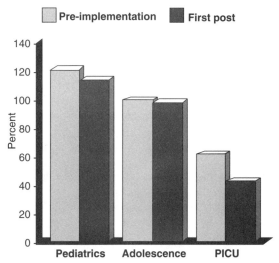

FIGURE 13-2   Length of hospital stay before and after implementation of the ProACT™ model. PICU, Pediatric Intensive Care Unit.

and nursing staff. The minutes were distributed to the staff within 2 days of the meeting; this validated that efforts were appreciated, suggestions reviewed, and problems resolved in a timely manner.

Other departmentally integrated meetings occur in order to support the model on an institutional level. The ProACT™ steering committee is an interdisciplinary group that meets monthly to discuss issues and trends related to the restructured work environment. It considers suggestions for change to ensure that every unit remains committed to the vision and objectives of the work redesign project. This ensures an institutional approach.

Nursing has several subcommittees to address the issues related to nursing case management and patient care delivery. One committee consists of the vice president of nursing, nursing directors, and head nurses. It meets monthly to focus on nursing issues and relationships. The committee continually strives to improve all work processes to enhance attainment of patient and family needs. Another subcommittee, which meets twice a month, is devoted to ongoing evaluation and refinement of the nurse case manager role. One meeting is a CCM business meeting, and the second is for CCM case presentations. The presentations provide a way to highlight the contributions the nurse case management program makes to the institution and facilitates continuous education and development of the role. The protocol subcommittee meets monthly to develop, review, and revise protocols. This assures the protocols consistently reflect the current practice and the case mix of RWJUH.

The essential work accomplished by the group illustrates that a supportive structure must exist. This structure perpetuates, innovates, and manages the highly complex relationships, concepts, and systems associated with a redesigned patient care delivery model.

■ FUTURE INNOVATIONS

In mid-1993, the steering committee conducted a ProACT™ retreat that involved many hospital departments. The objective of the retreat was to identify ways to further improve and innovate the delivery of services to patients using the coordination of present and future services in the ProACT™ model. Approximately 100 participants were involved, 75% of whom, representing every role, were front-line individuals with experience functioning within the model. The remaining 25% consisted of representatives from departments not currently in the model, including social service, radiology, respiratory, physical/occupational therapy, escort, admitting, home care, emergency, and quality management services.

Presently, a qualitative analysis of recommendations from the retreat is in process, and the steering committee will determine priorities for expansion and innovation. Certain departments, such as radiology, escort, and respiratory services, now want to formally integrate into the model. This will enhance the vision that the ProACT™ model represents the way the entire hospital organizes to deliver patient care and will further increase institutional commitment.

It is important to periodically examine how the model contributes to the achievement of institutional objectives to assure broad support and ongoing enthusiasm (Fralic, 1992a). In this way, the challenge of creating a contemporary and dynamic delivery system which meets RWJUH objectives will be met.

The author thanks these individuals for their invaluable contributions and assistance: Maryann F. Fralic, PhD, RN, FAAN, Senior Vice President, Nursing; Joanne Ritter, MA, RN, CCRN, Director, Critical Care Nursing; Maureen Bueno, PhD, RN, Director, Nursing Systems; and Kathy Soriano, RNC, MS, Head Nurse, Adolescent Unit.

▬ REFERENCES

Bower, K. A. (1992). *Case management by nurses.* Washington, DC: American Nurses Publishing.

Brett, J. L. & Tonges, M. C. (1990). Restructured patient care delivery: Evaluation of the ProACT™ model. *Nursing Economics, 8*(1), 36–44.

Fralic, M. F. (1992a). Creating new practice models and designing new roles: Reflections and recommendations. *Journal of Nursing Administration, 22*(6), 7–8.

Ritter, J. & Tonges, M. C. (1991). Work redesign in high intensity environments: ProACT™ for critical care. *Journal of Nursing Administration, 21*(12), 26–35.

Ritter, J., Fralic, M. F., Tonges, M. C., & McCormac, M. (1992). Redesigned nursing practice: A case management model for critical care. *Nursing Clinics of North America, 27*(1), 119–128.

Tonges, M. C. (1989a). Redesigning hospital nursing practice: The Professionally Advanced Care Team (ProACT™) model, Part 1. *Journal of Nursing Administration, 19*(7), 31–38.

Tonges, M. C. (1989b). Redesigning hospital nursing practice: The Professionally Advanced Care Team (ProACT™) model, Part 2. *Journal of Nursing Administration, 19*(8), 19–22.

Tonges, M. C. (1990, March). ProACT™: A positive response to the nursing shortage. *Echo,* pp. 26–27.

Tonges, M. C. (1992). Work designs: Sociotechnical systems for patient care delivery. *Nursing Management, 23*(1), 27–32.

Weber, D. O. (1991, July/August). Six models of patient-focused care. *Healthcare Forum Journal,* pp. 23–32.

Zander, K. (1990). *Differentiating managed care and case management.* Boston: The Center for Nursing Case Management, New England Medical Center.

Chapter 14

Caremap® and Case Management Systems: Evolving Models Designed to Enhance Direct Patient Care

MARIA HILL

Operational restructuring of care delivery systems is a highly significant activity occurring in health care institutions across the country. Improving the efficiency and effectiveness of patient care operations is the central focus of all restructuring projects.

Constant change in our health care environment requires more efficient and cost-effective alternatives in caring for patients. Two approaches are explained in this chapter. Also described is the production process (the system's purpose), the work to be done to move patients of a specific case type through the continuum of health care, the resources needed to accomplish this end, the outcomes (results) to be achieved, and the issues or systems inhibiting efficient care management. Explored are the reengineering of clinical processes through the CareMap® system and integration with variance analysis, continuous quality improvement, and case management.

The need for modifications in the delivery and management of patient care is complex. Such imperatives are driven by complex developments in medicine, shifts in economics and government regulations, and changes in demographics. During the past two decades we have witnessed unprecedented advances in medicine and technology, the appearance of epidemics such as acquired immunodeficiency syndrome, and threats posed by organisms such as methicillin-resistant *Staphylococcus aureus* and drug-resistant tuberculosis. Patients are also changing. As the population ages, there are increasing numbers of chronically ill patients. Patients are demanding access to a quality system of care at reasonable rates, despite a continuing decline in reimbursements. Many treatment avenues are shifting to alternate sites and models, such as subacute or transitional care, ambulatory care, clinics, surgical suites, and community-oriented health care programs. Length of stay for acute, inpatient care, and total number of inpatient days per year are decreasing. Hospital systems or networks are rapidly evolving because of diversification of services, mergers, and acquisitions. Such changes are broadening our awareness of the business of health care beyond traditional inpatient services. These factors contribute to the need for providers to restructure and redesign systems to promote effective and efficient management of patient care across the health care continuum.

▬REDESIGN FOR SYSTEMS IMPROVEMENT

CareMap® and case management systems are pragmatic and flexible clinical systems designed to span the care continuum and focus on cost and quality care outcomes. The systems were developed at the New England Medical Center (NEMC) in 1985 in response to 1) the inability of the documentation system to assist clinicians in integrating a plan of care into one working document, 2) the limited ability of diagnosis-related group (DRG) systems to accurately reflect the required resources for care delivery and its concomitant reimbursement limits, 3) the advancement of nursing knowledge without expanded skills and roles to support the knowledge, and 4) the experience of key administrative players at NEMC in a sociotechnical systems approach to work redesign (Zander, 1992).

CareMap® and case management systems have evolved over the past 10 years. The current goals of these systems include identifying patient/family needs, determining time frames necessary to achieve quality patient outcomes, reducing length of stay and inappropriate use of resources, and clarifying the appropriate environment, providers, and timeliness of interventions across the health care continuum. These systems serve as the major impetus to restructure and redesign projects, and in identifying core patient populations served, clinical needs demonstrated by the patient case type, and priority outcomes to be achieved along the continuum of care. They also pinpoint inefficiencies that inhibit the delivery of effective quality care, as well as work process duplication by various professionals. CareMap® and case management systems are exemplary models of care delivery restructuring and redesign that drive the delivery of high-quality, cost-effective care.

▬THE CAREMAP® SYSTEM

This system is designed to provide continuity to the plan of care and consists of four critical components: 1) the CareMap® tool, 2) variance analysis, 3) communication processes (eg, physician rounds, discharge planning rounds, patient/family conferences, change of shift reports, health care team meetings), and 4) collaborative group practices (Zander, 1992).

A strong infrastructure is necessary to implement a fully integrated CareMap® system (Zander, 1993). The structure which most successfully supports this system includes a central steering committee composed of top-level administrators representing operational and support services, a design team composed of clinical staff, collaborative group practices composed of professionals directly involved in care of specific patient groups, and a project manager.

Developing The CareMap® System

The *steering committee* provides clear direction and leadership of the process by overseeing program development, implementation, and evaluation; determining program goals; selecting case types; allocating resources; and establishing specific activities. The *design team* creates the standard templates for the CareMap® and variance tools and develops guidelines for their use. The team also identifies roles and responsibilities for clinicians as they interface with the CareMap® system and develops the new documentation system as the central focus of the patient's medical record. Roles and responsibilities of *collaborative group practices* include creating CareMap® tools; piloting these tools with specific patients and making appropriate changes after implementation; creating educational materials which complement the Care-Maps®; and aggregating, analyzing, and addressing variances. Teams use a continuous quality improvement (CQI) process to analyze variance data. The *project manager's* role is all-encompassing. He or she directs the work plan, serves as staff to the steering committee, leads the design team, facilitates CareMap® development, and establishes an office and library to support these systems.

The CareMap® tool consists of four key elements (Figs. 14–1 and 14–2): 1) the critical pathway, with the x-axis representing the time line and the y-axis representing multidisciplinary interventions incorporated into standard categories; 2) a patient problem or issues list; 3) intermediate goals which progress to clinical outcomes for each problem or issue identified; and 4) a variance record designed to capture chronological deviations from the norm (Center for Case Management, 1992a). Potential problems or inefficiencies requiring investigation and further process improvements are identified through variance analysis.

The CareMap® is created for specific patient case types by a team of professional staff (collaborative group practice) intimately involved in the delivery of care. To gain a consumer's perspective, a patient who has received care through the CareMap® system may be invited by the group to help evaluate the care. The case type identified for caremapping may be designated by DRG, ICD-9 code, procedure, or condition. Discussed and analyzed are priority problems, issues, concerns experienced by patients, and the cost of care for the case type selected. Patterns of care can be identified for each case type selected through chart review, evaluation of standard plans of care, comparison of clinical practice guidelines published by professional organizations, analysis of institutional policies and procedures, and reviews of physician orders.

Clinical outcomes are identified for each respective issue or problem. The team maps out the care delivered by preselected time intervals or phases of clinical progression. At this point in the process, the traditional aspects of care delivery are challenged. The group inquires why the test, task, or intervention is required. What can be changed without negatively impacting the quality of care delivered? Interventions democratically agreed on by members of the team are then listed in the appropriate cell of

(text continues on page 178)

COLUMNS: ER - DAY 3

DRG:

Prescribed LOS: 6 Days

Congestive Heart Failure CareMap®
CAREGIVER INTERVENTIONS
CRITICAL PATH
SECTION 1

ADDRESSOGRAPH

DATE																
INTERVENTIONS	**DAY 1** **ER 1-4 Hours**	N	D	E	**DAY 1** **Floor Telemetry or CCU** **6-24 Hours**	N	D	E	**DAY 2** **Floor**	N	D	E	**DAY 3** **Floor**	N	D	E
Assessments **Consults**	Vital signs q 15 mins Nursing assessments focus on lung sounds, edema, color, skin integrity, jugular vein distention Cardiac monitor Arterial line if needed Swan Gantz Daily weight Intake and output				VS q 15 minutes Repeat nursing assessments Cardiac monitor Arterial line Swan Gantz Weight I & O				VS q 4 h Repeat nursing assessments D/C cardiac monitor at 24 hr D/C arterial and Swan Gantz Weight I & O				VS q 6 h Repeat nursing assessments Weight I & O			
Specimens/Tests	Consider TSH studies Chest X-ray EKG CPK q 8h X 3 ABG if pulse OX:____ Lytes, Na++, K, Cl, CO2, GLU, BUN, Creatinine Digoxin: (range)_____				B/G				Evaluate for ECHO Lytes, BUN, Creat							
Treatments	O2 or intubate IV or Heparin Lock				O2 IV or Heparin Lock				IV or Heparin Lock				D/C pulse Ox if stable D/C IV or Hep lock			

FIGURE 14-1 Sample problem list, intermediate goals and outcomes.

COLUMNS: ER - DAY 3

DRG:

Prescribed LOS: 6 Days

Congestive Heart Failure CareMap®
Standard of Care
PATIENT/FAMILY OUTCOMES
SECTION 1

CareMap ® is a registered trademark of The Center for Case Management, Inc. 6 Pleasant Street, So. Natick, MA 01760, tel. 508-661-2600

ADDRESSOGRAPH

DATE

PROBLEM/FOCUS	DAY 1 ER/1-4 Hours	N	D	E	DAY 1 Floor Telemetry or CCU 6-24 hours	N	D	E	DAY 2 Floor	N	D	E	DAY 3 Floor	N	D	E
1. Alteration in gas exchange/perfusion and fluid balance due to decreased cardiac volume	Reduced pain from admission or Pain Free				Respirations equal to or less than on admission				O2 Sat = 90				Does not require O2			
	Uses pain scale								Respiration 20-22				VSS			
									Vital Signs Stable				Crackles at base			
	O2 Sat improved over admission baseline on O2 therapy								Crackles at lung bases				Resp 20-22			
									Mild SOB with activity				Mild SOB with activity			
2. Potential for shock	No S/S of shock				No S/S of shock				No S/S of shock				No S/S of shock			
													Normal lab values			
3. Potential for consequences of immobility and decreased activity: skin breakdown, DVT	No redness at pressure points				No redness at pressure points				Tolerates chair, washing, eating and toileting				Has bowel movement			
	No falls				No falls								Up in room and bathroom with assist			
4. Alteration in nutritional intake due to nausea and vomiting, labored breathing					No c/o nausea				Eating solids				Taking 50 % of each meal			
					No vomiting				Takes in 50% of each meal							
					Taking liquids as offered											

FIGURE 14-2 Sample critical pathway, multidisciplinary interventions.

the standard template. In addition, the intermediate goals, which drive clinical outcomes, are identified and listed for each time interval or clinical phase. Through this effort the team moves from current to best practice.

The functions of a CareMap® tool include coordinating the interdisciplinary plan of care over an episode of illness, focusing care delivery on outcome management, providing central documentation for the medical record, and establishing the standard against which to measure care delivered to a specific patient within an identified population.

Use of CareMaps® in Practice

When a patient is admitted, the appropriate CareMap® is selected. The tool is individualized to meet unique patient needs. For example, adding information for a secondary, active diagnosis facilitates individualization. This may include adding management of diabetes mellitus for an elderly patient recently placed on insulin therapy who is being treated for a primary problem of congestive heart failure. The CareMap® would identify information related to the management of insulin therapy, recognition of hypoglycemic reactions, the ability to follow a recommended American Diabetes Association diet, knowledge of skin and foot care, and the demonstration of blood glucose monitor use.

After the CareMap® has been individualized, health care team members directly involved in the patient's care use it to assist them in overall patient care management. Clinicians use the tool to manage the care delivered over specified time intervals for the entire episode of illness. In acute care and skilled nursing care facilities, CareMaps® are used 24 hours a day. In ambulatory care settings, they are used for same-day surgical procedures from admission through discharge and for visits to the physician's office, nursing center, or home care setting.

In all settings, nurses typically are the micro-managers of patient care, because they spend the most time in providing direct care. As micro-managers, nurses coordinate team efforts to meet the identified intermediate goals and outcomes at the appropriate times. However, every team member is expected to record information on the CareMap® tool, such as initial interventions, intermediate goals, and achieved outcomes (see Fig. 14-1). In addition, team members must identify, record, and respond to variances in a timely manner. Because of proximity, it is often the professional nurse who recognizes that a variance has occurred and mobilizes appropriate team members to create an action plan to address the problem or issue.

Variance Analysis

Variances occur when the unexpected happens. Variances can be positive, if a patient progresses ahead of the schedule identified on the CareMap®, or negative, if a patient does not progress as planned. This may occur if interventions are not completed, the patient does not meet the expected intermediate goals, or outcomes are not achieved.

There are four categories of variances: 1) patient/family, 2) clinician, 3) internal system, and 4) external system (Center for Case Management, 1992b). Patient/family variances occur if a patient's clinical condition changes or length of stay is negatively impacted because of lack of family involvement in the patient's care. Some examples are development of a gastrointestinal bleed, a lack of family support and ability to care for a patient after discharge, or failure of a parent to present for a scheduled teaching session on Hickman catheter care in the home. Clinician variances occur for many reasons. For example, a staff member may fail to consult expert resources available to assist in efficiently managing patient needs; there is a lack of timely response to a consultation or request to review a patient's condition; or a team member does not complete a key intervention as detailed on the CareMap®. Internal system variances occur if a department is overbooked; the appropriate medication, equipment, or ordered supplies are unavailable; or a scheduled procedure is canceled. External system variances may include inavailablility of an extended care bed. Another example would be a lack of home health care personnel to allow movement of a patient from an acute care facility into the home for continued care.

Variance analysis occurs at two levels: the concurrent or individual patient care level and the retrospective or aggregate case type level. As previously indicated, variance analysis is an essential component of a CQI initiative. It generally provides data that quality assurance programs have not successfully uncovered. The system provides data which is extracted directly from the clinicians delivering direct care to patients and families. This process of data collection and analysis provides opportunities to develop strategies for improvements in the overall delivery of patient care. It also allows management to determine where system inefficiencies exist and to effectively problem-solve to improve the care delivery process. These activities enhance quality clinical outcomes and minimize costs.

Data generated by a variance analysis system can be voluminous. It is imperative to ask several key questions before creating a structure for variance analysis: 1) What are the goals for variance analysis? 2) What information is needed to attain the identified goals? 3) What additional information is desired by the clinicians for specific case types? 4) Is a computer system available for data entry? 5) What resources are available for data entry? 6) What is the process for review of the data? and 7) Who should receive what data?

Some examples of results realized through effective variance analysis structures for the cardiac bypass surgical case type at Healthspan's Mercy and Unity Hospitals include creation of protocols for early weaning and extubation of patients in intensive care units; early and aggressive mobility programs in the intensive care and telemetry units; administration of prophylactic Inderal to prevent atrial arrhythmias, creating shorter intensive care stays; and alteration of strict use of the cardiac diet after surgery to encourage adequate caloric intake for the promotion of tissue healing.

Managing CareMap® Systems

The CareMap® is an extremely powerful management tool. It provides evidence of clinical outcomes achieved and allows professionals to focus narration on the identified variances. In addition, it targets interventions that have not been completed and outcomes that have not been achieved. It provides an accountability mechanism, enabling follow-up with the individuals who did not assume appropriate responsibility.

CareMap® systems can be integrated into any type of nursing care delivery system. Redefining the focus and role of the staff nurse is essential to the success of this system. Essential skills needed for clinicians to successfully direct and manage care include knowledge of the disease process and potential complications, repertoire of interventions to remedy the most commonly seen complications, strong decision-making skills, knowledge of when assistance of another professional is required and what resources are available, basic administrative skills, and an understanding of one's own level of authority. To accomplish this, staff must be educated on the aforementioned skills, encouraged to practice them in a risk-taking environment, and mentored to develop strong decision-making, conflict resolution, and negotiation skills. Because of this need, several institutions have implemented care coordinators who are responsibile for managing the CareMap® and variance analysis system for specified case types at the unit level.

Only with strong, innovative management can this system grow and prosper. Nurse managers must appropriately impart clinical and systems knowledge, delegate authority and responsibility, and create a network of health care team members and resources. It is also necessary to provide the required education and training and to create and support an environment of healthy interpersonal relations in which conflict is managed between staff members and patients or families, as well as between physicians and other professionals. In addition, managers must assist staff in the transition from intervention to an outcome focus, from shift-based to episode-based care, from sole patient proprietorship to a team network, and from a focus on the individual patient to understanding patterns of needs for particular patient populations. Finally, managers must assist the team in identifying which professionals are accountable for specific tasks and outcomes of care. It is necessary to focus on the above issues to eliminate redundancy of efforts occurring within and across disciplines. It is essential to eliminate the interventions performed at cross-purposes and to acknowledge the necessity of coordinating and prioritizing identification of problems, determining the interventions to be performed by specific disciplines, and reinforcing each others' efforts to achieve key patient outcomes. In addition, job redesign and restructuring of the division of labor can be more readily planned for and realized with good management.

CareMap® systems simplify and standardize rational planning through a strong team planning and management approach. The CareMap® tool serves as a quick reference on the history and status of the patient, because it is the core of the medical record and the primary system of documenting the process of care delivered as well as the intermediate goals and outcomes achieved (see Figs. 14–1 and 14–2). System inefficiencies and staff performance are readily assessed through the ongoing use and analysis of CareMaps®.

CareMaps® also foster the development of strong collaborative relationships among professionals. This provides an effective vehicle for developing multidisciplinary care teams. The 1990s will become the decade of team management of patient populations across the continuum of health care. The challenge will be to get the key players together and teach them to talk to one another and respect the knowledge that each member brings to the care of patients and families. Other challenges will be to outline the domain of accountability for each discipline within each case type, acknowledge the old agendas interfering with integration, and create new transdisciplinary practices (Porter-O'Grady, 1993).

CASE MANAGEMENT

Case management is a dynamic model that is constantly evolving. As the need for a system of care across the continuum rather than event-managed care (Berwick, 1989) and the need to maintain a balance between cost, process of care delivery, and desired clinical outcomes (Etheredge, 1989) are expected, clinicians from a variety of disciplines turn to case management as an optimal model. Programs of service coordination extend back to the turn of the century, at which time the focus was social and financial support for the impoverished. Models of public health nursing have always held coordination of services as a primary focus. The term "case management" now appears in the nursing, insurance, social work, quality control, and utilization management literature. The common elements of these programs are service coordination and care management.

The primary objective of case management is to coordinate care and services for patients and families requiring extensive interventions. CareMap® and case management systems are designed to focus on the achievement of patient outcomes, within effective and appropriate time frames, while making efficient use of resources. The primary emphasis of the CareMap® tool is continuity of the plan of care. However, in a case management model, the emphasis is on both continuity of plan and provider of care (Center for Case Management, 1992c). In addition, in a case management model, continuity extends beyond traditional geographic boundaries to the continuum of care. Case management focuses on the entire episode of illness, crossing all geographic settings in which the patient receives care (Zander, 1990). Several factors impact the focus of a case management program and practice. These factors include the theory or perspective of the educational training program of the practitioner (nursing, social work, medicine, physical therapy); issues that arise in the health care setting in which the professional practices (home, ambulatory, long-term, or acute care); goals of the case management program (insurance-, employer-, provider-, or family-based); and needs of the patient population served (maternal-child, mental health, gerontology, or acutely chronic and chronically acute).

According to Bower (1992), case management may be implemented as a strategy to 1) focus on the full spectrum of patient and family needs over the continuum of care, 2) coordinate care across disciplines and settings, 3) manage the cost of care by decreasing fragmentation and weighing the value of completion and timing of diagnostic tests and interventions performed, 4) merge clinical and financial outcomes, and 5) gain external market contracts.

Case management is often an additional expense, so the model should be reserved for select case types or outliers within particular patient case types. Programs may target high-volume, high-cost or high-risk populations. Examples are patients who are chronically ill with cognitive or moderate to severe functional deficits (eg, frail elderly with pneumonia and dementia, adults with chronic severe depression, women with multiple sclerosis); individuals with complex acute illness (eg, large pressure ulcer over coccyx, multisystem failure); and those complex, long-term, chronic illnesses (eg, AIDS, neonates weighing less than 1,400 grams, heart and lung transplant patients, children and young adults with cystic fibrosis). Patients who become recognized as outliers within a CareMap® system may also require case management. This may include patients who develop numerous complications following a procedure, are admitted with multiple active diagnoses, or evidence numerous variances from the CareMap®.

Systems Development
Designing case management programs and roles is an exciting challenge. Case management is a process, and there are many ways to structure a comprehensive program. Key issues to focus on when creating a model (Center for Case Management, 1992, p. 35) include

1. What patients will be case-managed?
2. What are the goals for the case management program?
3. What are the care needs of the patients and families requiring case management?
4. What is the trajectory of illness or health maintenance for the patient case type?
5. When in the trajectory should the population be case-managed?
6. What are the problems, issues, cyclical patterns?
7. Who should be included in the case management practice?
8. What services should be included in the network?
9. What are the resources available for case management?
10. Who would be the best case manager?

In addressing these issues, it is imperative that clinicians from multiple disciplines and settings discuss the complexity of needs, trajectory of illness, problems and issues, and services required. Collaboration and establishment of a network of services is essential to the success of the program. From the responses to these questions, the structure for a case management program is shaped.

Case Manager Role
The role of the case manager is critical to the model process. The role is directly affected by the patient population to be managed, the setting from which the case manager functions (home, ambulatory, acute care, social or insurance agency), whether the case manager is a coordinator or provider of direct patient care, and the scope of clinical and administrative management.

The primary functional categories of the case manager role include clinical expertise; administrative management and creation of a strong, expanded network; mentorship; and the promotion of self-growth. The specific functions of the case manager (Bower, 1992; Quinn, 1992) are to

- Case-find and screen clients appropriate for the practice;
- Comprehensively assess patient and family goals, health, emotional status, cognitive ability, functional ability including activities of daily living and instrumental activities of daily living, environmental status, formal and informal support systems, and financial status;
- Analyze and address the strengths and problems identified in the assessment;
- Develop, coordinate, implement, monitor, and modify a plan of care with the health care team, client, caregivers, individuals providing custodial services, and payors;
- Develop collaborative relationships with an interdisciplinary team representing the continuum of care and create a cooperative relationship with a network of quality service providers;
- Educate the patient, family, and community on appropriate health-related topics;
- Monitor the plan and the patient's progress towards the defined outcomes;
- Monitor the quality of activities performed by any contracted services; and
- Evaluate the program of care for all patients.

Case management has demonstrated effectiveness in reducing costs and improving client outcomes and satisfaction (Bair, Griswold & Head, 1989; Ethridge, 1991; Ethridge & Lamb, 1991; Quinn, 1992). Both CareMap® and case management systems demonstrate that when patient issues and outcomes are the focal points for health care systems, quality, efficiency, and effectiveness coexist.

▬OUTCOMES ACHIEVED USING CAREMAP® AND CASE MANAGEMENT SYSTEMS

The benefits realized from implementation of these systems are very exciting. Facilities that have developed a strong infrastructure and dedicated appropriate resources to these efforts (Healthspan's Mercy and Unity Hospitals, Montclaire Baptist Medical Center, Providence Medical Center, Scripps Institutions of Medicine and Science, and Tuscon Medical Center) have experienced some of the following outcomes:

- Cost savings through decreases in laboratory procedures, tests performed, interventions delivered, equipment and supplies used, and a decreased length of stay;
- Identification and monitoring of key clinical outcomes;
- Decrease in fragmentation of care by expanding the CareMap® tool and the work of case managers to span geographic locations;
- Impact on access to services by monitoring the use of emergency de-

partment services by specific patient populations and encouraging substitution with primary care sites;
- Improved patient satisfaction; and
- Enhanced communication on patient care issues between the patient or family and health care professionals.

▬THE FUTURE OF CAREMAP® AND CASE MANAGEMENT SYSTEMS

As models for health care reform unfold, it becomes apparent that systems which demonstrate enhanced patient care management are essential. These models span the continuum. They extend from the acute care setting to the ambulatory, transitional care, and home care settings for all case types. In addition, the focus must shift from an illness model to one of prevention and health maintenance for adults and children.

The CareMap® and case management systems provide a structure and process to better understand patient care needs, outcomes to be achieved, and the necessary resources to be allocated to achieve the desired outcomes. They will, after they become computerized, provide the foundation to link clinical and financial data and acuity/severity systems and to provide reports to monitor the cost of care delivered versus anticipated reimbursement on an annual, day by day, or visit by visit basis.

In addition, information collected through implementation of these systems may be used to restructure and redesign health care systems across the continuum. The structure of the hospital and hospital system will change dramatically. The bases for restructuring personnel, equipment, patient care, and information systems may be clustered by product line or by case type needs. Such needs may include the type and number of specific professional discipline services required, the type of equipment and supplies needed, the amount and level of investigational technology used, the length of stay in acute, subacute, or home care, and the level of case management services required on an ongoing basis. At United Samaritan Hospital, nursing staff follow several patient case types from the hospital to the home setting to more efficiently use nursing staff and enhance continuity of patient care (Donlevy, 1993). Healthspan's Unity and Mercy Hospitals have established a very successful cardiac product line using an integration of CareMap®, case management, variance analysis, CQI, and peer review processes (Henry, in press).

The implementation of these innovative systems will greatly assist hospital executives and nurse managers in understanding the needs of patient populations and in meeting cost and quality imperatives while reengineering clinical systems in this new age of health care reform.

▬CONCLUSION

Presented were two distinct patient care management systems, comprising the initial step in the process of restructuring care delivery systems. With respect to restructuring, these systems support the notions that form follows function and that the production process outlines both the function of care to be delivered and the basis on which the structure for care delivery should be built. The strength of these two systems is the merging of standards of practice (critical pathway) and standards of care (CareMap®) with a focus on patient outcomes realized as a result of care received. Emphasis on productivity and interdisciplinary team management and integration with a CQI process through variance analysis are central to the models' success. These programs require a total commitment from all members and disciplines in the organization. Total involvement of individuals within the organization and coordination among clinical professionals, both within and outside the organization, will be essential to the overall success of these systems.

▬REFERENCES

Bair, N. N., Griswold, J., & Head, J. (1989). Clinical RN involvement in bedside-centered case management. *Nursing Economics, 7*(3), 150–154.

Berwick, D. M. (1989). Continuous quality improvement as an ideal in health care, *New England Journal of Medicine, 320*(1), 54.

Bower, K. A. (1992). *Case management by nurses.* Washington, DC: American Nurses Publishing.

Center for Case Management. (1992a). *Definitions.* South Natick, MA: Author.

Center for Case Management. (1992b). *Variance management.* South Natick, MA: Author.

Center for Case Management. (1992c). *Case Management.* South Natick, MA: Author.

Cohen, E. L. (1991). Nursing case management: Does it pay? *Journal of Nursing Administration, 21*(4), 20–25.

Donlevy, J. (1993). Responsive restructuring: Part I. Acute care nurses provide home care visits. *The New Definition, 8*(3), 1–3.

Etheredge, M. L. (Ed.). (1989). *Collaborative care: Nursing case management.* Chicago: American Hospital.

Ethridge, P. (1991). A nursing HMO: Carondelet St. Mary's experience. *Nursing Management, 20*(7), 22–27.

Ethridge, P. & Lamb, G. (1991). Professional nursing case management improves quality, access, and cost. *Nursing Management, 20*(3), 30–35.

Henry, S. (in press). Integrating critical paths and case management into the product line management strategies at Healthspan's Mercy and Unity Hospitals. In P. Spath (Ed.), *Critical path implementation and applications in health care.* Chicago: American Hospital.

Porter-O'Grady, T. (1993). Patient-focused care service models and nursing: Perils and possibilities. *Journal of Nursing Administration, 23*(3), 7–15.

Quinn, J. (1992). *Successful case management in long-term care.* New York: Springer.

Zander, K. (1990). Differentiating managed care and case management. *Definition, 5*(2), 1.

Zander, K. (1992). Critical pathways. In M. M. Melum & M. K. Sinioris (Eds.), *Total quality management: The health care pioneers.* Chicago: American Hospital.

Zander, K. (1993). Toward a fully integrated CareMap® and case management system. *The New Definition, 8*(2), 1.

Chapter 15

The Vincentian Redesign Experience

MARY ANN DIMOLA   SISTER EILEEN DONOGHUE

TERRY KACMARYNSKI   KATHRYN KUWIK   SANDRA HAZEN

Health care reform is one of the most pressing concerns today, not only for hospitals but for society as a whole. As our nation moves toward universal access and the restructuring of the entire health care delivery system, community care networks, global budgeting, and managed competition are pressuring hospitals to become more innovative in the way they operate. Hospitals must offer a continuum of quality services at a fixed price to effectively compete for patients. Efficiently run hospitals that continuously improve organizational performance will have the greatest chance of success in a reformed system.

Given the political and social mandates for change, St. Vincent's Health System in Jacksonville, Florida, began looking critically at its continuum of care as well as its clinical roles and expectations, in an effort to maximize patient outcomes. This process began in the fall of 1988 and was driven at that time not by a government reform plan but by a response to professional staff shortages, most notably in nursing. A hospital-wide effort, funded in part by a "Strengthening Hospital Nursing" grant from The Robert Wood Johnson Foundation and The Pew Charitable Trusts, emerged to determine how to best use our human resources and other organizational assets to provide premium, integrated patient care which positively impacts the bottom line.

The outcome was a model of patient care delivery called "The Vincentian Program," in honor of St. Vincent DePaul, who devoted his life to service of the poor, sick, and aged. The mission statement of the program is outlined in Display 15-1. In the past five years, this model has evolved and been refined, but it still remains a work in progress to some extent. We realize that our experience has been a luxury that many other institutions will not be allowed. We had the opportunity to develop a concept with ample time and to test practices and redesigned clinical roles, make revisions, and evaluate outcomes without the pressures of impending reform and strategic urgency. It is our hope that this chapter of our history will help others who embark on a redesign project to accelerate their own successes.

Flarey, D: REDESIGNING NURSING CARE DELIVERY: Transforming Our Future

---

DISPLAY 15-1   Mission Statement of the Vincentian Program

The Vincentian program will design a model for delivery of care to patients stressing quality of service, cost-effectiveness, and efficiency while adhering to the mission of the Daughters of Charity which fosters respect and compassion for all.

St. Vincent's Health System comprises St. Vincent's Medical Center (SVMC), a 528-bed tertiary care center; Riverside Hospital, a 183-bed acute care hospital; St. Catherine Laboure Manor, a 240-bed long-term care facility, and a corporate structure with various community health care businesses. It is a member of the Daughters of Charity National Health System, the fourth largest health system in the nation.

PLANNING FRAMEWORK

An idealized model was used as a planning framework. This framework was popularized by Russell Ackoff, Professor of Systems Science of The Wharton School at the University of Pennsylvania and a health care and business consultant. We also experimented with scenarios ("If we could..., then we would...") rather than merely "fixing up" our current system.

Our planning was extremely interactive and occurred at all levels within the institution. Staff representing all disciplines and all positions in the organizational hierarchy were involved. The importance of this aspect of the process cannot be underestimated. Aside from creating a plan for innovation, the collaboration and enthusiasm generated were significant byproducts of the overall process. All participants had a stake in the outcome and some degree of ownership and acceptance of change. An advisory board was created as a consulting body and included top hospital executives, physicians, board members, and community leaders such as the dean of the University of North Florida, and the president of the Daughters of Charity National Health System. A smaller core team was composed of executive hospital staff: the chief executive officer, chief operating officer, vice president for nursing, chief of medical staff, and project director. This core team was the approving body and ultimate decision-making group. There were additional focus groups made up of physicians, staff, and patients.

A steering committee, which was the major working group, included representatives from all patient care departments and other key service areas such as finance, medical records, and education. Because this group was fairly large, some smaller, focused work groups were established. These often divided further into extended work groups, which added additional staff layers to the process.

Planning and implementing a redesigned practice model is a significant undertaking. This project raised the consciousness of not only administrators, nurses, and physicians but all employees regarding important aspects and outcomes of the care we deliver. Redesigned practice has enabled us to provide our staff with opportunities to develop new skills, refine old ones, and stretch talents to achieve new practice patterns. Although this growth has been difficult, it is rewarding to both the individual and the health care environment.

■ MODEL DESCRIPTION

Traditionally, many physicians practiced on a specific unit, and their patients often shared a common pathology. A typical patient was assigned to a diagnosis-related group (DRG) on the third day of hospitalization or at discharge. Patients were transferred up to five times during hospitalization, resulting in an average of 2,100 total transfers per month. There was a narrow range of patient acuity; as patients became more ill or improved, they were transferred to other units. The support services were totally departmentalized.

Before redesign, the traditional "team" seldom went on group rounds, and a patient interacted with up to 30 individuals a day. Nurses were very task-oriented and provided minimal direction to technical assistants. The courier/transport process was fragmented, and often nurses or other health care professionals provided this service.

The redesigned Vincentian units cluster patients who are admitted by certain specific physicians. The DRG is assigned on admission, and the patient remains on the unit unless critical care is required. Telemetry capability is available so as to limit transfers and enhance continuity of care. The range of acuity, therefore, is much broader.

The Vincentian model is patient-focused rather than department-focused. The support departments are integrated with all services on the patient care unit. Decentralization of professional and ancillary services to the unit level provides for greater efficiency in the delivery of patient care with a subsequent impact on the quality of service.

The Vincentian work redesign model sets up a patient care system that allows for a collaborative focus on patient care issues. Patient care is planned around the needs of the client, not the schedules of hospital departments. Allied health professionals are assigned to specific patient units, not departments. Their unit assignments are now consistent. The ratio of these professionals to units depends on patient type. For example, a respiratory therapist may be assigned to only one unit or may cover several units if the need is not as great. The full-time equivalents (FTEs) from various hospital departments, such as laboratory, electrocardiography (ECG), admitting, and environmental control services, are assigned to the appropriate units and provide services that are not performed by other team members.

Registered nurses (RNs) are empowered with more control over meeting their patients' care needs in a more timely way. Professional nurses act not only as planners of care but as managers of care, who identify and delegate appropriate tasks to ancillary and other professional staff. By mastering the art of delegation, professional nurses have time to provide professional services that only they can offer the patient, such as discharge planning, patient and family teaching, physical assessment, and multidisciplinary coordination. This facilitates quality patient care outcomes.

The Vincentian redesign project proposes nursing partnerships, in which a nurse and two new ancillary staff members agree to work as a team on a long-term basis. These new ancillary roles have been created to provide registered nurses with the support they need to deliver care. Although their primary functions are different, there is some blending of the roles to provide mutual support and cross-coverage if needed.

The ancillary care provider (ACP), is a multiskilled technician who can be a certified nursing assistant, paramedic, medical assistant, or licensed practical nurse (LPN). The scope of practice of the ACP is determined by the specialty unit to which the ACP is assigned and the training or licensure she or he holds. Skills for the nonlicensed ACP might include phlebotomy, 12-lead ECG machine operation, cardiac monitoring, housekeeping, and general nursing assistant skills. The licensed ACP (usually an LPN) provides additional clinical skills, such as starting intravenous (IV) treatments, performing blood glucose monitoring, and administering medications. The ACP works in partnership with the RN, who delegates and manages the care that is delivered to patients.

The second ancillary role is that of patient service attendant (PSA). The PSA has a background either in environmental service (housekeeping) or as a nursing assistant. Besides ensuring that patient rooms and surrounding areas are cleaned on a daily basis, the PSAs are also involved in simple nursing assistant skills, such as measuring intake and output, obtaining heights and weights, determining percentage of meal consumption, delivering ice, and transferring patients.

The incorporation of these roles within the unit allows nursing to better coordinate services with patient care needs. Blood work, ECGs, and starting of IVs can be planned around meals and physical care. The patients interact with the unit staff on a regular basis, thus providing greater continuity of care. The ACP who helps them with their baths may also perform blood work and obtain their ECGs. Patients feel the care providers are more familiar with their personal needs, and patient satisfaction increases.

The model uses a case management approach, which emphasizes discharge planning and patient teaching and incorporates the family into the care plan as much as possible. The case manager (CM) is responsible for tracking patient progress. The CM role was new for St. Vincent's and is still in its evolutionary stages. The concept of differentiating nursing practice at the RN level was foreign to most of our staff, and they were uncomfortable with the role delineation.

The CM is considered the overseer of care. Under the direction of the nurse manager, the CM assumes responsibility and accountability for the clinical management of patients in specific case groups for a specific episode of illness. The CM develops a case management plan that facilitates a progressive movement toward discharge within the designated DRG length of stay. Discharge planning, which starts at the time of admission, includes assessing for treatment and teaching needs as well as early identification of resources needed to facilitate a timely discharge.

The multifaceted CM role allows the CM to be a *collaborator* with all disciplines and an *educator* to both patients and unit staff, as well as a *clinical resource professional* if needed. Because the CM role is new, it is very important to differentiate its unique responsibilities from that of the clinical RN. For example, the CM may communicate an identified patient teaching need, but it is the RN's responsibility to see that patient teaching is completed. CMs are accountable for quality-of-care outcomes, clinical coordination of resources, and specific financial outcomes. They set goals that cover all aspects of care and regularly review measurable clinical results.

The roles that have been decentralized to the unit include pharmacist, registration counselor, and respiratory therapist. These professionals come to the unit with the skills and knowledge of their specific specialty. They however, must be oriented to the concept of the Vincentian patient care delivery model and learn ways of collaborating to provide quality care. For many, this is a new experience and requires continued learning and motivation.

Team rounds are made daily at a specified time. The team, as we have instituted it, includes the patient, the professional RN, the physician, the family, allied health professionals, and the ACP. PSAs provide guest services, and a registration counselor admits patients and provides financial consultation to families. In the Vincentian model, caregivers are limited, couriers are centralized, and the professional nurse is accountable for patient outcomes. Documentation is integrated; staff from all disciplines chart on the same form, and it is placed at the bedside. Families are strongly encouraged to actively participate in care, rather than being passive observers.

The model provided certain contrasts to our previous organization. For example, there were no assistant head nurses or charge nurses as we traditionally defined these roles. Instead, a daily team leader coordinated the patient caregivers, and RNs assumed more accountability for their professional practice. Nurses carried vibrating beepers to enhance communication, save steps, and reduce overhead pages. Telemetry capability in each room limited transfers and improved continuity of care.

The Vincentian program was prepared to accomplish the following recommended goals of reorganization:

- Eliminate some of the traditional boundaries between specialized departments, with the intention of satisfying patient care needs versus department needs;
- Make managers responsible for cost-effective, quality patient care outcomes; and
- Redesign work so that new patterns of staffing and care assignments emerge.

The components of the model are summarized in Display 15-2.

DISPLAY 15-2   Components of the Vincentian Model

- Patient-focused
- Multidisciplinary team
- Limited transfers
- Case management
- Emphasize discharge planning
- Multi-trained technicians
- Family involvement

IMPLEMENTATION ON A DEMONSTRATION UNIT

In December 1990, we implemented the patient-oriented delivery model on a former general medical unit. After evaluating our top Medicare DRGs, we realized that our impact would be greatest if we began our model with cardiovascular patients; in analysis, heart failure patients comprised our top DRG, with a length of stay that exceeded the national mean. Thus, any gains made in reducing length of stay while maintaining or improving quality would have major financial benefits to the organization.

IMPLEMENTATION ON A MEDICAL-SURGICAL UNIT

After 1 year of operation of the Vincentian model on the demonstration unit, 4-West was chosen to be the first fully implemented Vincentian unit. This unit was chosen because of its stability and because it had a similar patient population to that of the demonstration unit. The unit had 35 medical-surgical beds and no telemetry system. There was an identified need to maintain or increase the number of telemetry beds, so the addition of telemetry capability was a desirable goal.

The method of patient care delivery on 4-West was a modified total patient care system, with many RNs and few nursing assistants. The RNs on the day shift cared for an average assignment of four to five patients with some assistive support. The RNs were directly involved in providing physical care and taking all blood pressures. There was an assistant nursing manager (ANM) assigned to the desk during the day and evening shifts. The responsibilities of the ANM included 1) signing off on physician orders, 2) making staff and bed assignments, 3) calling pertinent data to physicians as needed, and 4) assisting the unit clerk with routine desk duties.

The 4-West RNs, previously medical-surgical nurses, had very high levels of anxiety related to the telemetry process. Physicians were also concerned about their lack of experience. This increased RN anxiety had further decreased their levels of confidence. The RNs also felt the new staffing ratios were unsafe and unfair. They had previously taken care of less acute patients with more staff and were now expected to care for higher acuity patients with fewer professional nurses and more assistive personnel. This feeling was exacerbated by the fact that they perceived other units in the hospital to have better staffing patterns.

▬INITIAL EVALUATION

Implementation of a redesigned model without an evaluation of its outcomes is like traveling in a foreign area without a map or compass. Our evaluation process began with the initial planning of the redesign initiative. At this time, the criteria by which successful outcomes would be measured were defined. These criteria are presented in Display 15-3.

Baseline data were collected, and ongoing, informal evaluations were done. After 1 year of operation on a 16-bed cardiac telemetry demonstration unit, and another year of implementing the model on a 32-bed cardiac telemetry unit, a comprehensive formal evaluation was completed. This evaluation confirmed the strengths and weaknesses of the program and the validity of our initial assumptions.

During the 2 years that informal evaluations were conducted, pitfalls and successes were identified and changes were made to improve the efficacy of the Vincentian program.

One pitfall which was particularly significant was the RNs' perception of their role. It was important for the RNs to differentiate technical and professional components of practice in the new model, as they had traditionally been placed under one job description. With the defined changes designed into the demonstration model, RNs were fearful and anxious about role transitions, delegation to technical staff, and the different expectations others might have of their new role. This made recruiting RNs to the model unit difficult and created challenges in implementing the differentiated roles. The nursing staff had no role models or previous experience with different practice models; specifically, case management. This was an anticipated obstacle, and a process was systematically implemented which included education, observation, consultations, and group sessions to define the concepts and associated behaviors of each role.

In the initial design, the cross-trained caregiver (ACP) was trained to assume all of the unit clerk activities of the unit. After a short time during the

---

DISPLAY 15-3   *Initial Evaluative Criteria*

- Quality
- Medical variances, falls, readmissions
- Length of stay
- Patient satisfaction
- Allied health staff integration
- Cost of care
- Revenue
- Staffing
- Increased professional accountability
- Role clarity
- Staff satisfaction with quality of care
- Team coordination
- Family integration

pilot, it was clear that this was not efficient or effective, and the unit clerk position was reinstated. It was also the belief that an administrative manager would be held accountable for the administrative activities of several units, a responsibility previously assumed by the nursing managers, and that functions previously handled by assistant nursing managers or charge nurses would be assumed by RNs. It was assumed that the clinical coordination of patient care would be the role of the CM.

Our first CM had previously been a head nurse. It soon became evident that the CM role was becoming diluted as administrative duties and clinical responsibilities merged. It also became clear that staff RNs were not prepared to assume the roles of self-scheduling and controlled shared governance which had been part of the original vision. A nursing manager was hired to perform the managerial duties and to assume more accountability and responsibility for administrative functions. This led to a clearer definition of the CM's role as patient care coordinator, educator, and consultant. A primary role of the nurse manager is to mentor the staff RNs in fulfilling the duties previously performed by assistant nurse managers or charge nurses. This empowered staff nurses to acquire more control over their units' operations and become more autonomous in clinical decision-making.

Two physicians participated fully in the demonstration model of the Vincentian program on the 16-bed unit. Except for patients requiring critical care, all of their patients were admitted to this unit. In the past, there had been significant problems with prolonged lengths of stay for these physicians' patients. Within the first 3 months of operation on the pilot unit, there was a significant reduction in patient length of stay for both physicians. This impact is detailed in Figure 15-1.

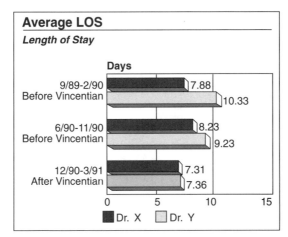

FIGURE 15-1 Average length of stay for physician X and physician Y before and after implementation of the Vincentian model.

■REDESIGNED ROLES AND EDUCATIONAL INTERVENTIONS

It is important that all redesigned roles, as well as their integration within a new practice model, be clearly defined (Fig. 15-2). Because job responsibilities have been somewhat altered, role confusion must be prevented. Comprehensive training programs were developed to meet the needs of our institution and the new model. St. Vincent's commitment to the success of the Vincentian program allowed us to provide the necessary time and support for the staff to develop positive behavioral changes in their new roles. We believed that the key to the success of cross-training staff in many tasks was adequate class time and a clinical preceptorship. It was through some initial negative training experiences that we learned that particular skills must be given special attention and nurturing in order to facilitate a competent, assured caregiver. Anything less leaves employees frustrated and unsure of their skills and capabilities. It is imperative that RNs become critical thinkers with a move away from task orientation and that their developmental training include the leadership skills essential to drive quality outcomes in patient care. Other special training requirements of the RN include time management, delegation, and conflict resolution.

The importance of a planned curriculum to address all of the educational needs should not be underestimated. The classroom instruction or didactic portion of the curriculum meets only a small portion of the educa-

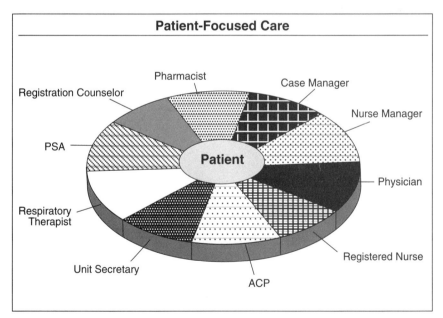

FIGURE 15-2 The patient care team as defined in the Vincentian model with the patient at the center and multidisciplinary staff interconnecting to provide quality service.

tional objectives. Skills sessions and clinical practicums are essential to the ongoing development of redesigned roles. Sample training schedules are presented in Table 15-1.

▬ IMPLEMENTATION ISSUES
Unit Selection
The unit selected for the pilot program is very important and ultimately drives the program's success or failure. The nurse manager of the unit should have a successful history of using sound management principles, be

TABLE 15-1   Sample Training Schedules

POSITION	REQUIRED EDUCATION	LENGTH OF CLASS/PRECEPTORSHIP
Registered Nurse	Vincentian orientation	1-day class
	Professional development (time management, delegation, conflict resolution)	1-day class
	Starting IVs	4-hour class
	Select RNs are trained in phlebotomy/ECG skills	4-hour precept.
Ancillary Care Provider (ACP)	Vincentian orientation	1-day class
	Housekeeping	3 days with housekeeping dept.
	ECG machine operation (select areas)	2-hour class 4-hour precept.
	Cardiac rhythm monitoring (select areas)	2-day class 1-week precept.
	Skills lab for licensed personnel in starting IVs, bedside blood glucose testing, and medication administration	
Patient Service Attendant (PSA)	Vincentian orientation	1-day class
Case Manager	Vincentian orientation	1-day class
	Professional development	1-day class
	Management development/DRGs	Determined by institution
	Phlebotomy	1-day class 3-day precept. with lab
	ECG (if specialty area)	2-hour class 4-hour precept. with ECG dept.

knowledgeable about the change process and change theory, have strong relationships with the staff, and have the time and interest necessary to provide the continuous, high-level leadership the staff will need. Additional traits are presented in Display 15-4.

Without high-quality leadership, the staff, especially in times of perceived crisis, tend to revert back to the traditional methods of patient care delivery. The staff must be supported through the ambiguity that may occur throughout the implementation process. This can only be accomplished through sound leadership.

The ability to tolerate chaos is extremely important. This chaos can't be taken personally or perceived as a sign of failure. It seems appropriate that the unit manager should solve all problems and restore order. However, by avoiding that, the staff learn to collaboratively solve their own problems. Obvious administrative issues have to be dealt with by the manager, but issues previously believed to be administrative can often be solved by the staff. For example, the patient care assignments and team delineations should be handled by the staff. During this transition time, staff can be coached to greater levels of performance by teaching them effective problem-solving skills and techniques.

Nurse manager flexibility is of the utmost importance. Nurse managers must be willing to drive changes to the program on a daily basis and revise the current system if needed. The most important managerial trait for the success of this kind of change is a total and unwavering belief that the program can work and that it will work. If this does not exist, every challenge along the way is going to cause an internal conflict with questions and doubts as to whether one is proceeding in the right manner. Staff and physicians will also recognize this, and will question the program's success and survival. The nurse manager's role must be defined from the beginning, especially if a project coordinator is involved. There must be a strong, collaborative relationship between the manager and the project coordinator.

DISPLAY 15-4   Required Nurse Manager Traits for Care Redesign

- Flexibility
- Ability to tolerate uncertainty and chaos
- Tendency not to personalize setbacks
- Sense of humor
- Faith in staff ability to solve issues
- Patience while they do
- Unwavering belief in the validity and success of the model
- Strong relationship with project coordinator
- Successful history of sound management practices
- Knowledge of the change process and change theory
- Strong relationship with staff
- Time to provide ongoing direction to staff

Their separate responsibilities must be identified, and agreement must be reached before implementation, or significant chaos can result. Other important considerations in unit selection include

- The level of preparation of RN staff to assume roles of increasing accountability for patient outcomes;
- Evidence of the staff's ability to work together as a team;
- The staff's comfort level in caring for the unit's patient population;
- Ability of physician stakeholders on the unit to accept and support change; and
- Ability of the nurse manager to manage the change process.

Staffing Patterns
Staffing patterns are based on patient acuity, required skill mix, and patient populations. They are negotiated with the vice president of nursing by the director and nurse manager of each unit. As staff become more efficient, a reduction in FTEs can often be made.

Role of the Licensed Practical Nurse
The Vincentian program attempted to solve something that was an institutional issue: the role of the LPN. The LPN had traditionally functioned in a broad, poorly defined role throughout the medical-surgical units. The Vincentian model called for the LPN to function as an ACP; however, the original 16-bed demonstration unit did not have any LPNs, so implementation of this redesigned role was not an issue. After the program was implemented on the larger unit, "what to do with the LPN" was a frequently asked question. There were approximately 50 LPNs in the institution and a strong commitment from administration to keep everyone employed. As job descriptions were being redefined, a reaffirmed decision was made to move LPNs into the ACP role, if they so chose. This meant that all aspects of the ACP role, including the ACP title and daily hygienic care, would be assumed by the LPN. They, in essence, would be practicing in partnerships with RNs.

Human Resource Issues
Because one of the major goals of our project was to change the skill mix, the shift to fewer RN staff and more ACP staff was created. Although it was felt that there would be a natural evolution into the roles and that everyone who wanted to be a part of the program would be accommodated, a bidding proposal for positions was established using competency criteria. This involved a change from our traditional method of selection, which was seniority-based. We were committed to a professional practice model which required competency and accountability in nursing practice. It was decided to base 50% of the decision on performance evaluations and 50% on seniority within the job classification.

Interdepartmental Involvement
All hospital departments directly involved in the new care delivery model were invited to participate on the planning committee. As the model was being planned and departments were asked to transfer FTEs to the demon-

stration unit, resistance was evident, and it became clear that many had not made the paradigm shift. In most cases, conflicts were worked out between the Vincentian coordinator and the department director. However, in some cases, involvement at the vice presidential level became necessary. This further emphasized the importance of the fact that support for the project must come first from management if the change is to be successful.

As staff were transferred from ancillary support departments into the nursing department, nurse managers were faced with the dilemma of managing services they knew little about. This was somewhat overwhelming as they realized their inherent accountabilities for the outcome of the new model. To assist nurse managers in this transition, each department participated in the development of the new job description, assumed responsibility for part of the employee's orientation and training, and provided input to the manager at the time of the employee's evaluation. In a sense, there was a modified matrix reporting system, but with the nurse manager assuming ultimate responsibility for management of the staff. The laboratory, environmental control, medical records, and food services departments were impacted through a reduction in their departments' FTEs as the patient care unit began to take on activities that had formerly been the responsibility of those departments (eg, phlebotomy, medical record breakdown, tray delivery and pickups).

Employee Preparation
Keeping all levels and departments of the Medical Center staff informed about the progress of the Vincentian program was a goal of the planning committee from the beginning. Discussion in staff meetings was encouraged, and forums open to all hospital departments were held periodically. Hospital publications contained Vincentian updates and, on occasion, publications devoted to the Vincentian program were distributed. Updates were also included at the department directors' monthly meeting. Directors were constantly encouraged to invite the Vincentian coordinator to their staff meetings, but few invitations were forthcoming until the specific department was affected. A similar scenario occurred with the nursing staff. After announcements were made as to which units would pilot the new delivery system, staff on those units became very interested in the project.

Unit Preparation
Plans for physical renovations of the pilot units were made early in the process. Items that were considered essential to the success of the program, as opposed to those that would be simply nice to have, were determined and budgeted for. We believed that nurse servers would be a key timesaver for the staff because medications and supplies were frequently not readily available under the old system. The nurse servers were designed to house basic supplies and medications in patient rooms.

Some additional equipment that was essential to the program's success included a desk, typewriter, and computer in the registration counselor's office and a round table, several comfortable armchairs, chalkboard, television, video cassette player, and flip charts for the patient/family education room.

To create the homelike environment that was part of the concept, the unit was freshly painted, and each room was upgraded to include bedspreads with pillow sham, curtains, a table lamp, an artificial plant, wallpaper border in the bathroom, and a bath mat and shower curtain. The cost of the room renovation, including the nurse servers, was approximately $3785 per room. A family galley was also provided on the original demonstration unit, but because of space limitations we were unable to provide this on the subsequent Vincentian unit. Other accommodations for families were made for coffee, but complete access to other amenities was not possible because of lack of space.

■EVALUATION

Two years after implementing the new delivery system on the two units, a formal evaluation of specific, important outcomes was completed. Our assumption in the beginning was that this system of delivering nursing care would provide better quality, more efficient, and more effective patient care and would improve the satisfaction of patients, physicians, and caregivers. At the time our redesign was initiated, we were not faced with immediate health care reform, but we are convinced that this redesign positions us favorably as we move into the future of a reformed health care system.

Satisfaction of all of our customers was critically important as we planned for a redesigned health care delivery system. Patient satisfaction was measured in two different ways. The Medical Center regularly conducts patient satisfaction survey interviews on all of the units. A comparison was made between a three-month period in 1991 (before implementation) and a similar period in 1992 (after implementation). Outcomes are presented in Table 15-2. The results of that comparison were very favorable, indicating that we were moving in the right direction. However, we were very interested in both the negative and positive impacts that the different components of the Vincentian program were having on patients. A targeted, internally designed questionnaire was used, and 30 patients were surveyed during a one-week period. Two raters were trained to use the interview tool and conducted all of the patient interviews. The responses of the patients were gratifying in that they identified some of the key issues related to the Vincentian program. For example, all those surveyed preferred having registration and discharge procedures performed in their rooms or on the

TABLE 15-2   Patient Satisfaction Survey–4 West for One Quarter of Each Year

	BEFORE VINCENTIAN (1991)	AFTER VINCENTIAN (1992)
Very satisfied	201	333
Satisfied	145	53
Somewhat dissatisfied	38	14
Dissatisfied	16	0

unit; some mentioned that the CM helped them to understand what was happening to them; and several felt that their care was less fragmented with fewer caregivers interacting with them on a daily basis. About 50% of those surveyed, who had been patients before, noted improvement in the promptness with which call lights were answered and that greater comfort care was available to them. Some (about 40%) noted that they were happy to see an increase in the number of staff members. In reality, there had been an overall decrease of FTEs, but a significant change in the mix of caregivers had provided more ancillary care personnel to respond to patients' basic comfort needs in a timely manner.

A physician satisfaction survey was conducted through interviews by one person. Of the fifteen physicians who participated, ten regularly admit to the Vincentian unit, and the other five sporadically admit depending on bed availability. The intent of the interview was not only to determine their level of satisfaction with the new redesign but also to get some comparative data from those who admit to other units in the Medical Center (Table 15-3). The results of this survey and staff input initiated some strengthening

TABLE 15-3   Satisfaction Survey–4 West (December 1992)

	POSITIVES	NEED IMPROVEMENT
RN	Increased interaction with MDs improves collaboration	Role of the case manager
	Cross-training meets patients' needs	Delegation skills
	ECG and lab results more timely	Assignment by acuity
	Registration counselor on unit	
	Pharmacist on unit extremely helpful	
Ancillary Staff	Patients see same staff for care (phlebotomy, ECG, daily care)	
	Self-improvement (ie, added skills)	
	Emphasis on team approach	
Physicians	Quality of care improved	Consistency of service on all shifts
	More collaboration with RNs	Continuity of care (12-hr shifts)
	Lab and ECG results more timely	
	Case managers	
	Patient care conferences	
	Interdisciplinary approach	
	Unit-based pharmacist	
	Admission and discharge process	
	Focus on patient by the team	

of the clinical resources on the evening, night, and weekend shifts, since a lack of continuity was expressed as a problem.

Staff surveys were anonymously written, one for the registered nurse and one for the ancillary staff. These were distributed in closed envelopes and returned in sealed envelopes within 10 days. The professional nurses and the physicians both identified improved and increased collaboration as a positive outcome of the Vincentian program. RNs perceived the role of the CM somewhat negatively. In retrospective analysis, it was thought that not enough education with staff nurses had been planned regarding the integration of the CMs. Other findings included some difficulty RNs had adjusting to the added responsibilities designed into their new roles. Ongoing role clarification is an essential component in the success of any redesign program and must be stressed repeatedly.

Quality improvement activities were monitored and compared with measures taken before implementation. There was a decrease in medication errors, attributed to the presence of the pharmacist for immediate intervention and clarification. Patient incidents in general decreased because of the renewed focus on the patient and because everyone on the unit was more responsive to patients' needs.

Financially, there were some efficiencies, although this was not the main objective of the patient care redesign. Cost per case was reduced from the pre-Vincentian level as a result of the change in mix of the staff. Although the FTE component was only slightly reduced, the overall staff mix changed, thus decreasing costs. Drug costs decreased with the intervention of the pharmacist making rounds with the physicians. Collections and reimbursements increased as the registration counselor, an integral member of the patient care team, developed helping relationships with patients and families and pursued reimbursement issues aggressively. The outcomes of all of these indicators helped us to identify more clearly the pitfalls and the areas needing improvement, but most of all they indicated that we were on the right road and were providing our patients with a higher quality of care and our staff with an innovative practice environment.

DIRECTION FOR THE FUTURE

We are currently in the process of planning and implementing the Vincentian program on our other six medical-surgical and telemetry units. Our goal is to have the Vincentian model of care operational on all of the units by spring of 1994.

During medical-surgical implementation, we have begun to focus on the specialty units and the form that the Vincentian model will take in those areas. Staff and physicians are now involved in planning and in adapting the model to meet the needs of intensive care, maternal-child, and mental health practice units. Our long-term goal is to implement the Vincentian model throughout the organization.

It has been said that the only constant in health care is change. The Vincentian program has required many changes that will assure our future success in health care. For us, the future is "Vincentian."

Chapter 16

Transformational Leadership: The Partnership of Theory-Based Practice and Work Redesign in a Nursing Care Delivery System

RUBEN D. FERNANDEZ   GEORGE J. HEBERT   JOANNE RIGGS

> *I can't help thinking of the Venetian Republic in their last
> half century. Like us, they had once been fabulously lucky.
> They had become rich, as we did, by accident. They had
> acquired immense political skill, just as we have. A good
> many of them were tough minded, realistic, patriotic.
> They knew, just as clearly as we know, that the current of
> history had begun to flow against them.
> Many of them gave their minds to working out ways to keep
> going. It would have meant breaking the patterns into which
> they had crystallized.
> They never found the will to break them.*
> —C. P. Snow

Health care is a consumer service—a commodity to some, a right and
necessity to others. At its core are service organizations in transition, redefining themselves and attempting to meet the challenges and demands of
health care reform. Essential to the survival of many organizations is the
need to restructure, right-size, downsize, and maximize the work force. Critical to this change process is the role that nursing service must play in work
redesign endeavors. Restructuring of nursing care is often haphazard, triggered by the rapidly accelerating pressure to reduce health care costs. Innovation, risk-taking, paradigm shifts, and planned change are actions that are
no longer optional but necessary for survival. There are no road maps to
follow as we traverse health care territory. As Meehan wrote, "It is clear that
we must adopt a customer orientation that is wanting in our current system.
Yet, whatever is done to improve customer service and competitiveness must
be undertaken within the context of efforts to contain cost" (Meehan, 1993,
p. 28). This calls for creative and innovative transformation of current policies and procedures.

Flarey, D: REDESIGNING NURSING CARE DELIVERY: Transforming Our Future
© 1995, J. B. Lippincott Company

The purpose of this chapter is to share with readers a visionary alternative that can transform an organization. The selection of the sociotechnical model for work redesign and Orem's "Self-Care Deficit Nursing Theory of Practice" was not by chance but the outcome of serious deliberations. Nursing administrators of Newark Beth Israel Medical Center spent many hours performing self evaluations, asking questions such as why do we provide this service, and what are our basic beliefs regarding human relations and the capacity of individuals to change and create when provided with an environment that allows them to be part of the solution and not part of the problem. Newark Beth Israel Medical Center is a 545-bed tertiary, teaching, urban, not-for-profit health care facility. The Department of Nursing is a recognized national leader in the utilization of theory-based practice as elucidated by Dorothea E. Orem's Self-Care Deficit Theory of Nursing.

Late in the spring of 1989, the New Jersey Department of Health provided the hospital industry with a wonderful opportunity. It made available to all New Jersey hospitals 20 million dollars through a competitive grant to those institutions willing to develop specific projects with innovative ideas to recruit and retain nurses.

At Newark Beth Israel Medical Center, we rejected quick-fix solutions and developed two major themes in the grant application: 1) theory-based nursing practice and 2) work redesign.

Theory-based nursing practice was not a new idea at Newark Beth Israel Medical Center. Approximately 2 years before the grant became available, we had committed ourselves to implementing Dorothea E. Orem's self-care deficit nursing theory as a framework for professional practice. The sudden availability of grant money gave this project an additional dimension; it was decided that one aspect of our grant proposal would include the computerization of self-care deficit nursing theory. Our plan was to install bedside computers on three nursing units initially, to be followed by all remaining nursing units in sequence. We also decided to use a software vendor, Nursing Systems International of Bordentown, New Jersey, which is the only company developing software based on Orem's nursing theory framework. This unique software package was developed by nurses for nurses; staff nurses from Newark Beth Israel Medical Center participated in focus groups that assisted in its development and design.

The second part of our proposal was to implement a house-wide work redesign program. We decided to use the sociotechnical model as outlined by our consultants, Lawrenz, Madden and Associates. They secured assistance from industry experts to further guide us in our endeavor. We selected this model because its focus was on systems problems, work flow, resource allocation and distribution, long-range planning, and teamwork, rather than on individual issues or people.

What do either of these two ideas have to do with recruiting or retaining nurses? From our experience and perspective, nurses want more than just money for their work. They want more time with their patients, more control over their work environment, and greater self-satisfaction.

▀ WORK REDESIGN

Work redesign is a multidisciplinary process of changing the way work is accomplished in order to improve patient care outcomes. The process creates greater efficiency, emphasizes shared responsibility, provides higher levels of job satisfaction, and improves productivity. An outcome of work redesign is the restructure of the work environment. "Work redesign is not merely shifting a few organizational components and people; it is the complete reorientation of the work and culture of the organization" (Drucker, 1991, p. 45).

The unique feature of this process is that individuals from all levels of the organization get involved in developing the design and formulating the recommendations, not just the experts or top managers. This approach provides more data, facilitates a way of doing something differently, involves those closest to the work, helps employees rethink how the work should be completed, and assists individuals in getting organized to get the job done, as well as creating a sense of strong commitment to change.

The sociotechnical model of work redesign integrates the social (human) and technical (skill) aspects of work, forming a unified whole. The model provides both the rationale and methodology for change. It acts as a filter through which all proposed changes are viewed. The end product is a well thought-out plan for change that has been distilled from many diverse ideas.

The social aspects of the model (Lawrenz, Madden and Associates, 1992) address the human contribution to the organization, including people's talents, relationships, values, culture, objectives, attitudes, dreams, and experiences. This system provides the organization with the ability to learn and adapt to the change.

The technical components of the model (Lawrenz, Madden and Associates, 1992) look at the tools, technique, knowledge, and methods people use to complete their work. In any work environment, the technical system includes the knowledge base people operate from, the processes for generating and using knowledge, and the procedures for sharing that knowledge and information. The effectiveness of this aspect of the system determines the ease with which work is performed.

From the beginning, the intent of this project was twofold. The first goal was to emphasize patient care rather than nursing care. With this in mind, we worked to make nursing part of a larger structure rather than isolating it in its own exclusive territory. This eventually had a big payoff for everyone and facilitated a collaborative environment. Our operating premise was that teamwork drives good patient outcomes. The second goal was to define nursing practice from a theoretical nursing model that not only defined, outlined, and structured practice but also expressed what the department believed about nursing. Although the theory is our framework, it alone is not enough. Nursing does not exist in a vacuum; nurses function within a larger system and must participate as a part of a team that is providing total patient care. It is imperative, therefore, that the entire system be reviewed. This is the purpose and function of work redesign.

The awarding of the Department of Health grant enabled us to bring together these two foundational elements, forming the keystone that supported the weight of all future change.

■ ESTABLISHING A STRUCTURE FOR DESIGN
The sociotechnical model involved creating a work-ready structure to facilitate the process (Fig. 16-1) as well as define the roles (Lawrenz, 1992) within the structure (Table 16-1).

In order for the structure to work, the organization must support what Lawrenz, Madden and Associates (1992) term the work redesign underlying principles:

1. Interdependent tasks need collaboration.
2. Whole tasks make work meaningful.
3. Knowing more than one task gives flexibility.
4. Flexibility and rapid response are needed in a rapidly changing environment.

Three-Tier Strategy

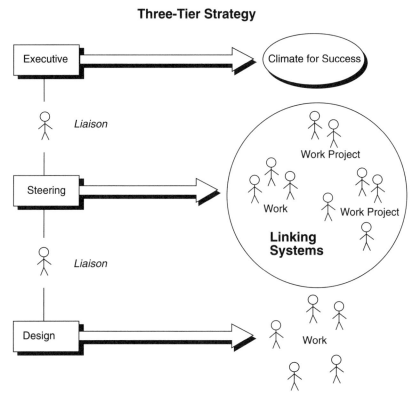

FIGURE 16-1   Three-tier structure of the Work Redesign Process—sociotechnical model—with related function.

TABLE 16-1   Roles and Responsibilities of the Various Members that Constitute the Organizational Structure of the Work Redesign Program at Newark Beth Israel Medical Center

	RESPONSIBLITY	CRITERIA
External Sponsor	• Takes the organization's vision and mission out into the community • Assures financial support for the project • Represents the work redesign effort in the community	• Recognized in the community as a leader • Willing to provide support and visibility to the project outside the organization
Internal Sponsor	• Provides political leadership/championship to entire work redesign project • Person who has ultimate authority and resources to initiate and legitimize change effort ■ Prevents staffing disruptions during the project	• Sponsor of work innovations (paradigm shifts) • Willing to support risks • Willing to provide support and visibility to project within the organization
Executive Steering Committee	• Represents all stakeholders • Determines vision and direction for total hospital • Sets mission, objectives/specifications for work redesign • Selects/authorizes and gives charge to the steering committee ■ Approves or modifies final recommendations ■ Communicates overall change efforts to entire organization ■ Provides leadership and evaluation to overall process and implementation ■ Models collaboration through partnership	• Multidisciplinary (all stakeholders in system whose support is essential to project's success) • Senior level physicians and administrators ■ Resource controllers ■ Policy influencers
Champions	■ Members of executive steering committee who act as conduits to champion design team recommendations ■ Members of design team ■ Ensures communication links	■ Senior level ■ Excellent communication skills ■ Willing to be spokespersons
Steering Committee	■ Manages the project ■ Drives mission values and objectives into the daily work of the organization ■ Integrates work design efforts with the overall mission of the organization ■ Collects and shares best practices among design team ■ Approves design recommendations under their control	■ Multidisciplinary ■ Resource controllers ■ Policy influencers ■ Excellent coordinators ■ Excellent communication and team skills

(continued)

TABLE 16-1   Roles in Work Design Change Process *(continued)*

	RESPONSIBLITY	CRITERIA
Steering Committee *(continued)*	■ Captures, documents, and evaluates learning from design processes into larger organization ■ Accountable to executive committee	
Design Team	■ Analyze current "work systems" ■ Recommends design/redesign of work system ■ Communicate with and represent needs of entire organization to peers ■ Educates self about work innovations/best hospitals	■ Multidisciplinary ■ Multi-level (people closest to work) ■ Ability and willingness to deal with ambiguity, with team, represent larger organization to peers
Facilitator Consultants	■ Advisory role to the organization ■ Suggests appropriate concepts/ methods to work with all teams ■ Process and team facilitator	■ Willing to challenge organizational assumptions ■ Experience with/knowledge of high performance systems/work innovations ■ Seen as "neutral" ■ Excellent communication and facilitation

5. Balancing relationships and work is the goal, not one at the expense of the other.
6. Boundaries include time and scope of work.
7. Boundaries for work units or departments need to be semipermeable.
8. The manager's role is to manage the boundaries.
9. Managing boundaries includes work inside, outside, and across groups.

The need for these underlying principles is predicated on a clear understanding of the direct and indirect care needs of the central figure: the patient.

▬DEPARTMENTAL STRUCTURE

Although many theories of nursing have evolved over the last two decades, only Dorothea E. Orem was found to have both a formalized definition of nursing and a proposed theory of nursing administration (Allison, McLaughlin, & Walker, 1991). Orem defines nursing administration in terms of identifiable elements or parts (Orem, 1989, p. 56). Collectively, it consists of those persons who, through their actions within a situational context, manage courses of affairs specific to the provision of nursing, both now and at future times, to described populations served by a formally constituted enterprise and, in so doing, exercise powers given them by the established authorities of the institution for purposes which are accomplished, in whole or in part, by the provision of health care in the form of nursing.

Allison, McLaughlin, and Walker support the view that nursing administration, "through the actions of nurse administrators, is responsible for ensuring a reasonable quality of the delivery of nursing services. It must also facilitate the work of nurses in the delivery process in a fiscally responsible way and create an environment that supports professional growth and development" (Allison, McLaughlin, & Walker, 1991, p. 73).

Orem maintains that theory-based nursing practice enables nursing administration to make explicit nursing's role and contribution to the mission and goals of the organization. "Nursing administration is enterprise oriented. The population to be served through the continuing availability and provision of nursing at this or that time is a service that is justified in terms of its relationship and contribution to the purpose of the mission of the enterprise" (Orem, 1989, p. 62).

Orem further postulates that nursing administration is nursing-oriented. This occurs through the "nursing administrators' dynamic knowing of nursing and through their ability to think nursing. Nursing administrators' judgments cannot be practical and rational unless these persons know nursing as a discipline of knowledge and practice both in relationship to their own work and to the work of nursing practitioners" (Orem, 1989, p. 62).

The nursing department's initial step was to clearly state its mission, vision, and objectives (Display 16-1). In addition, a revised organizational

---

**DISPLAY 16-1   Vision, Mission, and Behavior Statements
of the Department of Nursing at Newark
Beth Israel Medical Center**

VISION
To provide quality managed care that is responsive to the self-care needs of the patient.

MISSION
To provide patients with humane, ethical, safe, competent care. By making our patients' self-care needs our highest priority, each of us becomes part of this mission.

BEHAVIORS
To achieve our mission, I will:

1. Do for the patient what he/she cannot do for himself/herself.
2. Treat each person with whom I come in contact with courtesy and respect.
3. Accept responsibility to improve my job performance.
4. Perform my job to the satisfaction of the patient.
5. Be flexible enough to make changes to meet the patient's needs.
6. Make ethical decisions that respect the dignity and wishes of the patient.

OUTCOME
Upon discharge, patient and family will be more knowledgeable about their illness and treatment and will have received expert, professional, humane, and ethical care.

chart was designed to better exemplify the commitment to a patient-centered care philosophy (Fig. 16-2). After these guiding principles were established, the need to define nursing practice became more apparent. In this particular setting, nursing administration, after much research and dialogue, agreed that Dorothea E. Orem's self-care deficit nursing theory was most consistent with our values, our agenda, and what we as a collective team believed about nursing. Our basic assumption was that planned change would be the guiding force of our theory-based practice model, since it is the foundation of nursing. This concept defines who the nurse is and what the proper object of nursing is. As a result, it also defines the depth and breadth of nursing responsibility and accountability. However, this concept is deceptive in its simplicity, since we think we already know what nurses do. As long as the boundaries of nursing remain unclear, we will always be debating with other disciplines over the professional responsibilities of the role. This is not only a waste of time and energy but severely limits nursing's ability to control its own practice.

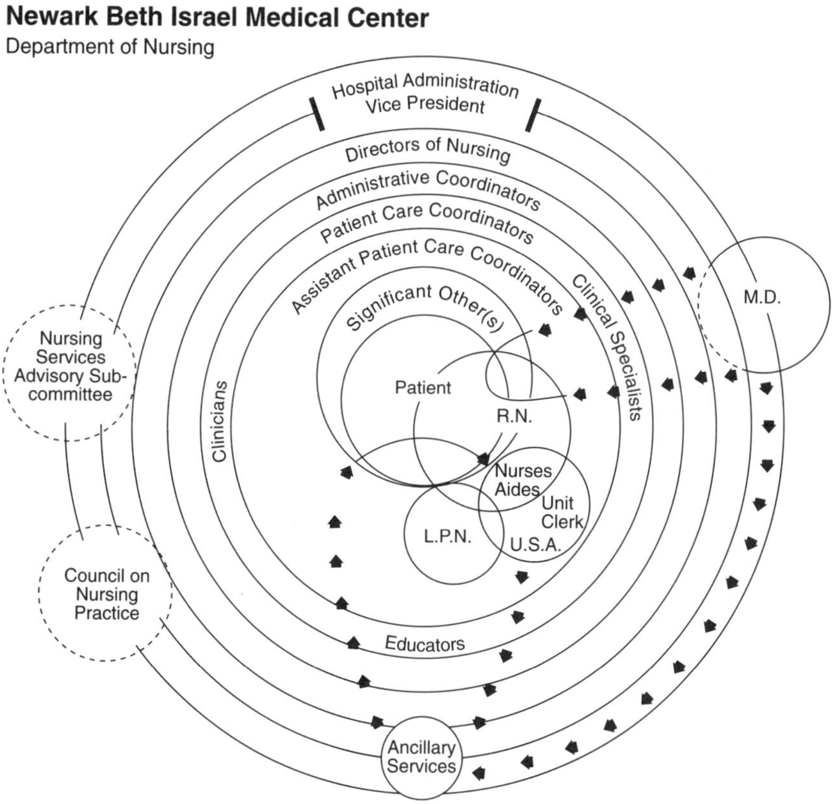

Newark Beth Israel Medical Center
Department of Nursing

FIGURE 16-2   Table of organization—Department of Nursing at Newark Beth Israel Medical Center.

The integration of work redesign principles into theory-based practice best describes our organizational design, in which work redesign is the organizational foundation and theory becomes the driving force for nursing practice.

▄ THEORY-BASED PRACTICE

A theory-based practice model for nursing provides the structure for understanding all the practice components of nursing service delivery. The model lays the foundation for nursing practice by providing a framework that organizes knowledge and delivery of care based on that knowledge, thus creating a bridge between nursing theory and nursing practice.

According to Fawcett, the usefulness of the conceptual framework comes from "the organization it provides for the nurses' thinking, observation, and interpretation of what is seen. It also provides a systematic structure and rationale for activities, gives direction to the search for relevant questions about the patient, environment, health and nursing that point out solutions to practical problems, and provides general criteria for knowing when a problem has been solved" (Fawcett, 1989, p. 2).

The need for practice-oriented theory and conceptual models for nursing practice has long been identified in the literature. However, actually implementating a conceptual model often creates some difficulties because of the incoherence of hospital systems, medical models superimposed on nursing practice, and a lack of understanding of the phenomenon of nursing.

Nursing is mandated by society to use its specialized body of knowledge and skills for the good of all people. The mandate implies that knowledge and skills must grow to keep up with the changing health goals of society. According to Meehan, "The traditional medical model, which failed to recognize the need for teamwork and patient involvement, is no longer working" (Meehan, 1993, p. 27). There has never been a time when creative and innovative ideas are more necessary. In order for us to survive, the future has to be our priority. Nursing must respond with new ways of organizing practice and evaluating outcomes.

Applying Orem's Self-Care Deficit Nursing Theory

In "Redesigning Our Future: Whose Responsibility Is It?," Sovie (1990) discussed the need to redesign care delivery to meet the needs of the future. She highlighted several aspects of structural and redesign theory to consider: patient care planning, delivery systems, manpower resources, and management systems. Organizing a nursing department through theory-based practice responds to the current and future needs of patients and nurses. Furthermore, it responds to the need to operate in concert while focusing on a common purpose. Orem's self-care deficit nursing theory best met the needs of the department because the model:

- Provides a common language;
- Identifies a framework based on concepts unique to the discipline of nursing;

- Directs nursing actions;
- Allows nurses to practice nursing as a learned profession;
- Reflects the values of the staff and the philosophy of the nursing department;
- Can be used to justify nursing actions;
- Provides measurable outcomes for which quality can be measured;
- Provides a structure that the nursing department can use to operationalize its action plan;
- Can cost out those interventions that are germane to nursing practice; and
- Provides a value system and practice identity that the staff can identify with, integrate, and interpret to others.

Nursing administration agreed that in order to make the project a success, certain investments were required (Fernandez & Wheeler, 1990): a dedicated specialist in Orem and nursing theory had to be hired as project facilitator; additional manpower resources had to be allocated for the purpose of education and implementation; collaboration with schools of nursing that use the model had to be increased; an Orem resource library had to be developed; and the nursing department had to become known locally and nationally as an Orem center of nursing excellence and practice.

The investment goals that we set were put into operation. An Orem coordinator was originally hired to spearhead the project; this position has now been replaced with an Orem consultant and facilitator. An action plan was formulated with a target date of 5 years to establish and integrate the model. At this point, the department is in an active phase of implementation, 5 years into the model. Nursing administration is conscious that this process is ongoing; yet, in order to evaluate goal achievement, time tables had to be established. Continuous quality improvement programs and staff development programs needed to reflect the totality of the model. Policies and procedures, as they were revised and updated, incorporated the concepts and principles of the self-care deficit nursing theory. An Orem Resource Center was created. In addition, the nursing department is committed to sponsor the Eastern Region Orem Self-Care Deficit Conferences, which are held biannually. The nursing department has been collaborating with national scholars in the field, including Dr. Orem, in planning the regional conferences. To date, four regional conferences have been held, as well as research symposia.

The vision and five-year plan called for developing Orem-based bedside computer system. The organization, through the New Jersey Department of Health Nursing Incentive Reimbursement Award grant and other sources, elected to sponsor and provide access to Nursing Systems International to assist them in developing the first Orem theory-based computerized nursing program. The nursing department is the first in the nation to contract services, provide data, and become a national testing demonstration center for the purpose of advancing the computerized development of the model. Beta testing efforts began in the fall of 1993.

At this point, the documentation system continues to be a manual one.

Current nursing forms used within the model are designed for use with Orem's theory. The goal is to have, by the end of 1994, four to six units computerized within the model. Upon completion of the two-year plan, all units will be fully computerized with the Orem program that is currently being developed.

In order for a theory-based practice model to effectively operate, a multi-level forum must exist through which ongoing evaluation, free discussion, and planning can take place. The communication process must encompass the unit level, the middle management level, and nursing administration. The overall concerns of the staff, the action plan, and the vision or mission must be clearly outlined and reiterated during each phase of the implementation process.

The implementation process (Fernandez & Wheeler, 1990, p. 77) includes, but is not limited to, five major phases:

Phase 1: The Identification Phase (2–8 months). This includes selection of a theory-based practice model.

Phase 2: The Education Phase (2–4 years). Although the process is ongoing, everyone in the department must be educated and have a good understanding of the model. This process includes educating departments and services external to nursing.

Phase 3: The Transition Phase (4–6 years). The staff has various levels of understanding and facility with the model. As they incorporate the theory into their daily activities, progress is made in documentation. Tools continue to be developed, expanded, and revised.

Phase 4: The Implementation Phase (6–8 years). The model is fully operational, and changes in practice and outcomes are evident. Tools of practice are near completion or completed. The staff practices according to the model, and true integration begins to occur.

Phase 5: The Evaluation Phase. Although the evaluation process is dynamic and ongoing, it is imperative that a thorough evaluation of the program be undertaken after completion of the implementation phase. This includes a review of compliance with preestablished goals, patient care outcomes, changes in practice, and movement toward theory integration. The theory is further refined by those staff members who understand it and have integrated it into their practice.

Adjustments to the Work Redesign Plans

Although our plans for the implementation of theory-based practice and work redesign were quite comprehensive, it became obvious that in spite of our best efforts something was missing. We decided to address this concern in a retreat day. In preparation, each director of nursing was asked to look at his or her own division as a part of the whole and consider what ought to be accomplished in order to more effectively synthesize our efforts.

Sometimes, through the process of review, "there emerges a dynamic glimpse of a way of knowing that is without question the right path at this particular point in time" (Rainville-Oliver, 1991, p. 41). It was the shared opinion of the director of the department of education and the assistant director of nursing for research that a dramatic change in the structure and function of the education department had to occur. Because this proposed change illustrates so clearly the type of redesign that must be incorporated into our health care institutions if we are to survive financially and successfully meet the challenges of providing nursing care into the next millennium, we have chosen to use it here as an example.

The primary focus of the redesigned department of nursing education and research is to meet the educational needs of the nursing staff. These needs are addressed through nurse orientation and continuing education. A majority of the department's resources are used in maintaining these services.

A secondary focus of the department is continuous quality improvement. Currently, problems that are identified through the continuous quality improvement process, by unit or medical center personnel, or by directors of nursing, are ultimately referred to the nurse manager of the unit involved for diagnosis and remediation. In reviewing the current investigative methodology, it can be found that some nurse managers are less skilled at diagnosing the clinical and practice deficits. At times, inappropriate intervention strategies, such as education, are requested for staff.

Department clinical support personnel are called "educators," which narrows their scope of practice as well as the expectations of the nursing staff, nurse managers, and directors of nursing. In order for the department to more effectively address the issue of quality nursing care, the scope and focus of the department must expand beyond the current limits of predominantly providing education. To this end, the creation of the department of nursing standards assurance and research (NSAR) has been proposed.

The director of NSAR will be a director of nursing. Three branches report to the director: 1) standards monitoring and investigation, 2) standards maintenance, and 3) research, (Figure 16-3). Personnel reporting directly include the coordinator of monitoring and investigation (CMI), standards assurance representatives (SARs), standards maintenance representatives (SMRs), and the assistant director of nursing for research.

The branch of standards monitoring and investigation will consist of one CMI and three SARs. The function of this branch will be to perform both selected standards monitoring and investigate deviations identified through the monitoring process.

The branch of standards maintenance will consist of nine SMRs. The function of this branch will be to provide orientation and continuing education to all nursing staff and to perform educational evaluation. The SMRs are assigned to specific clinical units for the purpose of providing the educational needs of those units.

The branch of research will consist of one assistant director of nursing. The function of this branch will be to facilitate grant writing and research within the nursing department and to act as a consultant to the SARs and nursing administration.

The restructure of the department of nursing education and research is an attempt to differentiate practice levels in order to respond more appro-

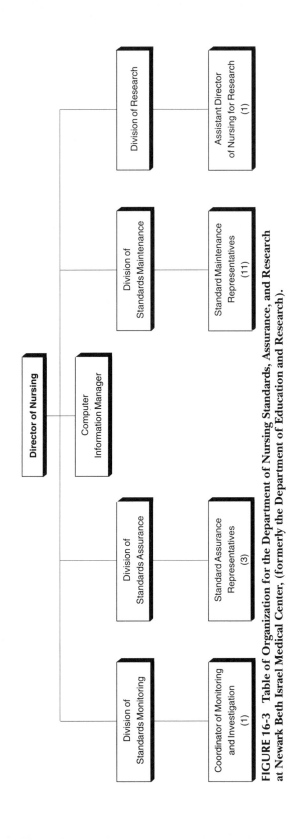

FIGURE 16-3 Table of Organization for the Department of Nursing Standards, Assurance, and Research at Newark Beth Israel Medical Center, (formerly the Department of Education and Research).

214

priately to the changing needs and requirements of the department of nursing. This restructuring is very much in concert with the overall redesign objectives of the organization.

▀RECOMMENDATIONS

If an organization is considering the implementation of work redesign and a theory-based model, we recommend the management staff be cognizant of several issues:

1. Work redesign efforts must be implemented before or simultaneously with the implementation of a theory-based model. The organizational systems that facilitate practice must be addressed first.
2. Any model represents an alternative system of care grounded in a nursing theory, and it is not to be considered the sole answer to defining and refining nursing practice.
3. If the organization is not truly committed, do not start the project.
4. Ultimately, the model must provide a mechanism to cost out that which is uniquely defined as the practice of nursing.
5. There is a need to validate through research some of the variables that the staff may identify as requiring further development and refinement.

The hospital is a complex organization. Its systems and the structure are not generally consumer-friendly nor based on the needs of the patients; rather, its policies and systems reflect the needs and convenience of the provider. According to Porter-O'Grady, "Policy, disciplinary and practice restrictions now appear to have less to do with protecting the public than they do with protecting the role of the practitioner. What we often see in many hospitals is a disciplinary siege mentality; one department against the other, with the clinical or critical problem that separates them acting as a battering ram swinging both ways, depending on who is wielding it at the time" (Porter-O'Grady, 1993, p. 7). Therefore, the restructuring of care to meet consumer needs must be the singular focus of concern in a competitive health care environment.

▀CONCLUSION

There is no question that the old systems will be able to meet neither our current demands nor those of the future. Paradigm shifts and change are inevitable. Let us take charge and control of our destiny rather than leave it to chance or to those with self-serving interests to become the architects of practice and health care reform. The old patterns must be broken, and, unlike the Venetian Republic, we have the will to break them.

▀REFERENCES

Allison, S., McLaughlin, K., & Walker, D. (1991). Nursing theory: A tool to put nursing back into nursing administration. *Nursing Administration Quarterly, 15*(3), 72–78.
Drucker, P. (1991). The discipline of innovation. *Harvard Business Review, 49*(5), 87–103.

Fawcett, J. (1989). *Analysis and evaluation of conceptual models of nursing* (2nd ed.). Philadelphia: F. A. Davis.

Fernandez, R. & Wheeler, J. (1990). Organizing a nursing system through theory based practice. In G. Mayer, M. Madden, & E. Lawrenz (Eds.), *Patient care delivery models* (pp. 63–97). Rockville, MD: Aspen.

Lawrenz, E. (1992). *Roles in work redesign change process.* Unpublished manuscript.

Lawrenz, Madden and Associates. (1992). *Concepts in work redesign.* Unpublished manuscript

Meehan, M. (1993). The nucleus of modern health care. *Health Management Quarterly, 15*(2), 25–28.

Orem, D. (1989). Nursing administration: A theoretical approach. In B. Henry, C. Ardnt, M. DiVicenti, and A. Marriner (Eds.) *Dimensions of nursing administration: Theory, research, education, practice* (pp. 55–62). Blackwell Scientific Publication.

Porter-O'Grady, T. (1993). Patient focused care service models and nursing: Perils and possibilities. *Journal of Nursing Administration, 23*(3), 7–8.

Rainville-Oliver, N. (1991). True believers: A case for model based nursing practice. *Nursing Administration Quarterly, 15*(3), 37–43.

Sovie, M. D. (1990). Redesigning our future: Whose responsibility is it? *Nursing Economics, 8*(1), 21–27.

▬SUGGESTED READING

Drucker, P. (1992). The new society of organizations. *Harvard Business Review, 92*(5), 95–104.

Fernandez, R., Lariccia, M., Alvarez, A., and Duffy, M. (1990). Theory-based practice: A model for nurse retention. *Nursing Administration Quarterly, 14*(4), 47–53.

Gilbert, G., Madden, M., & Lawrenz, E. (1990). *Patient care delivery models.* Rockville, MD: Aspen.

Hammer, M. (1990). Reengineering work: Don't automate, obliterate. *Harvard Business Review, 90*(4), 104–112.

Johnson, L. M. (1992). Structure, strategies and synthesis: The nurse executive as social architect. *Nursing Administration Quarterly, 17*(1), 10–16.

Nystrom, P. C. (1993). Organizational cultures, strategies, and commitments in health care organizations. *Health Care Management Review, 18*(1), 43–49.

Orem, D. E. (1991). *Nursing concepts of practice* (4th ed.). St. Louis: Mosby Year Book.

Porter-O'Grady, T. (1992). Transformational leadership in an age of chaos. *Nursing Administration Quarterly, 17*(1), 17–24.

Sorrentino, E. A. (1991). Making theories work for you. *Nursing Administration Quarterly, 15*(3), 54–59.

Chapter 17

Investing in Our Future

MARY JANE MADDEN   KATHY WILDE   SUSAN JESKA

The fall of the Berlin Wall and the collapse of the Soviet Union appeared to be surprise events, yet both were preceded by years of rumblings that created the context and climate for significant change. Likewise, in health care, the rumblings of increased costs, dwindling resources, lack of access, greater technology, new diseases, increased life expectancy, and ethical dilemmas are unsettling the environment and causing health care institutions across the country to struggle for change.

This chapter details the experience of the University of Minnesota Hospital and Clinic (UMHC), a publicly funded organization that came to face reality and recognize that the rumblings had reached a critical state. UMHC realized that over the next 3 years, its economic viability would be at stake. In response, the UMHC took a multidimensional approach to change. The efforts described here are projects initiated by nursing that focused on changes in nursing and service to patients. The project sites were, first, the bone marrow transplant unit and, later, all patient care units. These projects were not simple; they were not painless or smooth. But each effort has paved a piece of the path that we are walking today. As persons intimately involved in the projects, we describe how the University has and is responding to the continued, unfolding drama of reforming health care with fewer resources. The rumblings have not stopped. The course remains convoluted and sometimes disjointed, but with a clearer vision of a health care model for the future.

▀THE UNIVERSITY OF MINNESOTA HOSPITAL AND CLINIC

The UMHC operates within the metropolitan twin cities of Minneapolis and Saint Paul, Minnesota, primarily a managed care environment. The UMHC, affiliated with the University of Minnesota since 1911, serves a tripartite mission of service, education, and research. It is internationally recognized for innovations in patient care delivery including organ transplants, medical advances, and primary nursing. The tripartite mission and associated accomplishments present a special challenge in the face of current market realities shared by other academic institutions.

Although our mission has not changed over our 80-year history, our environment is radically different. Today, university hospitals across the country must meet obligations defined by both academic and marketplace criteria—and those two arenas can be vastly different. Our academic obligations say we must have patients from whom medical students can learn; the marketplace says we must compete for those patients with large private health care systems. University obligations say we must do research in highly specialized areas of medicine; marketplace demands say we must produce primary care practitioners. Academic standards can make us expensive; marketplace standards make it imperative that we be cost-competitive. So the question we face today is, can we manage to meet both university and marketplace mandates and obligations? (Hart, 1993, p. 16)

Can UMHC meet these mandates and obligations in one of the fiercest economic health care environments in the country? From 1982 to the present, more than 60% of the UMHC's metropolitan population of 2.2 million enrolled in managed health care plans. This majority is projected to reach 80% by 1996. The phenomenal change has produced stormy competition for existing patient care dollars and resulted in the closing of 18 metropolitan hospitals since 1961, including several hospital mergers into system-managed enterprises. The hard, cold reality of the managed care environment is that as the number of managed care enrollees goes up, the amount of reimbursement dollars for unmanaged health care goes down. Patient fees, although important to economic survival, have become increasingly less important. Reimbursement has shifted from a cost basis to a per capita basis. Not surprisingly, managed care plans have not reimbursed for costs associated with research or education.

The impact of managed care on the UMHC, although often perceived to have been sudden, has been gradual. Approximately 70% of all UMHC patients are now covered by a managed health care plan, thus reducing the profit margins substantially. Accompanying these inpatient trends has been a 17% increase in ambulatory clinic visits. Hospital admissions fell by 1,037 from fiscal year 1988–1989 to 1992–1993; patient days declined by 26,187; and length of stay dropped from an average of 8.4 to 7.4 days (Fig. 17-1). Occupancy today hovers around 65%.

One common assumption about university hospitals is that they are funded by state appropriations and thus are immune to economic trends in health care. This hospital relies predominantly on patient charges to fund operations (88.8%), with only 4.4% of support derived from the state. As the number of managed care patients has escalated, the Medicaid/Medicare population has remained at 25.6%, and only 16.3% of the UMHC patient population has carried traditional insurance or made traditional fee-for-service reimbursements. This changing managed care environment has resulted in a fixed amount of hospital income despite the escalating costs predominant in the industry (Fig. 17-2). Although a portion of this difference represents the impact of education and research, the marketplace demands that we reduce our costs.

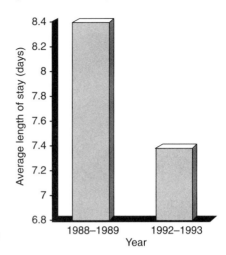

FIGURE 17-1 Comparison of lengths of stay.

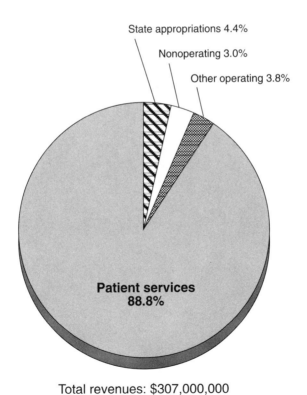

Total revenues: $307,000,000

FIGURE 17-2 University of Minnesota reliance on funds for patient care.

As health care dollars eroded over a five-year period, staff and physicians maintained the belief that the university would remain untouched. Hospital and medical school activities did not reflect the true picture of an eroding market share, shrinking capitated payments, and greater competition for research dollars. Actions were taken on a simplistic "as if" approach, based on stability rather than on change or systems thinking.

▬ A CRACK IN THE WALL

An initial "crack" in thinking came in the form of a challenge grant in 1989 from The Robert Wood Johnson Foundation and The Pew Charitable Trusts to strengthen hospital nursing. The grant provided an unprecedented opportunity to seek funding for the restructure of bedside care delivery. As recipients of one of the challenge grants, UMHC took this opportunity to explore the redesign of work on a bone marrow transplant unit.

Almost concurrently, other stimuli for change and awakening prodded UMHC. A second project was initiated to analyze and redesign the work of support services on three patient care units. A third project focused on the reduction of nonsalary expenses within hospital operations. The expectation for multidisciplinary involvement in all three projects prompted new movement among all disciplines. The commitment to change (action, not just ideas) varied from project to project, but the major impact of the three was, in the beginning, to "unsettle the settled."

Finally, in early 1992, the economic crisis became clear. Small, focused initiatives would not be enough to maintain the economic viability of UMHC in the foreseeable future. The hospital administration began a major strategic planning effort with the medical school to reduce costs and improve service while achieving demonstrable clinical outcomes. Open and frank discussions with the medical school, board of governors, and board of regents reinforced the need and desire for change to assure a viable institution. The managed care environment challenged UMHC to change, to anticipate the future, and to remain anchored in quality care while carrying out the missions of education and research. Although we felt there was no choice but to change, the significant task was deciding how to change. Changing patient care delivery became a hospital focus and, more specifically a nursing charge.

▬ REDESIGNING PATIENT CARE DELIVERY

The process for redesigning patient care delivery or adapting existing systems is the same. It is a process, never finished, that must be responsive to and harmonious with a continually changing and ambiguous environment. It requires the following:

- Being clear on the results you want and being passionate about them;
- Understanding your context, or your own situation, and the beliefs and paradigms you hold about it;
- Using an interactive process to discover how to get results; and

- Building into the redesign a process for continued learning, sorting, and growth, a process that makes it possible to avoid getting trapped with a fixed mindset in a changing world.

These processes were handled in various ways at UMHC.

Being Clear on Results and Passionate About Them

BONE MARROW PROJECT. "How to change" began with a return to our roots to see how we delivered patient care. We examined the earlier bone marrow project to find clues for redesigning on a larger scale. Each previous attempt to redesign work had prepared us for this larger leap with a broader scope. Although the specific results of the bone marrow project were not directly transferable to other patient care units, some of the process was. We clarified assumptions about the new design, stated targeted outcomes, and, in retrospect, we can review the actions taken. In the first phase of the bone marrow redesign, two of the outcomes needed were 1) to have pharmacy work done on the unit, particularly the mixing of expensive intravenous medications, so that patients had them when needed, and 2) to reduce the number of people entering a patient's room during the day because of the patients' risk for infection.

We decided that current operating assumptions were faulty in achieving these outcomes and that they should be revised. Assumptions underlying the redesign became the following: 1) costs can be lowered if predictable technical work is done by a consistent, appropriate person trained for the task, and 2) performing whole pieces of work focused on the patient results in work meaningful to the worker and less fragmented for the patient and family and decreases the number of persons working with the patient.

The actions taken to reach the outcomes were driven by these assumptions. We created a pharmacy medication assistant role to do unit pharmacy work under the direction of a pharmacist and in collaboration with nurse and physician. One patient care assistant now provides for environmental services, dietary needs, and activities of daily living for a consistent and limited number of patients.

HOSPITAL-WIDE REDESIGN. The fiscal goal of the bone marrow project had been to be budget neutral. Now we faced a redesign project intended to radically reduce costs. The challenge was to adapt this methodology to all units of the hospital and within all groups of professionals. Our goal of reduced costs had to ensure quality, be patient-focused, and take another look at how we did work. We established a patient care delivery task force charged with saving 8 to 13 million dollars in bedside care delivery, assuring that service standards were met, and retaining patients and families as the clear focus of our work. Co-chaired by hospital and nursing administration, the group dedicated the first 5 weeks of its time to reviewing the most recent literature on patient care restructuring (Lathrop, 1992; Weber, 1991; Hanrahan, 1991; Brider 1992; Henderson & Williams, 1991a,b; Gomberg & Miller, 1992). In addition, they acknowledged the lessons learned from the bone marrow project. In sifting out the pivotal themes and experiences of others working in the area, they found the following facts.

Nearly everyone has been restructuring care delivery, with projects varying in depth from the superficial to those involving deep value shifts.

The focus has been patient/family-centered care, with emphasis on viewing patients as customers.

Organizational roles have been under scrutiny, with an eye to eliminating work or shifting it to more appropriate job classifications.

Questions such as these are being asked: Who is doing what work? Why is this particular work being done? What could be eliminated? What could be done by someone else?

Multifunctional roles based on cross-training to new skills are being developed in all areas.

Skills are shifting from specialists to generalists.

Case management, instituted in a variety of forms, is becoming a common approach to managing patients and costs.

Services are being taken to the patient instead of patients being transported to services.

Patient care units are increasing in size—up to 80 beds but generally not fewer than 40 beds because of the inefficiencies of smaller units.

Major system changes are eliminating inefficiencies. These include such things as admitting patients on units rather than through a centralized admitting department.

Automation to improve communication, documentation, and coordination is spreading, and the target of a paperless organization is emerging.

Changes in patient aggregation, or how patients are grouped, are being examined as a way to improve efficiencies. For example, some units are being merged, but others are incorporating more beds, based on patient needs.

Most restructuring efforts are removing indirect activities such as passing dietary trays or preparing complex medications from bedside nursing duties.

Most hospitals are restructuring in budget neutral environments.

Most restructuring is occurring without an identified theoretical base or belief system, although many of the changes reflect change theory, systems theory, and transformational leadership concepts.

As we compared our experiences with the literature, it became clear that our redesign would be a deep cultural change, moving us from our traditional bureaucratic model to one based on interdisciplinary groups debating issues in a collaborative process. At the heart of the redesign was the patient. Although this sounds simplistic, we had to acknowledge that many of our systems served the systems themselves and not the patient. Contrary

to the past procedure of making cost reductions across the board, new reductions had to be based on assessment of all possible opportunities resulting from collaborative discussion and debate. This became reform through
collaboration, which required us to

- Stop seeing the work as rationally controlled;
- Set a tone and climate of reciprocity;
- Use others' energy; and
- Set ground rules on how to disagree.

This departure from customary operating procedures presented us with
a mixed bag of emotions: excitement, fear, anxiety, skepticism, hope. With
old rules obsolete, feelings of trust and security were replaced by trepida-
tion and questioning, not only of the process but also of the future itself. In
spite of these feelings, the commitment to patients and their care was passionate. We were determined to change on a broad scale and to examine
long-standing organizational practices.

Understanding Context, Beliefs, and Paradigms

Our next step was to clarify and accept our situation, what it was really like
and not what we wanted it to be. It was to tell ourselves the truth and to
explore the nature of the environment as it existed. We had to look closely
at our work and its fit with today's world, and we needed to understand
some of our past boundaries and choices. A solid data base of comparative
information relating costs, outcomes, and service underlies a true understanding of context. The unique medical and nursing needs of patients
shape the nature of work and the roles of caregivers. Realizing that these
needs had changed was essential to the next step of redesign, an intensive
work analysis.

Work analysis became our vehicle to identify major changes. We had to
develop a process that would hold individuals and units accountable for
thinking about their care delivery in dramatically different ways. Our success depended entirely on our ability to change our thinking, because only
then would we change our doing. Staff members providing patient care,
and not just a few selected specialists, carried out the analysis of their own
work. We believed that staff members had the solutions; we had to make it
possible for them to contribute them.

WORK ANALYSIS.   Work analysis is an interdisciplinary process designed to
provide information about the nature of a task and its function, with the
intent of identifying appropriate areas for changing work, eliminating it, or
redesigning it while maintaining quality, consumer satisfaction, and cost
containment. Work analysis provides an opportunity to redesign roles, reshape consciousness of providers, and redefine the rules by which patient
care is delivered. Principles underlying our work analysis include the following:

- Focusing on the needs of the patient and family;
- Eliminating nonessential tasks reduces costs;

- Persons working at their level of preparation and competence conserving resources, using knowledge, and enhancing job satisfaction; and
- Local decision-making, or decisions made by employees, increasing the potential for cultural change and employee satisfaction.

With this agreed set of principles, we moved forward to the next step of the process. Interdisciplinary unit teams, led by the nurse manager, used a structured questionnaire as a guide to assess the patient populations on their units and the staff knowledge and skills required to provide nursing care. Was the care given consistent with the patients' and families' needs? An effective work analysis asks very simple but basic questions about why a task is done and whose needs are being met by doing the task.

Through this process and discussion we identified

- Skills needed for caregivers on each patient care unit;
- Ways we currently assure staff competency;
- New knowledge and skills the nursing staff would require over the next 2 years;
- At least two nursing activities that nursing assistants could assume;
- Daily nursing practices, or rituals, that could be eliminated;
- Practice changes that could be piloted on each unit; and
- Ways to increase savings from salary dollars.

As each unit explored the nature of its work and the needs of patients and families, it recommended changes. Not only were we looking for unit-based changes, but we also wanted to have an assessment of broader systems changes that would help us meet our goals. Looking for "sacred cows," or things we do because "we've always done them that way," became the norm. Personnel from all disciplines wrote responses to the phrase, "What would happen if..." and posted them on large unit flip charts. One idea triggered another, and as creative ideas emerged, the process caught on.

People freed themselves to think differently. There was acknowledgment among some units that they had drifted from clear reasons for doing things and had added work for themselves: Why do we double check some medications? Why do we weigh diapers before using them? Why do we routinely check nasogastric tube placement when the tube is connected to suction and returns are noted? Why do we empty Foley catheter bags hourly and measure and test urine when the patient is stable? Why do change of shift reports take 30 to 60 minutes? The work analysis also challenged some sacred cows, such as who should transcribe a physician's order, who should check orders and how many times, and whether entering laboratory values on flow sheets and in the computer was really necessary.

In addition to patient care units' reviewing their own work, all active committees, councils, and work groups reviewed their goals, outcomes, and membership: How productive were they? Were all of the meetings really necessary? Was there a group goal, or had it long ago been met or avoided? If you could really make a change, how would you do things differently?

Themes began to evolve, and as the project leader analyzed responses from the staff, four major areas for potential cost savings became clear.

1. The skill mix and ratio of registered nurses (RNs) to assistants could change without jeopardizing quality.
2. Reducing the number of direct care hours could be done safely.
3. By changing what people did, we could use professionals and support staff more efficiently.
4. The charge nurse role could be refocused more closely on the patient, while supporting staff could meet the needs of the patient population.

No single idea could generate the savings required. We needed many ideas, and we needed to take the recurring themes and translate them into actions that were not too overwhelming to enlist support. The project director played a significant role in taking issues identified on several patient care areas and moving them into work groups formed for multidisciplinary problem-solving.

INITIAL WORK FLOW CHANGES. Unit staff members moved forward on implementing unit ideas to streamline work flow and make changes in their practice. By breaking the ideas into small actions, people felt they could participate and see progress toward their savings target. For example, they could reduce the number of steps in administering narcotics by eliminating the time required to obtain the narcotic key; with automatic dispensers, several minutes of nursing time per patient could be saved. In analysis, this came to 1 hour per nurse per shift, a significant cost savings. If we bundled several changes together, we could realize a cost reduction in staff hours.

Nearly all of the units began to eliminate work such as double-checking medications and triple-checking orders. They also increased the nursing assistant role in providing direct care to the patient. Delegation issues arose, and in some instances task-specific worksheets helped to clarify accountability for assistants. Two units combined their non-nursing work and shared an assistant on the night shift. The result was a reduction of one assistant position.

Desk functions, frequently performed by the charge nurse, moved to the unit secretary. The transport team of paraprofessionals expanded, resulting in a decrease in the time unit staff members spent off the patient care areas. The department of nursing alone realized a cost savings of 3.3 million dollars through the expansion of paraprofessional roles, a shift in the charge nurse role with clearer expectations and competencies, and a decrease in the number of direct care hours on each unit. In addition, the department identified new areas of knowledge and skills required for the future. These included charge nurse competencies in resource allocation and the development of a trusting climate. "Charge Nurse Adventures," a forum for exploring issues and developing skills, was part of the new structure. Advanced educational classes were offered for the development of new paraprofessionals and mentors, and planned opportunities offered unit staff nurses a chance to practice their new skills.

The work analysis within nursing demonstrated impressive cost savings. The outcomes were financial, structural, and personal. In less than 6 months, we had identified significant potential savings, developed an implementation plan, and put in place unit-based champions who were willing to be change agents. Skill mixes changed from 91% RNs on patient care units to 80%. The reduction did not impair ability to meet patient needs, and the new ratio of RNs to assistants compared favorably with local and national ratios. Most importantly, it was done by averting layoffs of RNs.

As a result of these changes, our productivity index per unit, a way to report patient classification, improved. Staff members changed the way they looked at tasks and problems, and these outcomes triggered work analysis projects in many other areas of the hospital.

Using an Interactive Process

One activity sparked another. People interacted within nursing and across departments, often spontaneously. Spanning the boundaries traditionally set up in our work was necessary to thinking differently. Revamping the way we did our work stimulated our growth in this area. We needed to talk about our experience and our assumptions about the university tripartite mission, patient care, research, and education. We needed to define and to debate the meaning of quality, to understand different ways of delivering care, and to understand better how to have employees contribute. We developed three major processes, in addition to work analysis, to bring about these results: 1) cross-functional retreats, 2) project teamwork, and 3) search conferences.

CROSS-FUNCTIONAL RETREATS. Retreats during which staff members could remove themselves from their daily work offered an opportunity to think, challenge ideas, and realize that all departments shared common problems and goals. Retreats were also held for nurses on nursing issues. Both types of retreats enabled heterogeneous cross-fertilization as well as homogenous idea-sharing and problem-solving. These retreats provided participants an opportunity to think together, to realize that their issues were "our" issues, and to move their thinking beyond the boundaries of what one person alone could do. There was healthy questioning of one another: In what situations do nurses need to do the bath? Why don't charge nurses care for patients? Why do nurses spend their time transcribing physician orders? The formula for successful retreats included meeting off-site, having a time period long enough to think (a minimum of 4 hours), beginning with a brainstorming period, breaking into unit-specific groups to consider opportunities for cost savings, identifying possible change strategies, and formulating plans. This formula fostered an increase in diversity of ideas and an acceptance of differences.

Storytelling became a strong component of our success. Units that had made significant changes (for example, having RNs successfully delegate to others) shared their stories, telling of problems along the way and how they had dealt with them. Successes and failures surfaced as honesty and trust grew. The interactive process reduced isolation, and exchange sessions became safe havens for sharing problems without feeling "dumb" or "wrong." One nurse candidly discussed how she couldn't trust the nursing assistant because she never worked with the same person; delegation was impossible. Another nurse realized that her perception of patient safety differed from the float nurse's. The float nurses considered it unsafe to have a lack of consistency between units on issues ranging from the place where supplies were stored to how assignments were made. "Sometimes," they said, "floating is like starting a new job every day."

After each retreat, staff nurse participants collaborated with their peers on the unit about the issues, ideas, and actions discussed. This feedback process enabled them to monitor, steer, and change course, if necessary. Feedback and exchange of ideas came in the form of notes, memos, comments, and formal meetings, so that they could assure input from all shifts and from both part-time and full-time employees. Staff nurses who participated in retreats became the unit change agents, fielding questions, responding to challenges such as "physicians not doing their part" and persuading "non-believers," who denied the fact of our changing environment and its impact on the hospital financial status. As the feedback process evolved, three or four consistent champions emerged on the units. Their enthusiasm, commitment to act, and courageous determination to change made the project work at the unit level. Without them, each unit would have been unable to achieve the cultural changes and the transformations in care delivery.

PROJECT TEAMWORK. Project teamwork followed the same format as cross-functional retreats except that the focus was on a specific issue or problem. Interdisciplinary collaboration became common. Pharmacists participated in solving one issue on the bone marrow transplant unit that appeared to be a nursing problem. Selected, costly medications required on-unit mixing because of the need to have them administered within a relatively short period. This was being done by the nurse and sometimes resulted in waste because of interruptions and other demands. As the cost to the patient became clear, the project team developed a pharmacy technician role for a pharmacy-based person to prepare the medications. The plan was quickly implemented, and the hospital realized a cost savings over 6 months of operation.

The scope of the organization-wide project required multiple work groups to examine concepts of multifunctional worker roles such as service, technical, and clinical partnerships. The primary nurse role, which embodied our values, had to change, and a case management system had to be developed and implemented. We used work groups to take the work analysis findings and change skill mixes. We now knew from our experience that we could reduce staffing without jeopardizing care. Other work groups took on the tasks of developing a more outcome-focused discharge planning process and of changing patient aggregates or groupings to decrease the number of small patient care units and subsequently increase flexibility in caring for patients. Today, we acknowledge project teams as a significant transformation in the way we conduct our business.

SEARCH CONFERENCE. A third effective interactive tool, especially for the bone marrow project, was the search conference. The search conference integrated ideas from the past, present, and future or went "back to the future." It looked at the culture as it existed and as it had developed to this point, and it traced themes and values. The conference was based on three assumptions.

1. You can transform the culture into what you want if you recognize what you have.
2. Every organization has themes, rituals, and heroes that repeat themselves over time and that symbolize and embody the history.
3. Culture shapes the behavior of members of the organization. It is the force that ties people together. It is neither bad nor good—it just is.

On one retreat, participants divided into three groups—past, present, and future. Before the search conference, each group prepared by collecting newspaper and magazine clippings describing events and trends from the past and present or trends they believed to be shaping the hospital's future. In addition, they brought photographs, brochures, and awards. As each group displayed its items, they told stories about them. In the process, they looked at the themes and discovered that they traced their history through significant milestones marked by medical advances. Nursing was noticeably absent from their lists of milestones, even though, in discussions, they acknowledged its significant contributions.

The search conference described by Weisbord (1990) made it possible to celebrate the past, to notice the present, and to draw conclusions for future transformation. Naming the events, norms, and themes of the culture that had brought us to the present freed us to begin affirming those that would serve in the future and to make new choices. As the total transformation effort unfolded, it became clear that we had made new choices about collective interaction and multidisciplinary problem-solving even though we were sometimes clumsy in our first attempts.

Building In a Process for Continued Learning, Sorting, and Growth

Work redesign is a way of doing business, a way of thinking that does not end. As a process, it enables the organization to keep its finger on the pulse of change and to respond quickly, to hear rumblings as they occur rather than after they reach cataclysmic proportions. Because of this, maintaining momentum, learning, and enthusiasm over time becomes an issue. Our project at the UMHC has been punctuated by a myriad of projects with beginnings and ends but has actually been in motion for 4 years. Three factors have kept learning and momentum strong: 1) identified leadership, 2) complete and continuous communication through multiple channels, and 3) systematic thinking.

IDENTIFIED LEADERSHIP. Leadership, both formal and informal, consistently has held the banner for redesigning work. The top leadership, as well as project leadership, has changed over the period we have been involved in work redesign. Still, we consistently have had hospital and nursing executives who supported the project and were advocates for patient care. In addition, full-time project managers with credibility and competence have led the project operations. To be effective, the latter have needed skills in organizational development, work analysis, and collaboration. The people in these positions have fielded doubt, handled unwillingness to confront turf issues, and managed subtle sabotage. They have presented unwanted news to physicians, administration, and staff. These are positions for the courageous and competent, for those people who are creative and who excel in getting things done. They are for those who can handle unique challenges, such as an unanticipated unionization effort by nurses that brought parts of the change process to a halt. During our work redesign, a full-time and skilled project director has kept momentum in place, despite the external forces that created an inability to fully proceed for several months.

COMMUNICATION. Nowhere is communication more critical than in a cultural change project in which everyone's job is affected and in which job security is the issue. Communication must be continuous, with opened channels throughout the organization. Several communication practices provided effective guidelines.

Communication is imperative; in the absence of information, people invent their own. As people work together in redesign, they think in new ways. During some periods of the project, it may seem as though nothing is happening. This was realized after we reached an impasse in our first attempt to design a case management model. To keep the staff informed, we issued a one-page, *Work Redesign News Flash*, with the intent of building and maintaining momentum. This biweekly news flash presented a visual image of sparks igniting and print flashing, and highlighted three or four bulleted items detailing updates on the project. We limited the text in an effort to assure that it was quick to read and informative. The success of this strategy was clear after the project director began receiving calls from managers asking to be on the mailing list or to receive additional copies.

People hear a message when they are ready. We found it necessary to repeat our message succinctly, frequently, and in multiple ways. We used *Nursing Links*, a weekly update to the staff, as well as monthly town meetings for all hospital personnel, staff meetings every 3 to 4 weeks, staff forums conducted by the director of nursing, and *Dollars and Sense*, a publication covering success stories often initiated at the grass roots. Often all of these channels carried the same message in different words, to different people, and at different times of day.

Communication is a visual tool as well as a verbal one. Visuals, including charts and graphs meant to demonstrate the acuity of the financial issues, helped sustain the message in a way that minutes, memos, or meetings could not. Drawings proved useful. To help staff members recognize that bone marrow patients did, in fact, have fragmented care, we asked two different multidisciplinary groups of four persons each to draw the process in the admission of a patient moving from clinic to hospital. The results substantiated our belief that visual descriptions can get the point across, especially if drawn by members of the staff we were trying to reach. The two drawings differed dramatically in the listing of steps, but they both effectively demonstrated the complexity and people involved in the process. This motivated a multidisciplinary group to collective action.

SYSTEMIC THINKING.   Our greatest challenge was helping people to understand that the interdependent functions form the whole of a patient's experience, rather than seeing the patient experience as a collection or accumulation of functions or tasks. Thinking systemically offers a realistic way to manage the challenge that results from change and ambiguity about the future. It moves us along the continuum from being reactive to becoming proactive. Learning to think systemically is unfamiliar and is a slower process than the more familiar, linear problem-solving represented in Gantt charts and work plans. However, to increase the likelihood of positive, long-term change, it is imperative that we move beyond the familiar to combine systemic with linear thinking.

We believe that learning to think systemically requires being able to experience systems at work in a place in which feedback is immediately possible. The feedback allows people to see the impact of their decisions and actions. To do this, we used a work simulation technique, during which participants constructed and sold space ships. The simulation showed the interdependence of systems and their complexity. Participants recognized in their experience of a faulty system that, although they could and did redesign it, there was no flawless design; the design of the system must be rooted in the intended results. Thinking systemically is an important quest. It requires us to live with issues as we search for patterns within them, rather than to come to quick solutions; it demands a new set of assumptions about how the world works.

Lessons Learned

We at UMHC continue to learn from others and from ourselves about how to build a learning organization in which we can reflect on the scope of our issues and the impact of our decisions. Some of our realizations include the following lessons.

GETTING STARTED.   Begin where you are, and begin with a small group of motivated staff members. Working to have all participants accept a change before its implementation is useless, since many people must see it work before they can grasp it. Positive modeling by a few respected persons is more powerful in getting others to participate than continuous classes and readings. The goal is team success, and it is through the team example that many learn what part they can play.

CRISIS.   Without a doubt, crisis or perceived crisis continues to be the single greatest motivator for change. We cannot ignore the fact that our initial efforts to change the system spread throughout the whole organization only after it was faced with a cataclysmic financial crisis. Until that time, change was valued, necessary, creative, fun—and for someone else.

ROLE CHANGES.   Most changes needed today are transformational; they are not reactive. People are hesitant and sometimes unable to see that another person in a different role might be able to do some of their work. The structure of roles in the patient care setting is driven by the care work and by the needs of the patient population. If the goal is to focus on what works best to meet patient and family needs, we must think deliberately about whether everything we do is consistent with the reason we are doing it. Many staff members are unable to make radical change instantly; they must be motivated and challenged to forge new paradigms.

MOMENTUM. Innovation and long-term change processes become tiring; participants become weary. Building and maintaining momentum—keeping each other energized in such a way that everyone can contribute—must be an integral part of the process. Maintaining momentum required the collective thinking of our creative people, the involvement and commitment of staff at the unit level, and the ability to juggle ambiguity if things did not work out as expected.

LEADERSHIP. The role of leadership in crisis, change, or transformation cannot be overestimated. It is paramount to the success of any endeavor for change. Those leading redesign efforts must be credible at all levels of the organization. They must be able to work with physicians and with technicians, within the bureaucracy, and within the political system of the organization.

▬SUMMARY

Reflecting on our work makes it clear that we often learned the most valuable lessons between projects, or between cycles of activity. There is no one way or right way to begin the transformation and redesign of patient care (Display 17-1). The goals we pursued over the past 3 years have not changed significantly. They became sharper, clearer, more personalized, and were pursued with stronger commitment, but never did they vary from our origi-

---

DISPLAY 17-1   Some "Truths" About Redesign

1. Systems thinking is not a typical way of doing business in health care.
2. Freedom without reprisal must be given if people are to think nontraditional thoughts.
3. Skill mix changes are rarely considered beyond nursing, yet everyone has opportunities for this.
4. Nursing remains the largest and most visible health care discipline; other disciplines are quick to criticize and offer suggestions for nursing and often project their own inefficiencies.
5. The perception of physician buy-in throughout the process is critical; however, most physicians have no experience in redesigning work and haven't a clue about how to contribute.
6. Something tangible must happen with plans for redesign; it cannot be business as usual.
7. External consultants are valuable when paired with internal consultants.

nal visions of reducing costs, ensuring the delivery of quality care, and increasing employee satisfaction. The experience of the UMHC affirms that there is no linear path to change and that projects are untidy and unpredictable, but that the stronger the commitment to the desired goals, the more likely we are to succeed. For us, change driven by crisis was stronger and provided more "ownership" than change driven by innovation alone. Redesigning the work of patient care provides us with a significant opportunity to chart a quality course for patients and health care providers that is fiscally sound and transforms the work environment.

REFERENCES

Brider, P. (1992, September). The move to patient-focused care. *American Journal of Nursing*, pp. 26–33.

Gomberg, F. & Miller, K. (1992). Focused care centers, decentralization, cross-training and care paths define "world class healthcare" at Florida's Lee Memorial. *Strategies for Healthcare Excellence, 5*(3) 1–7.

Hanrahan, T. (1991). New approaches to caregiving. *Healthcare Forum Journal, 34*(4), 33–38.

Hart, G. (1993, Summer). The University Hospital: A history, a vision. *Health Sciences*, pp. 15–17.

Henderson, J. L. & Williams, J. B. (1991a, July–August). The people side of patient care redesign. *Healthcare Forum Journal*, pp. 44–49.

Henderson, J. L. & Williams, J. B. (1991b, July–August). Ten steps for restructuring patient care. *Healthcare Forum Journal*, pp. 50–55.

Lathrop, J. P. (1992, May–June). The patient-focused hospital. *Healthcare Forum Journal*, pp. 76–78.

Weber, D. (1991). Six models of patient-focused care. *Healthcare Forum Journal, 34*(4), 23–31.

Weisbord, M. (1990). *Productive workplaces: Organizing and managing for dignity, meaning, and community.* San Francisco: Jossey-Bass.

Chapter 18

Project T.E.N.: Innovation Toward Excellence

LINDA SCHARF

Nursing restructuring and redesign of patient care delivery is often viewed as a time-limited project. With such perception, restructuring and redesign is often seen as a discrete set of tasks with few specified goals and objectives, a time-detailed table for completion, and easily identifiable beginning and completion milestones. In contrast, our view was to envision restructuring as an ongoing process of innovation that is dynamic and ever changing.

The impetus for the redesign of nursing care delivery at Millard Fillmore Health System was the invitation to submit a proposal for The Robert Wood Johnson Foundation/Pew Charitable Trusts planning grant, "Strengthening Hospital Nursing," in 1988. The Millard Fillmore Health System has two acute care, general hospitals. At that time, the hospitals were experiencing serious problems related to the national and local nursing shortage. Effects of the shortage included high vacancy and turnover rates among registered nurses (RNs), frequent use of temporary agency nurses to supplement staffing, increased costs for recruiting and orienting new RNs, reports of staff nurse dissatisfaction and burnout, and a general perception and consensus that the quality of nursing care had to be improved.

Organizationally, there had been attempts to deal with these escalating problems with strategies such as increases in RNs' wages and introduction of alternative work schedules. These strategies were reactions to suggestions and requests by staff nurses. Still, there were strong feelings by the administration and the nursing staff that these strategies were addressing symptoms rather than the underlying issues related to nursing and patient care delivery.

In order to address the issues and develop a proposal for the planning grant, a project planning team was formed. At that time, the organization was without a chief nurse executive. The planning team consisted of the hospital's chief executive officer, the chief operating officer, and a project director.

The team identified many major barriers to the effective delivery of patient care:

- Inadequate regard for nurses as professionals;
- Perception of nurses as assistants to physicians;
- Lack of structured opportunities for staff nurses to improve their practice, address interdepartmental conflicts, and problem-solve effectively with physicians;
- Head nurses who were inadequately prepared to function in an expanded management role;
- Lack of honest and open discussion between nursing and administration;
- Absence of nurse executive leadership and representation at the administrative level;
- Lack of full understanding by the nursing staff and hospital administration of the underlying issues affecting the delivery of high-quality, cost-effective care;
- Increasing patient acuities and shorter lengths of stay, intensifying the need for more nursing resources; and
- Inefficient communication systems within the hospital, characterized by overreliance on paperwork and cumbersome data collection procedures.

The grant application was a success, and the hospital received a one-year, $50,000 planning grant in 1989 (Strengthening Hospital Nursing, 1992). This allowed the hospital to develop and implement strategies to address the identified barriers by committing to a process of continual innovation which would foster excellence in patient care. Although the hospitals did not receive an implementation grant, a commitment was made to see the process through to a real transformation of care delivery.

The first step was to select a nurse executive who could lead the process forward. The next vital step was the selection and education of key stakeholders within the organization. The education task force included a board member, the project director, the newly appointed vice president of nursing, the vice president of medicine, and the chief executive officer.

Armed with newly acquired information and enthusiasm, the team returned to the hospitals and began the long journey toward innovation and transformation. The project was presented to the board of directors, medical staff, administrative staff, nurse managers, and staff nurses. General staff meetings were held, using such techniques as the nominal group process to identify areas related to patient care delivery requiring improvements. More than 250 staff nurses participated in this important process. The team decided that the project required a name to help members identify with its goals. The name selected was Project T.E.N (Toward Excellence in Nursing).

▄PROJECT T.E.N.

There were two major objectives of Project T.E.N.:

1. To redefine the roles, responsibilities, and tasks of the nursing staff and identify improvements in skills needed to deliver quality and cost-effective nursing care; to enhance nursing's sense of profession-

alism and job satisfaction; and to permit nurses to apply their knowledge and skills at the highest levels of performance possible.

2. To organizationally restructure nursing service to foster nursing
leadership, participatory management, enhanced communication,
collaboration, and quality patient care.

In order to accomplish these major objectives, two planning committees
were formed: a nursing practice committee, and a management and structure committee. These committees included the nurse executive, the project director, nurse managers, nurse educators, staff nurses, other hospital
administrators and managers, physicians, board members, and health care
consultants. It was important that the planning committees have representation of those involved in direct patient care delivery.

It was believed that a meaningful, working definition of nurses' roles and
responsibilities, as they are operational in practice, was necessary to move
the process forward. This working definition was developed in collaboration
with all organizational disciplines. Senge has stated that the creative tension
between the current reality and the future ideal can be used as a motivator
(Senge, 1990). Project T.E.N.'s definition of nursing is detailed in Display
18-1. The ideal was contrasted with the reality as a mechanism to identify
needed areas for improvement in nursing and the entire organization.

■ DESIGN TEAMS

The major vehicles used to implement the created innovations were design
teams. Design teams are multidisciplinary teams led by nursing representatives for the purpose of developing and implementing innovative strategies
for change. The design teams introduced many innovative changes that
transformed the structure and roles of nursing, improved patient care delivery, and resulted in measurable improvements in patient outcomes. Some

---

DISPLAY 18-1   Working Definition of Nurses

Nurses are patient care providers responsible for defining patient needs,
planning, coordinating, and participating in the delivery of care while
evaluating its effectiveness.

Nurses are communicators and teachers of health and wellness and focus on
patient capabilities and skills necessary for self-care. They serve as family and
patient advocates and assist patients in attaining maximum wellness. Nurses
are professional colleagues of physicians.

By applying their knowledge and experience, they make discretionary
decisions, perform, coordinate, facilitate, and delegate the process for the
overall delivery of patient care.

Nurses are leaders and members of therapeutic teams with unique
responsibilities for treating patients in collaboration with all other members of
the health care team. In addition, they are responsible for constant
communication and documentation of essential patient-related information to
all members of the health care team.

of the major redesign and restructuring accomplishments of design teams are detailed in the following paragraphs.

REDEFINITION OF NURSING MANAGEMENT ROLES. The introduction of the role of vice president for nursing meant an expansion of the functions of the nurse executive to include broad visibility and access to the highest administrative levels of decision-making. A level of nursing supervision between the nursing director and unit-level nurse managers was eliminated. The traditional role of head nurse was redefined to nurse manager. Nurse managers were acknowledged as having full management authority and responsibility on the nursing units, including budgetary and employment decisions and the development of practice standards.

CHANGING THE STRUCTURE OF NURSING MANAGEMENT. The formation of staff nursing practice committees occurred at both facilities. The committees were composed of staff nurses from each nursing unit. The commitment to seek staff-level perceptions and involvement in nursing department policies and practices meant seeking the committees' recommendations on such issues. Issues involving scheduling and financial support of continuing education activities were topics tackled by the staff nurse practice committee.

The chairmen of the two staff nurse practice committees served on the executive cabinet, the policy-making agent of nursing service, along with nurse managers, nursing directors, and the nurse executive.

The results were profound and measurable. There was a feeling that long-standing issues were being addressed and solutions were possible. There was a dramatic reduction in RN vacancy rates (from 13% in 1988 to 7% in 1993), and the corresponding reduction in RN turnover rates (from 14% in 1988 to 4% in 1993) resulted in significant savings in RN recruitment and orientation costs. With the reduction of RN turnover and vacancy rates, dependence on temporary agency utilization ended in 1990.

INTRODUCTION OF NURSING RESEARCH. As part of the attempt to emphasize the professional aspects of nursing practice, a design team identified appropriate research questions and approaches. Since 1990, the Millard Fillmore nursing service has sponsored three conferences on topics related to research in nursing practice. A team of 20 nurses completed a research study of nurses', physicians', and patients' perceptions of important nursing care activities. These initiatives resulted in local and national presentations as well as two published articles.

INTRODUCTION OF CLINICAL CAREER LADDERS FOR STAFF NURSES. In order to address the staff nurses' feelings of lack of respect for bedside nursing, clinical ladders were introduced. This was implemented to recognize and reward expert bedside nurses. The project was led by a steering committee of staff nurses. They based their clinical career ladder, from novice to expert, on Benner's theory of expert nursing practice (Benner, 1984).

Clinical career ladders allowed financial rewards for expert clinical practice and encouraged staff nurses to view bedside nursing as a lifetime career.

Some nurses voiced fear that this was an elitist endeavor that would not benefit the average nurse committed to practicing at the bedside. In fact, the unrest led to an unsuccessful attempt to unionize the RN staff.

The steering committee spent time orienting the staff with open presentations, a resource book on each unit, and the provision of nurse-to-nurse coaching to help applicants in portfolio preparation. Their commitment has had tangible results in a year and a half; more than 30% of the RN staff have advanced within the career ladder system.

Improvement in Nursing Documentation Methods

A team of nurse managers and staff nurses redesigned nursing documentation. This resulted in the introduction of flow sheets for general medical-surgical and critical care. The system of documenting nursing diagnosis and traditional nursing care plans was also redesigned.

Improving Communication

In order to mitigate feelings of alienation and lack of information, various communication strategies were attempted. Such initiatives included a nursing newsletter, "Nursing Advocate." High visibility of nursing and hospital administration and regular staff meetings have gone a long way in improving communications.

Improvements to Nursing Care Delivery

From the beginning, it was apparent that the way nurses delivered care to their patients had to change. Originally, a redesign team introduced some limited changes, such as the elimination of the charge nurse position and pairing of a nurse and a nursing assistant as a caregiving team. Although some improvements were seen, all of the defined goals were not met.

As an outgrowth of the original planning for Project T.E.N., nursing service received a 1.5 million dollar grant from the New York State Health Department in 1991 to introduce innovations in the delivery of care toward increased productivity. This project resulted in the introduction of nurse case managers and cross-trained workers on two demonstration nursing units. The nurse case manager's primary role is to coordinate and facilitate medical and nursing care, in order to decrease length of hospitalization and increase patient satisfaction. The cross-trained patient care assistants were paired with professional nurses and assumed expanded duties in the areas of phlebotomy, simple respiratory treatments, vital sign assessment, and other patient care tasks.

▬CLINICAL DESIGN TEAMS IN ACTION

One of the most successful clinical design teams was led by a clinical nurse specialist. This team was committed to reducing the prevalence of pressure ulcers which developed in hospitalized patients. A multidisciplinary team was convened. Membership included physicians, nurses, educators, dieticians, and others. Using the principles of total quality management (TQM), the team documented the current care process, designed and implemented an improved process, and measured its effectiveness. The newly designed care process included advanced training in the prevention and care of pressure ulcers; designation of a staff nurse in each unit as a resource nurse for pressure ulcers; introduction of a documented, comprehensive assessment for skin integrity at the time of admission and every 3 days afterward for all patients; and formal treatment protocols for all grades of pressure ulcers, from Grade 0 (prevention for high risk of developing a pressure ulcer) to Grade IV (treatment of deep ulcers involving soft tissue, muscle, and tendons).

The results were remarkable. The prevalence of pressure ulcers decreased by more than 80%. Resource nurses were proud of their accomplishments and were acknowledged by hospital staff. The actual hospital-wide utilization of special equipment used in the prevention and treatment of pressure ulcers decreased in cost by $86,400 annually. These accomplishments were highlighted at hospital presentations as well as local and national meetings and led to a long-term relationship with a manufacturer of special therapeutic beds to investigate innovative treatment methods and protocols.

▬MOVING FORWARD

The spirit of innovation and leadership has become part of the nursing culture, yet no one sees the process as complete. Despite the pains of change, the hospital is committed to moving ahead with more innovative projects, with the ultimate goal of transforming the entire organization. The changes in nursing care delivery, involving nurse case managers and patient care assistants, are being expanded throughout the facilities. Innovations require a tremendous commitment of energy. Great amounts of time have been devoted to communication. Still, everyone acknowledges that the process is far from complete. Effective communication is still problematic at times.

▬CONCLUSION

Introducing any change or innovation in a large, complex institution can be difficult. Project T.E.N. has made continued innovation part of the essential culture of nursing. It has emphasized the pivotal nature of nursing in all patient care activities. It acknowledges that to be successful, the professional nature of nursing must be fostered and celebrated. It has demonstrated that an empowered and energized nursing staff is a tremendous force for achieving excellence.

Nursing has served as a primary change agent in this organization. Nursing can lead the way in organizational transformation. There is commitment that the concepts and experiences introduced by nursing will disseminate throughout the organization over time and result in an organization-wide transformation.

The innovation and progress experienced would not have been possible without Dr. Harry Sultz, Project Director, Project T.E.N. Excellence in nursing is an ideal. The dedicated nurses, managers, and other staff at Millard Fillmore Health System make it a reality daily by their commitment to patient care.

■ REFERENCES

Benner, P. (1984). *From novice to expert.* Reading, MA: Addison-Wesley.

Senge, P. (1990). *The fifth discipline: The art and practice of the learning organization.* New York: Doubleday Currency.

Strengthening Hospital Nursing Program, National Program Office. (1992). *Strengthening Hospital Nursing: A program to improve patient care.* St. Petersburg, FL: The Robert Wood Johnson Foundation and The Pew Charitable Trusts.

Chapter 19

The Support Assistant: Key to Work Redesign in a Professional Practice Model

LAURA J. DUPRAT   MAUREEN P. McCAUSLAND   LESLIE J. AJL

EILEEN M. KEEFE   PATRICIA M. LYDON   PEGGY J. REILEY

The health care delivery system in the United States is under increasing pressure to improve quality of care, measure patient outcomes, reduce costs, and provide satisfying work environments for professional and support staff. Hospital and nursing leaders are seeking new organizational designs and roles that permit physicians and nurses to deliver professional care in an efficient and cost-effective manner. Reengineering and work redesign are being touted as strategies that allow hospitals to become patient-focused and more efficient. Successful reengineering and work redesign efforts build on a base of core organizational values and are congruent with the organizational climate. This chapter describes one work redesign effort at Boston's Beth Israel Hospital. The work was supported, in part, by a grant from The Robert Wood Johnson Foundation and The Pew Charitable Trusts, "Strengthening Hospital Nursing: A Program to Improve Patient Care" initiative.

▬ CARE DELIVERY SYSTEM

Primary nursing was instituted as a nursing care delivery system in several hospitals during the 1970s (Manthey, Ciske, Robertson, & Harris, 1970). Nursing professional practice models were introduced in the late 1970s and refined throughout the 1980s (Clifford & Horvath, 1990). The professional practice model at Beth Israel is multifaceted. Primary nursing is the nursing care delivery system. Primary nursing is characterized by accountability of the nurse for patient care, continuity of care between the primary nurse and patient, and collaboration among nurses, other providers, and hospital administration. It is supported by strong, decentralized management; opportunities for professional growth, recognition and advancement; and strong

Flarey, D: REDESIGNING NURSING CARE DELIVERY: Transforming Our Future
© 1995, J. B. Lippincott Company

clinical and support services. The professional practice model is satisfying to patients, families, nurses, and the organization.

Core values of Beth Israel Hospital are articulated in the hospital's mission statement (Beth Israel Hospital, 1983) and through communication to employees from the executive vice president/hospital director. The major mission of Beth Israel Hospital is to deliver high-quality patient care, in both scientific and human terms. This mission is carried out within a framework of financially responsible management. Interpersonal relationships are extremely important at Beth Israel Hospital. The nursing service has consistently focused on nurturing the nurse–patient relationship and the nurse–nurse relationship.

The core values led to strategic and operational decisions that supported the implementation of primary nursing and the evolution of the professional practice model.

Fifteen years ago, before implementation of the professional practice model, the focus of care was not the patient but rather the accomplishment of tasks. For those of us who were there, we cannot forget what our practice was like. We were assigned to rooms and to tasks. In the former, there were patients who represented little more than a collection of assignments: morning care, specimen collections and perhaps on occasion, teaching. In the latter were a set of activities completed for the unit or team, such as checking vital signs, medications and dressing changes. When discussing patient care the major issue addressed was the status of tasks assigned. There was no recognition of the concept of continuity of care or of its importance. Continuity of care was not necessary if the totality of your work was measured by tasks. One can complete those tasks on any patient in any setting in an isolated eight-hour shift. Floating was an outcome of this perspective, and nurses would be sent from one area to another to be "task masters" (Liston, Dick, & Greenspan, 1990, p. 59).

Increasing complexity of patient care, coupled with decreasing lengths of stay, has led us to develop new roles in the institution in which continuity, efficiency, and patient and employee satisfaction are core features. The current work redesign initiative is guided by the same values that led us to primary nursing. The focus is on providing patient care, not on substituting unlicensed personnel for the professional nurse.

ROLE DEVELOPMENT

In response to cost-containment pressures, hospitals have taken a greater interest in focusing on efficiency of operations. This was a major impetus to the development of a new role. The initial goals of the role were to 1) decrease the number of support workers coming into contact with patients; 2) enhance job enrichment for support service personnel; and 3) continue to support the role of the clinical nurse.

We formed a committee with members from the departments of nursing, environmental services, transportation services, and nutrition services to discuss the creation of this new role. Later, staff from human resources joined the group.

▬THE PROBLEM

The first priority of the group was to identify the major problems with the current system. We knew that on any given day, up to 30 employees entered a patient's room. This parade of people made it difficult for patients to rest, impinged on their privacy, and did not fit with our philosophy of personalized care.

Recognizing that the current system did not work well for the patient, we then examined how this centralized system worked for employees in support roles. Environmental service workers, on average, cleaned 13 rooms each on the day shift. They rarely, if ever, spoke to patients or other staff. They sometimes ate lunch in the tub room on the unit rather than in the lunch room with the nursing staff. Staff in the transportation department worked out of a central office with a dispatcher. Because of the large number of areas the transporter visited, working relationships were difficult to develop with patients and staff on patient care units. The nutrition staff, hired to deliver trays to patients, went from unit to unit delivering and removing meal trays from patients' rooms throughout the institution. Again, the transient nature of the work made it difficult for nutrition staff to develop meaningful relationships with patients and other employees.

Finally, it was determined that the current system was not consistent in providing effective, quality services. For example, the nutrition tray passers were often seen waiting at the elevators for the cart with meal trays to arrive. After the meal trays were delivered to patients, the nursing staff would often find the tray on a bedside table that was out of the reach of the patient.

Similar efficiency and quality issues were also evident in the work of environmental services and transportation staff. Because the staff in these departments were not directly involved with patients, it was difficult for them to understand patient needs. The problem of down time was evident in these departments, just as it was in nutrition services.

▬CREATING A SHARED VISION

According to Senge (1990), "the practice of shared vision involves the skills of unearthing shared 'pictures of the future' that foster genuine commitment and enrollment on the part of those involved, rather than compliance" (p. 9). As the committee discussed the realities of the current system, the direction for the new role became apparent. The role would be designed directly around the needs of patients. We restated the goals for the role as follows: 1) decrease the number of staff that patients come in contact with during their hospitalization; 2) reengineer support services to more effectively aid clinical nurses in their work; 3) make it possible for staff who work in a support capacity to become a part of the health care team; and 4) improve the quality and efficiency of support services provided to patients.

There was consensus among all committee members that the identified goals were the right goals and that they were possible and realistic. The decision to incorporate the work of environmental services, transportation services, nutrition services, and some tasks that nurses' aides had been doing into one role was based on a brainstorming exercise completed by the planning group. We brought the list of tasks generated during the exercise to various departments for feedback. Consensus as to which tasks would be combined to redesign the new role came easily. We titled the new position "support assistant." The decision to have the support assistant be unit-based, not centrally based, seemed to follow naturally.

The committee members next developed a comprehensive job description for the new role. The unit-based support assistant would be accountable for meeting the needs of patients by cleaning and maintaining the environment, distributing and collecting patients' meal trays and assisting them with their meals, transporting patients to other departments for diagnostic tests, performing other related transport functions, and performing a few tasks that have traditionally fallen under the domain of nursing, such as weighing patients, ambulating patients, and recording intake and output.

It was obvious to the group that everyone would benefit by this role redesign. The patients would have familiar staff with them throughout the day performing tasks that would normally have been carried out by several individuals. The support assistant would become more a part of the health care team in an expanded and enriched role. Nurses would benefit by having better quality services supporting their practice. The hospital would stand to benefit as well by increasing the satisfaction of patients and those providing services to patients. The committee had a goal of implementing the program in a cost neutral manner. Plans were formulated for a six-month demonstration that would take place on a 46-bed general medical unit.

▬ SUPPORT ASSISTANT PROJECT COORDINATOR

The work of education, orientation, and providing ongoing feedback to the support assistants was assumed by a clinical nurse on the demonstration unit. The selection of this project coordinator occurred early in the planning phase of the project. The nurse manager of the demonstration unit chose the coordinator. The decision was based on several factors: this nurse was a senior clinical nurse with recognizable advanced skills in leadership and communication; the positive relationships she had developed with nurses on the unit, as well as staff from all areas of the hospital, were noteworthy; and, she could easily identify, model, and support the values and culture of the unit. She worked in concert with the nurse manager to facilite the implementation of the support assistant role.

The project coordinator did not have direct patient care assignments for most of the six-month demonstration period. This was possible because of grant funding. A strong message was thereby sent that nursing supported this endeavor and valued its potential for improving patient care. In addition, the support assistant committee had specified that close collaboration with nursing was crucial to the successful outcome of the project. Committee members wanted the support assistants to have more involvement and a greater sense of self-identification as members of the unit and the health care team. This connection would be facilitated through the development of collaborative working relationships with clinical nurses from the demonstration unit.

▬PLANNING FOR CHANGE

As people were interviewed and hired, the project coordinator elicited suggestions and support from nursing staff on the demonstration unit, continually engaging them in the overall plan for change. Meetings were held on two occasions to discuss feelings about the role of the support assistant and potential problems that clinical nurses might encounter. The clinical nurses raised many important concerns at the meetings: What should we do if we observe that a support assistant cannot do his or her job? Who will be the support assistants' supervisor? Who will provide them with feedback? How is feedback best given? How should we facilitate the support assistants' ease of transition in interacting with the rest of the staff? How does it feel to share space with another group of people? During the meetings several staff members demonstrated interest in and support for the project. These individuals have subsequently become more involved with the support assistants than the other clinical nurses. They have helped facilitate acceptance and growth of the role. The pivotal person in the integration of the support assistant into the staff, however, remained the project coordinator. She established a strong working relationship with all of the support assistants. By her example, the issues from the nursing staff cited above were eventually resolved.

▬INFORMATION SHARING

Employees learned about the demonstration through the weekly hospital newsletter, from the hospital president, and from their work team leaders. There were many informal discussions between support assistant committee members and hospital staff.

It was through our experience as an interdisciplinary work team that we learned how important it was to present the role to the staff currently working on the demonstration unit, and to those potentially interested in the role, in an interdisciplinary way. The committee members planned a series of get-togethers for interested employees from the departments of nursing, nutrition, environmental services, and transportation to learn about the support assistant role. These coffee sessions took place on the demonstration unit. Committee members presented themselves as a cohesive work team to stress both the nature of a unit-based role and the importance of an environment in which people in different roles can work together to provide better patient care.

Initially, the coffee sessions were somewhat uncomfortable, with prospective support assistants on one side of the table and committee members on the other side. Nurses from the unit would gradually trickle in to spend a few moments as a way of lending support to the new role. As committee members became more comfortable, they were less formal, more welcoming, and better able to address questions and concerns that people had. The concerns were realistic: Will we still have our jobs if the role is not success-ful? If we don't like the role, can we return to our previous jobs? Is this new role the way of the future for the entire institution? Who will be my manager in the new role? Will I be earning more money? What hours will I work? The issues that emerged from the discussion were brought back to the commit-tee. In short, the questions helped to further shape the role of the support assistant.

SELECTION

Managers in nutrition, environmental services, and transportation helped interested staff recognize their potential for the role. We were looking for staff from each of these central areas for the demonstration, as each would bring some area of expertise to the new role.

Some individuals were encouraged by their managers to consider the new role. Others came forward on their own. Applicants were screened by a recruiter in human resources who was aware of the unique characteristics needed for the role. Applicants with a history of strong work performance, ability to work with others, and ability to communicate effectively in English were hired into the role. Problem-solving, flexibility, and some reading skills were other required qualifications. These were felt to be essential qualities for the support assistants, given the nature of their relationship with acutely ill patients, families, and professional staff.

Those individuals with proper qualifications were jointly interviewed by the nurse manager of the designated unit and the clinical nurse who spear-headed the role implementation. In keeping with the committee's goal of developing the role as an interdisciplinary effort, a manager from either transportation, environmental services, or nutrition services also met with the candidate. This enhanced the sense that a team was involved from the beginning.

A total of eight full-time people were selected. Each brought a variety of skills to the new role. Support assistants came from nutrition services, envi-ronmental services, and transportation services. There was one person hired from outside the institution who had previous patient care experi-ence.

The demonstration was planned for a six-month period. Each employee was informed that this was a temporary position pending results of the dem-onstration. Each employee's previous position was held open in case the support assistant was unable to fulfill the expectations of the role or was not happy with the new role. This provided a safety net for all.

EDUCATION AND ORIENTATION

Committee members realized that an effective orientation and training pro-gram was essential to the success of the role. The program included

- Training the support assistants to perform the tasks of environmental services, nutrition tray passing services, patient transportation services, and some basic patient care activities, such as obtaining patient weights and tracking patient intake and output;
- Enhancing the ability of people in the role to communicate with staff, patients, and families;
- Teaching techniques for task prioritization, problem-solving, and time management; and
- Guiding support assistants in their efforts to be accountable to each other, to patients, and to nurses.

The support assistant project coordinator, with help from two other nurses, developed an orientation manual. The manual was a synthesis of materials from the centralized departments' training programs. The department of nursing is the only department to offer a competency-based orientation; therefore, materials from the other departments had to be reworked to conform with the nursing department's format. Case studies were developed for teaching purposes. A hospital-wide scavenger hunt helped orient the support assistants to areas in the hospital that they may not have been familiar with, unless they had worked for transportation services. A unit scavenger hunt oriented them to equipment they would be using on the unit.

The four-week, competency-based program was conducted on the demonstration unit. The program focused on skills acquisition, integration of the support assistants into the culture and staff of the unit, defining relationships among support assistants, patients, and peers, and celebrating the new role.

The project coordinator did not have skills in environmental services, transportation services, or nutrition services that would enable her to conduct the training herself. She worked with the central departments to provide training specific to the work in their areas. This arrangement promoted the interdisciplinary approach of the demonstration. Each week of orientation focused on a specific skill area. Initially, persons from the transportation department oriented and trained support assistants to the role of patient transporter. Following that, environmental service supervisors taught procedures for cleaning a patient's room. Finally, nutrition services provided information and training about patient diets and meal tray delivery.

The project coordinator spent time working with support assistants on interpersonal skills. She also worked with them on learning modules which focused on different patient populations. The modules included information about geriatric patients, confused patients, patients with aspiration precautions, and patients with safety issues (eg, potential for falls). Support assistants attended educational sessions which focused on topics such as universal precautions, common infectious diseases on the unit, and body mechanics for moving and assisting patients. Constant guidance by a nurse provided an opportunity for informal education as issues and questions arose.

▬ MANAGERIAL CONSIDERATIONS

During the initial phase of the demonstration, there was no decision regarding who would manage the support assistants. We visited other hospitals to see how they had redesigned their support services. It was apparent that significant time and energy would be required by a manager to implement this new role on the unit.

We knew the nurse manager would be key to the evolution of the role and integration of the support assistants with other staff on the unit. The nurse manager assumes 24-hour accountability for patient care, personnel management, and standards of practice on the unit. It became evident that the nurse manager was the most appropriate person to manage the support assistants.

The support assistants were managed from a perspective that was new to them. They were now part of a decentralized unit. The decision-making process was at the unit level, where it was viewed in context of the central focus, the patients on the unit. Decisions regarding the hours of coverage, how many patients they would be assigned, who would do the sharable tasks, and appropriate times for breaks were some of the issues which emerged. As long as the group focused on the needs of the patient, recognizing the complexity of some needs and the value of continuity, the solutions were readily evident.

Support assistants required regular feedback; otherwise, behaviors seemed to regress. Committee members recognized that there were too many operational issues associated with the demonstration for the nurse manager to attend to them all effectively. During this transition, direct supervision was provided by an environmental service supervisor, who continued to do quality assurance monitoring and helped monitor work practices. This allowed the nurse manager to focus attention on managing the support assistants' development and integration on the unit.

The preferred management style of the unit was primarily one of consensus building. Support assistants were included but needed to develop skills that would enable them to work problems out collaboratively. A psychiatric liaison nurse developed team-building exercises for the support assistants. For example, there were certain tasks that were a shared responsibility for support assistants but were not being done consistently. One of the tasks was delivering routine specimens to the laboratories within an acceptable time frame. Since these tasks were not associated with any particular patient, they were, at times, ignored. The issue was brought to the support assistants as a group for problem-solving. The need for the timely completion of these tasks was emphasized and recognized. The group worked out a solution that was acceptable to everyone. A sign-up sheet for assuming responsibility for tasks was implemented. The solution that the support assistants designed dissipates responsibility to everyone and has significantly improved the work environment.

The development of cooperative working relationships among the support assistants and with others required ongoing nurturing. Discussions with the manager, staff meeting discussions, and biweekly lunch meetings with the psychiatric liaison nurse helped to develop the relationships.

▬ EVALUATION

In evaluating any restructuring and redesign effort, we need to ask the question, Is this new structure better than the old one, and if so, how do we know? To address this issue, we reviewed the purpose of developing the program. In our institution, the goal of redesigning the support service role was to improve the quality and efficiency of care that we were delivering to patients. We were concerned about service quality for several reasons. We had received several letters from patients, including one from a member of our board of trustees, that identified support functions that could be improved. For example, a former patient described the frustration of having a tray delivered to his room and then waiting for missing condiments. The dinner was cold by the time they arrived. Another letter addressed how impersonal it felt to be wheeled through the corridors to multiple tests by employees who, though they were very polite, knew nothing about their needs. As mentioned earlier, a study by nursing services had revealed that it was not unusual for more than 30 different people to enter a single patient's room during an eight-hour period.

Finally, we felt that restructuring the support service role would enhance the role of the support service worker and improve working relationships between nursing and the support services departments. The relationships had at times been stormy, and there were not well developed systems in place to promote effective communication. Although attempts were made to have the support roles relate to one or several units, there was no strong sense of belonging to a unit among the support workers, and nurses were not "invested" in these employees.

In evaluating the new role, we conducted focus groups with nurses and support assistants to determine their perceptions regarding the change. We also interviewed patients to determine their satisfaction with aspects of their care that were provided by support assistants, such as room cleanliness, tray delivery, and transportation functions. Finally, we talked with personnel from the departments most affected by the change; we asked staff in radiology, which is the area to which most patients on the demonstration unit were transported, nutrition services, and environmental services whether standards were being maintained in their respective areas with the new role.

Perspectives of Support Assistants

Support assistants have been consistently positive about their role. They feel their work is more satisfying because they have a stronger relationship with patients and can identify more readily the value and impact of their jobs on patient care. Diversity of the role has also been identified as a positive outcome from the perspective of support assistants. The ability to provide diverse role functions has allowed for the development of new skills in prioritization, communication, and problem-solving.

As with any change, there have been some problems with the new role from the perspective of the support assistant. Trying to balance competing demands for their time continues to be a challenge. Also, it has been difficult at times to manage the unpredictable nature of their new roles. They cannot plan their day in the same way they did in their traditional roles.

Perspectives of Nurses

The nurses working on the demonstration unit perceived the change positively. In a recent focus group, the most positive aspect of the role that nurses identified was the impact on patient care. They discussed how much more patient-focused the new support assistant role is.

Another positive outcome from the perspective of nurses is that relationships between nurses and support staff have improved. Support assistants and nurses are now members of the same team, rather than members of separate departments. There is the recognition that when they are working as a team, patient needs can be anticipated in a way that was not possible in the past. Nursing time is saved, because nurses do not have to look for or call people from different departments when they are needed; they are there on the unit.

One problem identified by the nurses was the inability of support assistants to set priorities. Nurses acknowledged, though, that they have a responsibility for helping support assistants sort out which tasks need to be done immediately and which tasks can wait. Training from the nursing staff will ultimately help support assistants develop prioritization skills.

Patient Perspectives

We knew early in the project that patients viewed the role positively. We received four unsolicited letters and notes from patients. The patients acknowledged how helpful the support assistants were to them during their hospitalization. One letter was reprinted in a weekly newsletter to all employees from the hospital president. "The newly implemented support assistants on Feldberg-6 are wonderful. Everything is clean and smells wonderful. The people involved are a breath of fresh air."

We also conducted patient surveys to obtain their perspective on how the role was working. We conducted face-to-face interviews with 35 patients. They were asked to rate how satisfied they were with the various aspects of the support assistant role, such as food readiness, room cleanliness, and comfort during transports.

We asked patients if they had needed assistance with getting their meals ready, and if so, had they received it. One hundred percent of the patients said that they did receive assistance. We also asked if they had received condiments that were missing from their tray (sugar, butter, etc.) in a reasonable amount of time. Only one individual responded negatively to this question. Finally, we asked patients how often their food, when it arrived, was the right temperature. One hundred percent of the patients answered that it was always or often the right temperature. The majority (76%) told us that food was always served at the right temperature.

In evaluating the transportation function of the role, we asked patients if they had been informed about where they would be going if they had a test or procedure. Again, 100% of patients responded that they often or always had been informed (91% responded, "Always"). We also asked if they had been satisfied with the amount of time they had to wait to be returned to their rooms after the test or procedure was completed. All but one patient responded that they were satisfied.

Finally, we asked patients how satisfied they were with the cleanliness of their rooms. All but one individual responded that they were satisfied. We then asked patients some open-ended questions about their perceptions regarding services. The information obtained from these questions provided a better understanding of the positive outcomes of the new role. For example, we asked patients if there were any individuals who had been particularly helpful to them during their hospital stay. As expected, the patients' primary nurse was often mentioned, but often support assistants were identified as well. Some examples include, "I love the support assistants," "The support assistant went out of her way," and "Support assistants do a great job."

Perspectives of Other Departments
Department managers from transportation, environmental services, and dietary services have been very pleased with the new role. Each of these departments does quality monitoring and has found that the work of the support assistants meets or exceeds their standards. Colleagues in radiology initially were concerned about having support assistants transport patients for radiology procedures, because if patients do not arrive on time, the entire system backs up. We worked closely with the department to develop systems that would facilitate the timely arrival of patients. Employees in the department have been very pleased with the program and have commented often on how good the support assistants are with patients.

Cost Issues
The program has proven to be less costly than the centralized system on weekends. During this time, there are the same number of support personnel as there were environmental service personnel, yet the employees perform additional functions. It has been more difficult to demonstrate a cost savings during the week. This is because of the large number and unpredictable nature of the transportation functions. We are continuing to evaluate this and are developing methods to make the transportation function more efficient.

CONCLUSION
As hospitals redesign from departmentalized institutions to patient-focused institutions, it is important to include input from and consensus by those who are affected by the proposed changes, including patients. Development of the support assistant role at Beth Israel Hospital has helped pave the way for other patient-driven redesign efforts. The process described in this chapter can be used as a template for organizational redesign that reflects the needs of patients, employees, and the community we serve.

REFERENCES
Beth Israel Hospital Board of Trustees. (1983). Expanded Mission Statement. Boston: Beth Israel Hospital.
Clifford, J. & Horvath, K. (1990). *Advancing professional nursing practice: Innovation at Boston's Beth Israel Hospital.* New York: Springer.

Liston, E., Dick, K., & Greenspan, M. (1990). The evolution of nursing practice. In J. Clifford and K. Horvath (Eds.), *Advancing professional nursing practice: Innovations at Boston's Beth Israel Hospital.* New York: Springer.

Manthey, M., Ciske, K., Robertson, P., & Harris, I. (1970). Primary nursing: A return to the concept of "my nurse" and "my patient." *Nursing Forum, 9*(1), 64–83.

Senge, P. (1990). *The fifth discipline: The art and practice of the learning organization.* New York: Doubleday Currency.

Chapter 20

Integrated Patient Care Delivery System: A Patient-Centered Model

DOREEN DANN   PAMELA GENTZSCH   CAROL PIERSON

MARILYN HOBBS   BARBARA MILLER   ANITA MAHONY

In keeping with the mission and values of the Sisters of St. Joseph of Orange, St. Jude Medical Center and St. Joseph Hospital, two Southern California hospitals within the St. Joseph Health System (SJHS), collaborated in early 1989 to establish alternate care delivery systems within both settings. This project was initiated in response to the many indicators of rapid revolutionary changes in the health care environment and the need for an innovative and creative means of delivering patient care. These changes necessitated focusing on efficient use of resources without reducing service level, quality of care, or patient satisfaction. Factors affecting future care delivery included caring for patients with increasingly complex problems, decreased availability of health care personnel, reduced reimbursement for services provided, decreasing length of stay, increasing shift to outpatient services, and a new focus on managed care. Because the SJHS is committed to four core values—dignity of person, management of excellence, opportunity for service, and pursuit of justice—it was critically important that this quality initiative integrate these values in the process, design, and outcomes of the overall project.

▬ PROJECT LEADERSHIP

A plethora of articles on organizational restructuring, work redesign, and self-directed work teams is available in the literature (Goldsmith, 1989). To facilitate improved outcomes, St. Jude Medical Center and St. Joseph Hospital appointed multidisciplinary staff members to an SJHS Alternative Care Delivery System Steering Committee, chaired by the corporate vice president for patient care services. Each hospital appointed a project coordinator responsible to the respective vice president of patient care/clinical services. To meet the identified requirements for providing comprehensive, sensitive, and cost-efficient care centered on the patient and family, it was

Flarey, D: REDESIGNING NURSING CARE DELIVERY: Transforming Our Future

determined early on that this could not be a nurse-driven model but must be a collaborative effort of all disciplines involved, from admission through discharge. With this realization, each hospital agreed to initiate internal processes for model development which would best address the culture and organizational needs for each site, thereby assuring successful implementation system-wide. This chapter presents the experience of St. Jude Medical Center, a 347-bed, full-service, not-for-profit, community tertiary hospital located in Fullerton, California, and the outcomes of the SJHS steering committee.

▬ PROJECT PLANNING

The initial work of the SJHS steering committee was to develop goals and objectives for the system redesign. These are presented in Displays 20–1 and 20–2. Each hospital established a project team with representation from all major disciplines. The St. Jude Medical Center team consisted of the project coordinator (who was also the director of education), the vice president of clinical services, the assistant administrators for both ancillary and support services, the director of medical/surgical/rehabilitation nursing services, the department managers from laboratory, dietary, environmental, and respiratory care services, and representatives from the two patient care units selected to pilot the new model. Planning by the project team focused on the following steps:

- Creation of an open forum for all staff, managers, educators, and physicians associated directly and indirectly with the two participating patient care units. This forum addressed the economy, forecasted changes for health care, and looked at the need to proactively restructur ? the Medical Center's patient care delivery system to meet the four primary objectives (see Display 20-1);
- Establishment of a multidisciplinary task force of volunteers from the pilot units and associated departments to develop the model following a

---

DISPLAY 20-1   *Goals and Objectives for System Redesign*

GOAL
To develop a model which provides patient-centered care with efficient resource utilization through professional collaboration.

OBJECTIVES
1. To increase patient satisfaction by developing a model which increases accessibility and is "user-friendly."
2. To decrease cost per patient-day and optimize productivity.
3. To increase satisfaction and enhance retention of all professional and support personnel.
4. To increase physician satisfaction by developing a model which provides patient-centered care with efficient resource utilization through professional collaboration.

DISPLAY 20-2   Purpose Statement for the St. Joseph Health System Steering Committee

1. Facilitate project development within the two institutions, using staff and management in a cooperative effort.
2. Assure continuity with the goals and philosophy of the health system, hospitals, and models.
3. Ensure and enhance communication between and among all constituents involved in the project.
4. Develop a forum for consultation and discussion to evaluate progress.

---

detailed assessment of patient care needs specific to each patient population served; and
- Identification of specific educational, licensure, and skill level requirements to meet the assessed needs.

The SJHS steering committee supported the overall project and system redesign within each site through the following techniques:

- Identification of tools to measure patient, physician, and employee satisfaction before and after implementation;
- Selection of quality control measures and fiscal indicators with which to evaluate the impact on the primary objectives of the model;
- Standardization of interviewing tools and processes;
- Development of an educational curriculum for restructured roles, including retraining and competency validation;
- Establishment of an internal and external marketing plan; and
- Coordination of training and education with an affiliated school of nursing to promote entry into practice experiences for interested students.

▬SELECTION OF PILOT UNITS

A 40-bed surgical-orthopedic unit and a 30-bed medical unit were selected as pilot units. Reasons for selection included stable management, strong physician support, and opportunities to improve service quality, satisfaction levels, and cost containment. The delivery model on the general surgical-orthopedic unit was consistent with that of nursing services, namely, total patient care by registered nurses (RNs) and licensed vocational nurses (LVNs). The nurse manager had accountability for multiple patient care units with assistant nurse managers working 12-hour shifts. The medical unit had a similar management structure but had moved away from total patient care to a team nursing model.

▬NEW MODEL DEVELOPMENT

Multidisciplinary groups from each pilot unit convened and, using nominal group processes, identified viable alternatives to the current department-focused care delivery system. Their goal was to identify an integrated approach to care delivery that would incorporate patient care needs across the continuum. Participants were divided into three small groups and were challenged to develop patient-centered models and share their outcomes with the entire group. This same process occurred at St. Joseph Hospital. Surprisingly, each hospital group identified similar structures and designs on which to base the new delivery system.

The essence of the alternative delivery model ultimately focused on patient-centered care, managed by a professional nurse who had 24-hour accountability for a designated group of patients from admission through discharge. The professional nurse would be accountable for coordinating, planning, and evaluating patient care activities. In addition, this same nurse would be responsible for an associated health care team of technical and support personnel. The RN would consult and collaborate with physicians and other health care team members and consultants to ensure quality patient outcomes through coordination of resources.

In the final analysis, five levels of unit staff positions were identified by the project team and approved by the SJHS steering committee for both hospitals' pilot projects. The positions were further refined by the model development team of each pilot unit. The positions included 1) patient care manager, an RN with a BSN preferred (an exempt position); 2) patient care nurse, licensed as an RN or LVN; 3) patient care technician (PCT); 4) unit hostess, a volunteer position which was explored but not implemented; and 5) unit assistant, a position piloted on only one unit.

Each position consisted of multiple functions, resulting in a progressive clinical career mobility system. Emphasis was placed on the inherent value of each level of this health care team. The role components were used to define position descriptions and titles. Technical and support staff included monitor technicians, clinical/clerical technicians, unit secretaries, and patient care consultants (eg, social workers, respiratory therapists, pharmacists, psychologists). Congruent with the proposed goals of the new delivery system, the SJHS steering committee subsequently renamed the model "Integrated Patient Care System," or IPCS as it was commonly called.

Selection of Unit Personnel

Patient care manager positions were selected first. This was accomplished by a specially designed application form which included the opportunity for the applicants to express their capacity for creative thinking. Packets consisted of IPCS information, the application form, and a list of questions to be asked by the interview panel. The interview panel consisted of the vice president for clinical services, the assistant administrator of ancillary services, the clinical director of the unit, the respective educator or clinical nurse specialist, the project coordinator, a physician, and a unit staff nurse. Before interviewing the candidate, each member of the interview panel perused the application, the preassigned questions, and the rating scale to be used. Questions were based on management, leadership, mentoring, critical thinking skills, and congruity with the Medical Center's mission statement and values. The selected candidates were photographed and publicized in the Medical Center newsletter with a short biography. The stage was then set for each patient care manager to conduct interviews and select, according to preapproved budgeted positions, their new health care team. Patient care managers were also supported through shared educational and collaborative sessions with the newly designated patient care managers from St. Joseph Hospital, Orange.

Educational Preparation

In designing a curriculum to prepare the RN for the *patient care manager* role, the following skills were analyzed:

- Coordinating and collaborating to assess the appropriate use of resources;
- Using critical thinking and problem-solving skills to achieve quality clinical outcomes;
- Managing a health care team of varying skill mixes based on acuity, intensity, and work design; and
- Managing the material and financial resources associated with achievement of defined outcome goals.

A patient care manager educational curriculum was designed based on this defined skill set. In addition to the initial training program, educational needs assessments are performed and ongoing educational offerings continue to be provided for patient care managers.

The *patient care nurse* delivers care in accordance with the state's Nurse Practice Act. The role focuses on participation in patient care delivery and collaboration with all team members. The patient care nurse can be an RN or an LVN, as determined by patient needs and competency requirements. Core features of the educational curriculum to prepare patient care nurses to practice in the new model included overview of IPCS, scope of practice, principles of delegation, team problem-solving skills, phlebotomy, patient medication coordinating, and obtaining a 12-lead electrocardiogram (ECG).

The PCT provides general patient care with associated phlebotomy and ECG components. Initially, the PCT position required previous experience in entry-level positions such as nursing assistant, emergency medical technician, student nurse, cardiology technician, or phlebotomist. The skilled individual received additional on-the-job training for areas in which they did not have previous experience, including the delivery of technical care. Evaluation of the position revealed that basic nursing skills were necessary as a foundation for the multiskilled PCT. Currently, certified nursing assistant or student nurse status is required for the position.

The laboratory and cardiology departments were an integral part of PCT curriculum design, clinical supervision, skills validation, and quality control. In addition, curriculum design was consistent with the California Code of Regulations, Title 22, and based on College of American Pathologists guidelines for preparing phlebotomists, which requires a minimum of 10 hours of didactic and clinical practicum. On successful completion of the St. Jude Medical Center course, the student received an institutional certification specific to adult venipuncture signed by the medical director of the laboratory. The total PCT program included 8 hours of didactic and a minimum of 40 hours of clinical training for the phlebotomy component, and 2 hours of didactic and 4 hours of clinical instruction for the ECG component. Education and training programs and skills validation are ongoing and are developed with input from the laboratory and cardiology departments.

The PCT role, or that of assistive personnel in general, has been questioned by many nursing groups and supported by others. In 1991, the California Nurses Association notified the State Board of Registered Nursing about the use of unlicensed personnel. According to the board's executive officer, Catherine Puri (1991), state law and past opinions from the attorney general indicated that health care functions requiring a substantial amount of scientific knowledge or technical skill may be performed only by a registered nurse. Puri (1991) also acknowledged that technical tasks such as drawing blood are seen by the board as part of the usual and common practice of the nurse. Technicians, unlike nurses, are not educated to notice subtle changes in patient conditions. In response to these concerns, the American Organization of Nurse Executives and the American Hospital Association provided a joint position statement recognizing that differentiated practice can serve to maximize nursing resources by differentiating roles according to competence, experience, and education. They also encouraged identifying a care delivery system that was congruent with this philosophy (Ehrat, 1991).

■INTEGRATION OF THE MODEL THROUGHOUT THE HOSPITAL

After the pilot project on the initial two units had been fully implemented, the steering committee began deliberation on which specialty unit should implement the delivery model. In order to meet the goals of the model, the most cost-effective strategy was to expand the system throughout the acute medical-surgical and rehabilitation clinical divisions.

Rehabilitation Patient Care Unit

The selection of the rehabilitation patient care unit coincided with a recent in-depth consultation conducted on the overall strengths and weaknesses of the entire rehabilitation product line. The recommendation was to structure services into a programmatic approach, (ie, stroke, brain injury, and spinal cord injury). Another recommendation, consistent with the model, was to have an RN responsible for the integration of services for all patients within a continuum of care. This RN would be the nursing representative on the interdisciplinary team that coordinates the patient's care. This would be accomplished by collaboration with physicians and other health care team members in assessing the use of resources, formulating a plan of care, and evaluating patient outcomes.

Based on the consultant's recommendations and the goals and objectives of the IPCS model, in October 1991, the model was implemented on the rehabilitation unit. A matrix relationship was then established with the vice president of rehabilitation services and program directors of rehabilitation services. Along with the development of this matrix relationship, organizational changes occurred in nursing services. These changes included having a clinical director responsible for the multiple units and the patient care managers for each of the three programs. This structure enhanced the integration and effectiveness of the new delivery model.

Training for PCTs on the rehabilitation unit was different from that for medical-surgical PCTs. The rehabilitation nurse clinician developed a 40-hour course with an emphasis on activities of daily living. This program was presented by all of the rehabilitation disciplines. This educational series included formal didactic sessions, practice labs, and skills verification.

Oncology Unit

The oncology unit was selected as the next area for implementation of IPCS. Before implementation, the 32-bed oncology unit was geographically subdivided into two separate patient care units—22 beds for oncology and 10 beds for medical-surgical telemetry—with 6 "swing" beds if further telemetry was required. As the model was implemented, a new clinical director was hired.

The new director soon realized that for the model to be successful, the unit had to become more integrated and more open to change. A plan to facilitate these goals was developed and implemented on the unit. In an attempt to proceed with implementation of the model, weekly unit meetings were held for the staff. These meetings redefined the core features of the model and helped establish solid working relationships between all health care team members.

Within a six-month period, team members were ready to implement the model. The team members held weekly meetings and redefined the geographics of the unit. The unit was equally divided into two areas of 16 beds each, and one cost center was created. It was believed that a patient care manager could follow this number of patients and provide optimal case management. Individuals were interviewed for the position of patient care manager. Collectively, it was decided to continue with three key nursing personnel. One patient care manager would work 5 days a week, 8 hours a day, and the other two patient care managers would job-share, working three 12-hour days. As this had been the previous situation with the assistant nurse managers and nursing personnel felt it was effective, the clinical director agreed to the proposal. Along with the established curriculum, the patient care managers oriented with other patient care managers already in the role, from within the Medical Center and within SJHS. This was a unique opportunity for these professionals to implement what they had learned from their educational sessions.

Patient care nurses had difficulty in delegating tasks to other patient care nurses and PCTs. This continued even after they had participated in the educational component for this position. The patient care managers and the clinical director identified this as a group dynamics issue, because total patient care had been the delivery system before implementation of IPCS. In order to assist the nursing staff to become comfortable with delegation and trust each other, weekly meetings were continued with an emphasis on team building. Each patient care manager met with the staff and discussed strategies for team building, communication styles, and role expectations. Monthly, the teams shared this information among themselves. Over a period of 4 to 6 months, these issues were actively addressed and the team focused on strategies for resolution.

Cardiac Unit

The IPCS model was implemented in January 1992 on a 30-bed cardiac telemetry and rehabilitation unit. Total patient care had been the nursing care delivery model, with a nurse manager and one assistant nurse manager on each 12-hour shift. The preparation for the implementation of this model was similar to that on the other patient care units. Weekly meetings were initiated to redefine the staffing mix, with a keen focus on the goals and objectives of the model.

Located on the cardiac telemetry unit was a monitor bank which provided 24-hour cardiac monitoring observation by monitor technicians for up to 64 patients dispersed throughout four patient care units. Training for the monitor technician consisted of a basic arrhythmia course and 72 hours of clinical orientation to the monitor bank. Because of the lengthy shifts (12 hours) and the repetitiveness of continuously watching the monitors, it was decided to cross-train the monitor technicians and the nursing assistants. These individuals now rotate their responsibilities; that is, they work 6 hours as monitor technicians and 6 hours as nursing assistants.

Phlebotomy training for the IPCS model was not implemented initially on the cardiac unit; rather, it was agreed to evaluate the initial success of the model before full implementation.

■ EVALUATION

The evaluation components of the redesigned delivery system were based on the goals and objectives for model development. Because the model was based on a patient-centered approach, it was critical to choose a patient satisfaction survey that would capture essential indicators. Before redesign, the Medical Center had its own patient satisfaction survey which focused on the services provided by the institution. This survey did not provide a sound comparison of St. Jude with other medical centers having the same bed capacity or similar patient care units. Additionally, this survey did not address essential nursing issues. After these facts were determined, the director of patient representatives and the clinical services administrative team researched many different satisfaction surveys and determined that the Press Ganey survey would best meet the needs of St. Jude Medical Center. This survey tool was implemented 6 months after the model was put in place and, therefore, preimplementation data was not obtained. Postimplementation data on patient satisfaction, however, was measured. Initially, postimplementation data revealed a high level of satisfaction with nursing service, with the exception of phlebotomy skills. This was a result of a lack of experience among the PCTs. Satisfaction surveys 3 months after implementation demonstrated an increased level of patient satisfaction. This was attributed to the trust established by the PCT with the patient and the improved skill level for phlebotomy.

The second goal for our redesign project was meeting the needs of patients while containing costs. A comparison grid was developed to assess progress through a same month/year data analysis. Costs per patient day were collected and analyzed by the initial two patient care units. Cost reductions were not initially realized because of the start-up costs associated with orientation and training. These programs were not anticipated in the original financial allocations. In year 4, the analysis of the skill mix changes on the two pilot units in comparison to the preimplementation year of 1989 demonstrated an 8.8% salary expense savings for the surgical-orthopedic unit and a 6.3% savings for the medical unit (after adjusting for inflation). Skill mix comparisons are presented in Figures 20–1 and 20–2.

Our third goal focused on employee satisfaction. It was anticipated that employee satisfaction would enhance retention of all professional and ancillary support personnel. Analysis of turnover rates before and after implementation demonstrated a lower rate of turnover on the surgical-orthopedic unit (from 4.4% to 1.48%) and a higher turnover rate for the medical unit (from 1.8% to 2.9%). This, we believe, was directly related to the initial attitudes toward the new model and the extent of employee involvement in developing and implementing the model.

The patient care nurses on the surgical-orthopedic unit were very positive about the model. They felt it provided more accountability to the bedside nurse, created a career mobility program for the certified nurse assistant, and increased communication between the shifts. The patient care nurses on the medical unit were less satisfied. They identified a lack of sup-

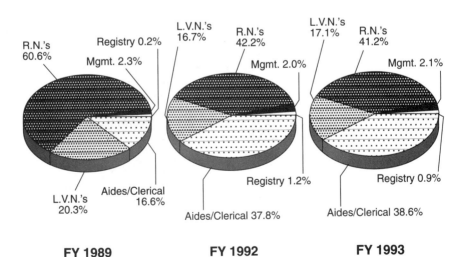

FY 1989   **FY 1992**   **FY 1993**

FIGURE 20-1   Skill mix—surgical ortho. Integrated patient care.

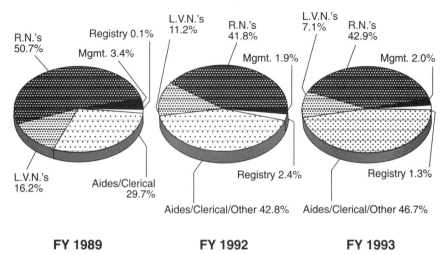

R.N.'s 50.7%
Registry 0.1%
Mgmt. 3.4%
L.V.N.'s 11.2%
R.N.'s 41.8%
Mgmt. 1.9%
L.V.N.'s 7.1%
R.N.'s 42.9%
Mgmt. 2.0%

L.V.N.'s 16.2%
Aides/Clerical 29.7%
Registry 2.4%
Aides/Clerical/Other 42.8%
Registry 1.3%
Aides/Clerical/Other 46.7%

FY 1989   FY 1992   FY 1993

FIGURE 20-2   Skill mix—medical. Integrated patient care.

port from the PCTs, resulting from their increased phlebotomy and ECG responsibilities; they believed that patient care was fragmented. The patient care managers, however, supported the project and were willing to invest adequate time and resources to make the model successful. What became evident from the experience of these two patient care units was the need for strong nursing support at the initiation of the project, the need to set specific selection criteria for personnel, and need for consensus and clarity on role definition. Once these critical issues were dealt with, focus was placed on uniting the nursing staff on the other units as the orientation to the model proceeded.

Physician satisfaction indicators were based on expectations of the nursing staff to meet their patients' needs. The physicians indicated an increased level of satisfaction with consistent availability of a patient care manager who possessed the most current nursing assessment and knowledge of patient/family needs and awareness of the patients' responses to treatment. Improvement continues to be demonstrated in the area of communication and collaboration between physicians and the nursing staff.

■SUMMARY

The development of an integrated patient care delivery system was an SJHS collaborative process. This model was generated from the anticipated changes in health care focusing on financial issues as well as service.

Differences between the two facilities in the health system directing this project were identified in the environment and culture of the employees and in the selected patients. The philosophy of this model in both medical centers reflected the philosophy of SJHS, but because of differing culture and organizational goals, the implementation process for the model reflected each institution uniquely. Regardless of the process, the key concept was patient-centered care.

The goal to design a patient-centered care model was the impetus in creating the roles of patient care manager and multifunctional skilled team member. Nurses in these two roles continue to be the essential care providers in the redesigned system.

Now in its fourth year, the integrated patient care system is fully implemented throughout the medical, surgical, rehabilitation, oncology, diabetic metabolic, cardiac telemetry, and neonatal intensive care units, with planned expansion to perinatal, pediatric, and gynecology services. Our findings are consistent with those of Dr. Tim Porter-O'Grady: "Substantial outcomes cannot be expected from system redesign and work refocus which involve a wide variety of folks, for at least five years.... Work in redesign is not merely shifting a few organizational components and people; it is a complete reorientation of the work and culture" (Porter-O'Grady, 1993, p. 8). Throughout our ongoing evaluation, it is apparent that consistent focus on improved patient outcomes from a multidisciplinary perspective must be maintained to assure the continuation of appropriate work redesign strategies.

At St. Jude Medical Center, several core issues on the patient care units were identified after implementation. One of these issues centered on the characteristics of the patient care unit. The unit staff must be involved in the evolution of the project to facilitate the change process. The unit staff must have a comprehensive understanding of the process as well as the format for change. Another issue is the characteristics of the individuals within and associated with the unit. Patient-centered approaches necessitate rethinking the traditional roles of nursing and focusing on change from a nonterritorial perspective. The final issue addresses the educational levels of the individuals working within the system. Basic preparatory levels, as well as advanced levels of education, need to be identified and evaluated as the patient care unit progresses through the change process to a new delivery system.

A coordinator for the delivery system redesign and a health management information system are essential to the redesign of a patient care delivery system. Unfortunately, at St. Jude, they have not been consistently planned for. Thus, many aspects of the model have not been well substantiated. The coordinator is important for providing the leadership necessary to ensure attainment of the goals and objectives of the project. It is this professional who assists with the implementation of a redesigned delivery system on other patient care units.

One year after implementation, the SJHS steering committee determined that, although the model design implemented within the two site hospitals may not entirely meet the culture, organizational, or patient care needs of other institutions, the following five critical factors are essential to a patient-centered redesign project.

A patient-centered system that provides continuity and enhances patient participation and satisfaction is critical.

Goals must be defined early and communicated, along with methods to identify, measure, and evaluate cost-effectiveness. This must include the evaluation of quality outcomes as well as the evaluation of goal attainment.

The case management role is critical to reduce length of stay, impact resource utilization, and effect positive patient outcomes.

A team approach to patient care delivery, using multiskilled workers to support professional nurses in the delivery of care, is essential to the success of the new model.

The RN role is pivotal for the effective coordination of care delivery in a redesigned system.

The following outcomes were realized after implementation of the redesigned IPCS:

- Increased networking and a sharing of resources between sister hospitals within the SJHS;
- Establishment of a career mobility system within and between the SJHS hospitals, through the initiation of various multi-trained technical and support roles;
- Improved patient satisfaction through care coordination and by daily interaction with one patient care manager throughout the course of hospitalization;
- Improved patient care processes with decreased wait times and increased turnaround of laboratory and ECG results;
- Enhanced physician satisfaction with the consistency and knowledge of patient care assessment and outcomes by the nursing staff;
- Improved case management through collaboration with the patient care manager, utilization management, and social services;
- Increased collaboration between nursing services and ancillary services;
- Improved collaboration with affiliated academic institutions; and,
- Integration of the successful aspects of primary, team, and total patient care delivery systems into one integrated system that is patient-centered, physician-sensitive, and employee-oriented.

The IPCS successfully met its overall goal and four primary objectives. Patient satisfaction demonstrated consistent improvement. Physician needs for continuity of care were met through the consistency of the patient care manager role. Employee satisfaction was enhanced through the career mobility offered in role redesign, flexible scheduling, provision of orientation and training, and willingness to adapt the model to meet ongoing identified needs. Cost containment goals, although exceeded in the first year, demonstrated a 7.4% overall salary reduction in year 4 of implementation compared with preimplementation data for all participating patient care units.

▬ REFERENCES

Ehrat, K. (1991). The value of differentiated practice. *The Journal of Nursing Administration, 21,* 9–10.

Goldsmith, J. (1989). The hospital as we see it is too costly, too unwieldy, and too inflexible to survive. A radical prescription for hospitals. *Harvard Business Review, 67*(3), 104–111.

Mayer, D. (1991). California Nurses slam hospitals' use of unlicensed staff. *Healthweek News, 5,* 8–9.

Porter-O'Grady, T. (1993). Patient care-focused care service models and nursing: Perils and possibilities. *The Journal of Nursing Administration, 23*(3), 7–15.

Index

Accountability
  in organizational redesign, 62
  for patient outcomes, 105
Ackoff, Russell L., 29, 187
Ackoff's model of interactive planning, 6, 7, 154
Activities of daily living (ADLs), in redesign process, 122
Acuity system, in redesign process, 117
Administration. *See also* Executives; Management
  organizational analysis of, 144
  in patient-centered framework, 18
Administration, nursing. *See also* Leadership
  and organizational restructuring, 48
  in patient-centered redesign, 132–135, 137–138
  in redesign process, 113
Admissions turnaround, evaluation of, 53
Admitting procedures, and patient-care restructuring, 96–97
Allison, S., 208
Ancillary care providers (ACPs), in Vincentian program, 189, 195*tab*
Ancillary staff, in Vincentian Program, 200–201
Assessment. *See also* Evaluation
  in redesign process, 112–113
  in restructuring process, 24, 25
Assistant nursing managers (ANMs), in Vincentian Program, 191
Associate nurse, role at SVH, 111
Assumptions, in model for redesign, 114
Automation, 11
Availability/affordability dilemma, 36

Belief systems
  and patient-centered care, 24
  and redesigning patient care, 223
Benchmarking, in organizational restructuring, 42, 49
Beth Israel Hospital, Boston, MA, 240
  core values of, 241
  creating shared vision at, 242–243
  evaluation of support assistants at, 248–250
  information sharing at, 244–245
  management at, 247
  planning for change at, 244
  role development at, 241
  selection of support assistants at, 245
  support assistant project coordinator at, 243–244, 246
Bone marrow project at UMHC, 221
Booz-Allen and Hamilton, Inc., 93
Brainstorming sessions, 110
Bridging the Leadership Gap in Healthcare (Healthcare Forum), 60

Cardiac unit, in IPCS model, 259
Cardiogenic shock, RCP for, 86–87*app*
Care. *See also* Patient care; Standards of care
  managed, 9
  patient-centered framework for restructuring, 17–24
Care delivery. *See also* Delivery systems
  affordable, 4
  patient-focused vs. department-focused, 188
  operational restructuring of, 173

265

Empowerment
and changing nursing role, 136
of employees, 61–62
in patient-centered redesign, 134, 138
in planning for redesign, 8
Environment
for innovation and change, 95, 107
patient-centered, 18–19, 22
in ProACT™ model, 167–168
Evaluation
of administrative outcomes, 51–52
and change, 107
of clinical outcomes, 50–51
of IPCS model, 259, 260*fig*-261*fig*
of patient-centered framework, 23–24
of ProACT™ model, 168–169*tab*, 170*fig*
in restructuring process, 26
of service outcomes, 52–53
of SHNP process, 33
of STAR model, 158–160*tab*, 161
of Vincentian Program, 199*tab*-200*tab*, 201
Executives, nurse. *See also* Administration; Leadership
necessary competencies of, 57–63
and organizational redesign, 57
skills necessary for, 35–36
and VHA Hospitals' redesign project, 67–68*app*
Expert practice, Benner's theory of, 236

Fall Festival, at VBMC, 84
Families
in patient-centered framework, 18
in STAR model, 159*tab*
Finance Department, interaction with clinical staff of, 44
Financial analysis, in redesign process, 50
Financial skills, need for, 36
Focus groups
content analysis of, 23
in planning for redesign, 7
Function, vs. process, 59

Goals, in patient-centered approach, 21
Gross Domestic Product, health care spending in, 54
Gross National Product (GNP), health care spending in, 47
Group norms, in model for redesign, 114
Guest relations program, 82

Hartford Hospital, 128
changing nursing role at, 136–138
environment and culture of, 129
patient-centered redesign program at, 129–132
Health care consultants, in restructuring process, 142
Health Care Financing Administration (HCFA), 82
Healthcare Forum, 1992 study of, 60
Health care industry
nursing services in, 15
redesign efforts in, 16
Health care organizations
building shared visions within, 58
nurse executive's evolving role in, 57
and systems thinking, 7
Health care reform, 16, 46, 54, 186
Healthspan's Mercy and Unity Hospitals, 179, 184
Heparin protocol, 84
Hospitals. *See also specific hospitals*
delivery problems in, 5
operating budgets of, 56
and patient-centered framework, 23
in SHNP programs, 29
and SHNP implementation, 31–32
Human Resources, in Vincentian Program, 197
Hypoglycemia protocol, 84

Iacocca, Lee, 46
Implementation
in redesign process, 115
in restructuring process, 24, 25